Doctor, Will You Pray for Me?

Doctor, Will You Pray for Me?

Medicine, Chaplains, and Healing the Whole Person

ROBERT L. KLITZMAN, MD

Professor of Psychiatry

*Vagelos College of Physicians & Surgeons and
Joseph Mailman School of Public Health*

Director, Masters of Bioethics Program

Columbia University

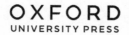
OXFORD
UNIVERSITY PRESS

OXFORD
UNIVERSITY PRESS

Oxford University Press is a department of the University of Oxford. It furthers
the University's objective of excellence in research, scholarship, and education
by publishing worldwide. Oxford is a registered trade mark of Oxford University
Press in the UK and certain other countries.

Published in the United States of America by Oxford University Press
198 Madison Avenue, New York, NY 10016, United States of America.

CIP data is on file at the Library of Congress

ISBN 978-0-19-775084-1

DOI: 10.1093/oso/9780197750841.001.0001

Printed by Sheridan Books, Inc., United States of America

To the men and women who shared with me their views and experiences for this book, and to Charlie.

Between "there is a God" and "there is no God" lies a whole vast tract, which the really wise man crosses with great effort.

Anton Chekhov, *Notebooks*

Every man takes the limits of his own field of vision for the limits of the world.

Arthur Schopenhauer

Paint the visible and the invisible.

Leonardo da Vinci

Contents

Acknowledgments

This book could not have been possible without the help and support of several people—first and foremost, the individuals with whom I have spoken over the years about these issues and the participants in several studies I have conducted, especially the chaplains who generously offered their time and insights into their work. I am immensely grateful to all of them. For their input and suggestions, I am also deeply indebted to Stacy Schiff, Rick Hamlin, Alice Truax, Will Schwalbe, Patty Volk, Paul Rauschenbush, Melanie Thernstrom, Royce Flippin, Tim Duggan, David Harris, Amy Amundsen, Kristine Dahl, Wendy Strothman, Linda Golding, Mychal Springer, Amy Amundsen, Lizzie Leiman, and Rubén Kraiem. I would also like to thank my research assistants Jay Al-Hashimi, Gabrielle Di Sapia Natarelli, Elizaveta Garbuzova, and Stephanie Sinnappan for their help coding the interviews. In assisting with preparation of the manuscript itself, I want to thank Beverly Gu, Timothy Keith Hung, Jiseop Kim, Amanda Shen, Gabriella Smith, and most especially Patricia Contino. At Oxford, I am grateful to Madison Zickgraf and Teddy Reiner, and once again owe immense thanks to Peter Ohlin for his enormous and invaluable support. As cited in the book, several sections of the text appeared in different form in *Academic Medicine, Patient Education and Counseling, Journal of Religion and Health, Social Science and Medicine—Qualitative Research, Journal of Health Care Chaplaincy, Journal of Pastoral Care and Counseling, BMC Palliative Care, The New York Times* and CNN.com. I am grateful for permission to reprint this material here.

PART I
IN THE FOXHOLE
Patients facing crises

1

"Disappearing into clouds of smoke"

Confronting threats to life

Carol was one of the first patients I treated as a medical intern. Breast cancer had invaded and now riddled her body. We started her on chemotherapy, but didn't know how long she would survive—perhaps only a few months. The drugs crippled her ability to fight infections, so we now confined her to her room. She lived in "isolation" to prevent any germs from entering. Other doctors and I, along with nurses and visitors, had to don special light-blue paper-tissue hats, gowns, masks, and shoe covers, and rubber gloves in order to enter her room. She was, essentially, a prisoner.

As part of my training to become a psychiatrist, I first had to work as a medical intern, treating hospitalized patients severely sick with serious physical diseases like cancer. I was the doctor whom Carol saw the most. Over the first few weeks, every morning, her sparkling blue eyes looked up at me with hope. She was 24, with soft skin and long, wavy, light-brown hair. Her mother visited her every day, and sat close by her side. Both women wore tiny gold crosses. At the foot of the bed, an embossed card of Jesus in a bright crimson cloak hung, Scotch-taped to the wall. Pointy gold rays beamed from around His head.

After a month, her cancer had shrunk only slightly. Her bangs now clung to her forehead, sweaty from fever. Most of the day, she now lay on her side, tired or staring at the wall. Other times, her nose and forehead scrunched in pain. The card of Jesus had begun to slip down the wall—the Scotch tape had mostly peeled away. No one had bothered to replace it.

I felt badly that I could not offer her any better treatment, and wondered whether to call a priest. I had no idea whether or when to call a priest. No one had ever told me. I didn't know what it might mean to her if I broached the topic. I feared that she and her mother would feel that I was giving up on her.

Through my medical training, I had never received a single lecture about religion or spirituality. Professors never mentioned these topics. Occasionally, on hospital elevators and wards, I glimpsed priests in white collars and rabbis

Doctor, Will You Pray for Me?. Robert L. Klitzman, Oxford University Press. © Oxford University Press 2024.
DOI: 10.1093/oso/9780197750841.003.0001

in yarmulkes or black hats, but other doctors and I ignored them, never speaking to them. Usually, they exited patients' rooms when we entered, or they entered when we left. They operated in an entirely other world.

Yet as I now cared for Carol, I wondered whether to ask my supervising resident about whether to contact a priest. I felt uncomfortable doing so, trying to fit into my new profession, and feeling obliged to follow what the doctors around me all seemed to be doing—standing apart from patients' internal existential struggles and maintaining a strong wall.

Yet despite the chemo, she continued to worsen. Her fevers became more frequent; she sweated more and lost all her appetite. One afternoon, tears welled up in her blue eyes. I wondered: Didn't I have responsibility to help her as much as possible?

Finally, one morning on rounds, I asked my supervising resident, trying to be casual, "By the way, do we ever call a priest?"

He looked at me coldly, askance: "Huh?" He contorted his face, eyeing me as if I were nuts—as if I had suggested consulting a voodoo doctor. Apparently, calling a priest was simply not something that we, as physicians, did. In the world of scientific medicine, even broaching this subject was out of bounds.

I felt awkward, sensing Carol's terror and psychic pain, which we all just sidestepped. A few days later, though, hurrying by her door, I spied a priest in her room and felt relieved. Two days afterwards, I again spotted him, heading to visit her.

The next morning, I thought she looked calmer, more relieved than I'd seen her in weeks. Still, she had unremitting fevers. Sadly, she died a few weeks afterwards, never having left the room.

But I saw how this clergyman had aided her in ways that my medical treatment had not—how religion and spirituality had comforted her as we, as physicians, had failed to do.

I still regret my silence, which has continued to haunt, embarrass, and disturb me. Yet it made me wonder about the roles of religion and spirituality in patients' and families' lives.

Medical training encouraged us to see the human body as mere flesh, and numbed us to the human sides of suffering. As doctors, we were now supposed to be tough, inured against feelings of closeness to our patients, and able to literally stand back and apart from them, thinking of them not as people per se but as compilations of organs. Increasingly, however, I saw countless patients and their families, especially when facing the prospect of death, wanting and needing something more—to make sense of the experience.

Linguistically, health and spirituality are inextricably linked. The words "health," "heal," "holy," and "wholeness" all derive from the same German and Old English roots for "whole" and are all related. Today widening discussions in popular media about "holistic medicine" that address not just the biological parts of a person, but the *whole*—the mind and spirit as well—reflect this historical and psychological interconnectedness between wholeness, healing, and holiness. Most of Jesus' miracles involved healing—curing leprosy and blindness and even raising the dead. Maimonides, in the 12th century, probably the greatest Jewish theologian ever, was also a physician.

For centuries, hospitals in the West had close religious affiliations. The names of many prominent institutions reveal these origins—Presbyterian Hospital, Methodist Hospital, Baptist Hospital, St. Jude's, St. Luke's, St. Barnabas, St. Claire's, St. Elizabeth's, Mount Sinai. Yet, in the late nineteenth century, spirituality and medicine began to diverge. Louis Pasteur and other scientists discovered that many diseases in fact result from viruses and bacteria. In 1928, Alexander Fleming found that mold produces penicillin that kills bacteria, thereby triggering the development of antibiotics. Western medicine pushed to distinguish itself from quackery by being more scientific—and, in doing so, became increasingly antagonistic to spiritual, holistic, and existential aspects of healthcare.

My medical school classes were all strictly scientific, never mentioning religion or spirituality. In the rapidly expanding medical center, all the new shiny steel and glass buildings, money, faculty, prestige, and jobs focused on science alone, not on any spiritual, religious, or existential aspects of what doctors did. Science was where all the new discoveries occurred, generating all the excitement, energy, media attention, and money—billions of dollars yearly in National Institutes of Health grants. Science had answers about our bodies and conquering disease. Spirituality and religion didn't seem to fit.

Over the past century and a half, religion has also become increasingly controversial. Karl Marx famously decried religion as "the Opiate of the Masses." In *The Future of an Illusion*, Freud argued that religion was a form of neurosis. Darwin, Einstein, and quantum physics all accounted for marvels of creation—trees, animals, and humans—that religion had once uniquely claimed to explain.

America's spiritual and religious landscape is, in addition, dramatically changing. In the past few decades, scandals have convulsed churches. Across major faiths, attendance numbers at mainstream religious institutions have been plummeting.[1] Bestselling books like Richard Dawkins' *The God Delusion*, Christopher Hitchens' *God Is Not Great*, and Sam Harris's *The End of Faith* argued that religion is merely a dangerous myth that we should abandon and eliminate.

As a medical intern, I was not especially religious. My grandfather, two great-grandfathers, and a few of my great-great-grandfathers were all Orthodox rabbis. In Lithuania, my great-grandfather had told one of his students, "*You* will marry my daughter," and that young couple moved to America and became my grandparents. My father's oldest brother, Abraham, became the president of my grandfather's temple—The Sons of Israel—in Belmar, New Jersey.

But, born a decade after his older brother, my father preferred playing football to sitting in synagogue, and fought bitterly with my grandfather about it.

The year I was born, my grandfather died. A handful of times, usually for the funerals of a relative, my parents took my sisters and me to his synagogue. The women all sat in the back, behind a dark wooden screen, or upstairs in a dark wooden balcony, and wore hats or veils. The men all wore plain black satin yarmulkes. The wooden pews were hard, and the dark brass chandeliers created a somber, dim atmosphere. The services droned on for hours, almost entirely in Hebrew, which I didn't understand—part of a distant, odd, ancient world that felt utterly irrelevant to me and my life.

Growing up on the Upper West Side in Manhattan and then in Huntington, a Long Island suburb, my family and I had attended a Reform temple, where I was bar mitzvahed; but science, not religion, soon attracted me, and seemed more exciting, able to explain the mysteries of life and the cosmos. In junior high school and high school, physics showed me how atoms made elements. Chemistry revealed how these elements created molecules. Biology taught how we breathed—how cells made tissues that formed organs that pumped blood and sucked oxygen from the air into our blood. The Bible claimed that God created plants, fish, birds, animals, and people in seven days, but Darwin and DNA research supplied far more detailed and accurate explanations.

In college, I thought of myself as an atheist, which was also considered "cool" among my classmates. When I learned that a few classmates regularly attended church together on Sundays, it seemed odd that they would spend time doing that every beautiful sun-soaked [or stormy] Sunday morning.

After my medical internship, treating Carol and other patients, I became a psychiatrist, and in the 1990s, began to conduct research on how patients coped with diseases, such as HIV infection. I focused, overall, on other, medical and psychological aspects of disorders, rather than on the roles of spirituality and religion.

But then, my life dramatically changed.

On September 11, 2001, my sister Karen died at the World Trade Center. At 8:40 a.m. that day, my mother called me at my medical center office to tell me a plane hit the World Trade Center where Karen worked.

"I'm sure she's fine," I said, unsure what to do with this information. I assumed she was OK. Newspaper stories about disasters, shootings, and wars invariably involved *other* people—not me.

Still, after hanging up, I tried phoning Karen and got her voice mail.

I had to hurry to attend a meeting, for which I was now late. But at the building's front desk, a guard sat gaping at a TV. Orange and black flames poured out of the sleek World Trade Center tower. My heart froze.

At the meeting, we talked only about the attack. Colleagues suggested I go downtown to see if my sister was in any hospital there. I took the subway, surprised it was still running, and unsure what I would find. In front of St. Vincent's Hospital, hundreds of crisply uniformed medical personnel stood in rows, waiting for patients to arrive. Inside, a staff member told me that Karen had not been admitted there. He gave me a list of ten other hospitals to call or visit. A surgeon arrived from the crash site, covered with dust. "We're not finding any bodies!" he told me. "They've all been vaporized!" I tried calling the other hospitals, but now had trouble getting a dial tone on my cellphone. When I did, most numbers were busy. One hospital wouldn't give me any information about any patients over the phone.

I wondered why we had not yet heard from Karen. Maybe her phone wasn't working. But my hopes were slowly sinking. I drifted out onto the street along with other stray family members. Some had already visited every hospital in town. We hovered, our phones in our hands, tears in our eyes, with nowhere else to go.

That night, I couldn't sleep. The next morning, my phone started ringing. Each time, I thought it might be Karen or news of her. But the callers were friends and relatives, asking if we had heard from her. At my mother's house, relatives started arriving, bringing bagels, brownies, and cookies—as if for a shiva, when, in Judaism, mourners gather at the home of the deceased's family. I was confused, unsure whether to mourn. I looked around my apartment at framed photographs of Karen, smiling, and couldn't believe she might be dead. She was always confident, defiant, strong; nothing in her pictures said *dead*. I had seen her a few weeks ago, and she was fine. And there was no tangible evidence of her death. Officially she was not dead—there was no death certificate, and legally there couldn't be one without a body. She had seemingly disappeared in a cloud of smoke.

The following morning, a heavy rain fell as my older sister, Susan, and I decided to trek to the Armory to register Karen as "missing person." I hadn't been downtown since the day of the crash and was astonished to see flyers posted on every phone booth, displaying color photos of "missing" people staring out, with a phone number to call if we saw them . . . as if they might be wandering around lost and unable to identify themselves—which made no sense.

At the Armory, we sat at a small, collapsible table with a worn and scratched wooden top, waiting for a police detective. Beside us sat a wet and haggard couple, talking to a cop. The woman's hair was straggly, the man unshaven. They looked as if they hadn't slept in days, either. The Red Cross handed out sandwiches—bologna on white bread with mayonnaise. I devoured three of them.

We registered Karen and walked back out into the heavy gray rain, still hoping that she might somehow be alive.

"I know she's dead," my mother said the next day. "We should schedule a memorial service."

"I'm not sure," I said, still wishing, despite the mounting evidence, that we could somehow escape the horrific finality of such a loss.

Yet reluctantly, the next day, we planned her funeral.

The morning of the service, I felt awful, empty. My head pounded. I felt nauseated—the first time I ever had, when not physically sick—and dreaded getting through this day, as never before.

Karen's identical twin sister, my older sister, my mother, and I arrived at the temple early, and met with the rabbi. We passed around a bottle of Extra-Strength Tylenol and all gulped some down.

In the service, I said I loved Karen and would always miss her. She had spent years working all over the world, conducting research to help emerging nations develop energy resources. She had determination, verve, and wit. I said I was trying to understand her death, but couldn't. A jumbo jet, hijacked by Arab terrorists from the Middle East, had hit her while she was sitting in front of her desk computer. I had trouble grasping it. I wondered if she had tried to jump from the World Trade Center's 101st floor or if flames had burned her alive. None of the atrocity made sense.

Over the following weeks, we turned off her telephone and divided up her belongings and books. I took her texts on how to learn Chinese. In the first page of each she had printed her name in bright blue ink.

The TV company took back the cable box from her apartment. I ran out of toothpaste, so took her tube, indented by her fingers, from her bathroom. Each morning at home, I further squeezed the half-empty container. She had bought this tube with her two hands—now gone. I began to use up the container and felt sad anew.

Then, my body gave out. I had no energy, felt hollow, and couldn't get out of bed. A dull weight hung over me. Work seemed meaningless. When I tried to move, my muscles ached. Even my eyelids felt scratchy and hurt. I had to force myself to read books, even watch TV or listen to music. Only between the cool sheets of my bed did I feel comfortable. For several weeks, I did not feel like going to work and just stayed home.

I thought I had the flu, and was surprised when a psychiatrist friend said, "No, these are symptoms of grief and depression." I soon realized he was correct, but I was amazed how the experience was far more physical—bodily—than I would have thought. The loss of my sister and the attack on the city had been more than my brain could process. My mind and body had just collapsed from under me. The horror lay beyond words, or emotions I could identify. Many psychiatrists implicitly look down at patients who complain of bodily symptoms, rather than only verbally expressing their feelings. We say these patients "somaticize," converting psychological symptoms into physical ones. They are not being "psychologically minded," as if they are psychologically less developed or sophisticated. But I realized how powerful, real, and automatic these corporeal symptoms were, and how little we knew or appreciated what these individuals experienced—how much physicians did not understand. Indeed, new research is now showing how neurochemicals are involved in our emotions and affect the body, too.

I went to psychotherapy but still felt depressed. For hours, I sat in Central Park, just staring out over a lawn. In my busy life, I never sat as long doing nothing. I assumed that being a psychiatrist would help me, but it did not.

The city offered to ferry family members to Ground Zero on a boat, since wrecked buildings and debris still blocked the surrounding streets. One cold late autumn morning, we gathered in a chilly wind on a bare wooden dock in the West 20s and boarded a rusty red tugboat. Police gave us yellow hard hats to wear. Volunteers handed out flowers and small stuffed brown teddy bears to hold. The stuffed animals seemed childish, but I took one. As we approached the site, a smell of burning electrical wire and dirt stung my nostrils. The dusty gray wreckage smoldered over several blocks, far more vast than I imagined. All around us, mounds of black and lead-gray debris rose five or six stories, still smoking. We slowly wended into the wreckage, all tightly clutching our teddy bears.

I felt dazed and bewildered, unsure how to make sense of the war zone all around us. I glanced up. Somewhere in the sky above us she had worked, yet nothing remained. The whole World Trade Center and my sister had vanished. It was too much to take in. I couldn't move and began to weep.

As I stood there, and over the weeks that followed, I wondered even more why my sister had been one of them, and why my family had been one of the unlucky ones, singled out, while the vast majority of people didn't have to endure this pain.

Gradually, I began to accept my sister's death more, but in many ways, as the city lowered its estimated number of 9/11 deaths, life became harder— not easier. Why us?

A few months after her death, I attended a synagogue, but felt little comfort. I tried going to a Presbyterian church and even a Buddhist service, where a red-robed priest rang bells as we walked in a circle around the room. I visited a psychic who claimed to communicate with Karen, though I was dubious.

One afternoon in the park, as I sat on a bench, a gentle wind began to blow. The tiny blades of grass shivered nervously, struggling to remain upright. But ultimately, they all bowed together in the breeze, the green blades suddenly flashing white in the sun. The invisible breeze rolled across the silent grass like a wave.

Nearby, on a small pond, sunlight sparkled. Tiny wavelets shimmered, dark green, blue, and white. A weeping willow tree lay flat on its side, downed by a storm several years earlier. Small, thin shoots now fingered upwards from it toward the sky. Though crashed to the ground, the tree had struggled and survived. Larger forces of Nature and the universe beyond us, I saw, somehow continued on. I felt it was a sign—as if her spirit, too, would somehow continue on in some form. I sighed, and began to feel a sense of gratitude to whatever forces lay beyond us, and the need to keep going on as best I could. I was, after all, still alive. I felt a connection to the extraordinary power and beauty of Nature. Yet these thoughts were untied to any religion per se.

A few days later, I returned to work, but the subway stops and hospital buildings all seemed strange—I felt disappointed that they were unchanged, as if nothing had happened. The world seemed just to move on, oblivious of my family's and my own thoughts.

Over the next few months, I began to ponder more how other people faced such existential, spiritual, and religious crises. I wondered, too, how other doctors did so—how, after a medical or emotional crisis, they looked at their prior training, and what, if anything, they now learned or unlearned. I searched the medical literature, but found little. A handful of doctors had written a brief article or chapter about their individual case, but no one had tried to examine how doctors as a group responded and handled the vast chasm between strictly scientific approaches and these other, human realms that they now faced.

I embarked on a journey to find out, and ended up interviewing in depth 75 such physicians who became sick with severe illness, and writing a book, *When Doctors Become Patients,* about what I saw.[2] What I discovered astonished me: Similar to what I'd experienced, they almost all found themselves grappling, often for the first time, with larger existential, spiritual, and religious questions about life, fate, meaning, purpose, and the universe, though in varying ways, and were usually surprised to do so.

As one elderly physician with cancer told me, "For years, patients used to say to me, 'Doc, will you pray for me?' I'd say, 'Yeah, yeah.' But I'd pooh-pooh it." He brushed the remembered request away with the side of his hand. "Then, I became a patient myself, and realized how important spiritual issues are." Not until he became ill did he seriously contemplate these realms. These doctors described a range of spiritual journeys they undertook as they dealt with their disease.

I became more sensitive, too, to how other patients and their families also struggle with profound spiritual and existential questions, striving to make sense of their disease, to grasp the cause, seek solutions, and gain some feeling of control, and grapple with scientific knowledge, though it is frequently uncertain and incomplete. Given these gaps, many patients wrestle with deep existential quandaries about what will happen to them, what the ultimate meaning of their life is and will be, and "Why me?"

Even when they have a genetic mutation, patients confront such quandaries and look to metaphysics and spirituality. Patients whom I interviewed as part of research studies on responses to genetic testing for various disorders pondered larger cosmological questions as well.[3] As one man in his late 30s told me, "I know I have Huntington's disease [a severe neurological disease] because of the mutation. But why did God give the mutation to me, and not to my sister?" When I explained that it was due to chance—the flip of a coin—he shook his head back and forth slightly, unmoved and unconvinced. This explanation didn't feel emotionally satisfying to him.

A woman who learned she did *not* have the genetic mutation, though her mother and sister did, similarly asked me, "Why did God give the HD mutation to my brother and not to me?" The fact that the cause of our death may result largely from random chance is very hard to accept. Even Einstein, I thought to myself, famously argued that "God does not throw dice."[4] In studying decision-making about infertility treatments and assisted reproductive technologies, patients (and their loved ones) also wondered whether God had intended for them to have or not have a child.[5]

I saw how frequently patients and their families grappled with these conundrums, yet how poorly we as doctors were trained or equipped to address these topics.

Though Freud argued that religion is merely a manifestation of neurosis, recent studies show that most religious people are not mentally unwell, but rather happier than others.[6] Viktor Frankl, a Nazi concentration camp survivor and psychiatrist, argued that humans all seek a sense of meaning and purpose.[7] People yearn not only to obtain the necessities of life, but also to feel connected and fulfilled in some way. Overall, belief in a "higher power" of some sort appears to offer certain psychological benefits.[8] Religions can provide, too, a sense of security, increase feelings of self-esteem and well-being,[9,10] and create a moral community.

Recent neuroscience and psychological research as well shows how religious and spiritual beliefs and practices aid people and are in fact *hard-wired* into the human brain, associated with neurobiological changes. We feel calm because of neurochemicals, released or suppressed by the presence or absence of certain external stimuli. Scientists have measured resultant electrical waves, and oxygen use and activity in the brain, and found that people who say religion and spirituality are important to them, compared to those who have depressive negative emotions or fear God, have thicker layers of neurons in portions of their brain and more "neural reserves" to draw on. These neural reserves help people disengage from negative emotions and ruminations, enhancing well-being, empathy, altruism, coping, and resilience against depression and anxiety. Several studies have found such neurobiological differences between individuals praying versus not praying, or reading religious versus secular texts.[11] Mindfulness, too, has been associated with variations in brain structure and function, including alterations in the thickness of the cortex, the density of gray matter, and the amount of atrophy in the hippocampus—part of the brain involved in memory and learning. Mindfulness can affect regulation of attention and emotions, though more research is needed to elucidate what mechanisms might be involved.[12] Religious and spiritual coping has also been found to be associated with decreased risk of certain diseases—for instance, of hypertension in African American women.[13]

Conversely, stressful life events exacerbate religious and spiritual struggles, especially for people who feel isolated, angry, and anxious about death.[14] In one study of patients over 50 years old, for instance, those with depression were more likely to have no religious affiliation and to be "spiritual but not religious."[15] Intrinsic religious beliefs also predict shorter time in overcoming depression, partly because religion provides community support.[16]

Critics who aver that religions are all simply pernicious delusions fail to grasp the forceful strength of these deep neurobiological and psychological impulses—profound human needs for purpose and larger understanding—that occupy vital spaces in our lives and society, and provide unique and necessary solace to millions of patients and their families, helping them cope and serving as forces for good.

Indeed, all human societies have created and worshiped gods, looking upward toward some notion of superior, divine beings. The ancient world created a pantheon of deities, including Zeus, Jupiter, Neptune, Apollo, Venus, and Athena, and demigods such as Gilgamesh, Pharaoh, and Hercules. Among the most ancient extant human structures, from around 3800 BCE, are tombs and monuments of massive stones, in Newgrange, Ireland and elsewhere, often decorated with arrays of powerfully chiseled spirals and concentric circles—rich symbols believed to hold religious and spiritual meanings. For millennia, in most cities across the world—from Luxor, Jerusalem, Athens, and Rome to Chichén Itzá, Delhi, Beijing, London, and Paris—the tallest buildings were religious.

Yet the modern world faces religious, spiritual, and existential conundrums. In medicine, new technologies have redefined the beginning and end of life, posing new challenges. Machines pump the hearts and lungs of brain-dead patients who will never recover and will die if the machines stopped. A colleague jokes that we spend millions of dollars keeping dead people alive in hospitals—brain-dead patients with no chance of recovery. Doctors, patients, and families therefore face excruciating choices about when to turn off the machines—whether to "play God."

The COVID-19 pandemic made these dilemmas ever more acute. Suddenly, hundreds of millions of people were getting sick, and millions were dying, frequently alone, isolated in bare sterile hospital rooms, if they were lucky to get one, separated from their loved ones. Generally, people cope with stress by spending time with family and friends and going to churches, restaurants, bars, theaters, and gyms. But COVID-19 stymied these activities and connections to others. Locked down, curfewed, quarantined, masked, and socially distanced, billions of people now feared disease in themselves and their families and felt distraught, confused, and desperate. Not surprisingly, studies showed that during the pandemic, half of Americans suffered from symptoms of depression.[17]

Many healthcare providers had to put their own lives at risk. They had to hide behind paper face masks and plastic shields and tried to spend as little time as possible at patients' bedsides, scared of catching the virus themselves. They soon felt overwhelmed and burned out. As the media reported,[18,19] a superb physician at my own hospital, Dr. Lorna Breen, after trying to treat scores of COVID patients and seeing them perish, committed suicide herself.

Billions of people, seeing friends and family get sick and die, began to question the meanings of their daily routines, work, relationships, and goals—what was truly important in their lives—and reset their priorities, adopting a new perspective of "YOLO"—you only live once. In past epidemics such as the Black Death, people turned to religious institutions. But now, many religious institutions moved online, reduced to electronic screens that lacked vital human touch.

While critics have rightly attacked corrupt religious institutions, as a doctor I have increasingly witnessed how patients and their families seek and struggle to find sources of meaning, purpose, and hope. While Dawkins and other recent bestselling authors insist that religions are merely dangerous delusions, I saw how these authors have failed to appreciate the forceful strength of psychological impulses toward religion—human needs to find meaning and endure, especially when facing death and dying.

But I have observed, too, how patients and their families, especially when confronting imminent threats of death, grapple with these issues, reimagining, redefining, and reconceptualizing their views in manifold ways.

Due in part to globalization and social media, beliefs are taking new forms. Patients reveal how much *we are in fact living in an age of enormous religious and spiritual transformation.*

Atheism and agnosticism have spread, and most traditional religious institutions have lost members. Much of America has become more secular. In response, fundamentalism and evangelicalism have vigorously pushed back and burgeoned, with recent bestselling books such as *Heaven Is Real* and *Proof of Heaven* insisting that God and Heaven definitely exist. In 1966, a *Time* magazine cover story provocatively asked, "Is God Dead?"[20] Today in the United States, religion seems to be alive and well, but changing. Religion clearly isn't dead, though some traditional institutions are dying.

Still, at the same time, between these two extremes of atheism and evangelicalism, growing numbers of individuals, when asked whether they are Catholic, Protestant, Jewish, other, or "none of the above," check the last category and have thus been dubbed "Nones." They constitute the fastest-growing category in the United States. From 2007 to 2014 alone, the number of religiously unaffiliated Americans rose over 40% (from 16.1.% to 22.8%), while the percent of self-identified Christians fell.[21] Christians made up 85% of the so-called Silent Generation (born 1928–1945) but only 56% of Millennials (born 1990–1996).[21] Though rising numbers of people consider themselves to be "spiritual but not religious," I have found that they interpret this phrase in vastly different ways. Indeed, half of Americans who "have no religion" still believe in Heaven, and about 40% believe in Hell.[22]

While public discourse and debates have focused on whether religion is simply "all good" or "all bad," more balanced and nuanced perspectives are needed. In our pluralistic society, we need to move beyond arguments about whether religion is simply good or bad or whether Heaven and Hell exist—binary questions without clear answers. Instead, the major challenges are *how we struggle to make sense of life crises, and construct narratives that make sense for ourselves, and how we face, view, frame or reframe notions of spirituality and higher powers.* People need meaning and hope in their lives, but increasingly vary in how they seek and find these. I saw how religion and spirituality are critical in medicine and countless areas of contemporary society, yet are often misunderstood.

For many patients and families, religion and spirituality are vital, especially when encountering serious disease and possible death, but their clergy, if they have any, are far away and/or can't visit them in the hospital. *Hence, the field of chaplaincy has come to fill this vacuum.*

The term "chaplain" derives from the Old French *chapelain*, from the medieval Latin *cappellanus*, from *cappella* or "little cloak." The priest who oversaw a relic, kept by the Frankish kings, of St. Martin of Tours' cloak, half of which he had given to a needy beggar, was called a *chapelain*. In the mid-fourteenth century, the term came to mean "minister of a chapel."[23]

The field is also known as *pastoral care*, from the Latin word for shepherd, reflecting the notion, especially in Christianity, of a minister caring for a flock. Pastoral care has come, however, to include the entire realm of religious, spiritual and nonreligious beliefs. Chaplains exist in other types of institutions as well, notably prisons and the military. Away from their own local clergy, individuals in all these varied settings commonly lack religious support.

Over the years, medical chaplaincy has evolved. In the United States, prior to the Civil War, hospitals were often built by Protestant organizations and cared largely for the poor. In the latter half of the nineteenth century, as masses of immigrants arrived from Southern and Eastern Europe, Catholic and Jewish organizations constructed hospitals as well, and patients came from more varied faiths.

Hospitals for soldiers and veterans have long recognized needs for chaplains. In 1865, Abraham Lincoln established the first national homes for disabled war veterans, hiring chaplains, who were paid "$1,500 per year and forage for one horse."[24] In 1945, the Veterans Administration established chaplaincy services in all its hospitals.[24]

In recent decades, chaplaincy has burgeoned, but also changed, shaped partly by outside economic, social, and religious trends.[24] In 1940, chaplains were all white Protestant men;[25] starting in the 1960s, however, chaplaincy gradually started becoming more diverse in gender, race, and ethnicity. Beginning in the 1980s and 1990s, financial pressures led many hospitals to merge or close. New technological advances, including artificial life support, extended the quantity, but not necessarily the quality, of life for severely sick individuals, raising profound bioethical and religious dilemmas about whether doctors, patients, and families should pursue such interventions, including futile care and keeping alive comatose patients who will never recover. Partly as a response, various needs arose for more attention to religion and spirituality in healthcare. Since 1992, The Joint Commission on Accreditation of Healthcare Organizations (JCAHO), which accredits hospitals, has mentioned the need to address patients' spiritual needs, especially regarding end-of-life and other types of care.[26] Chaplaincy also began to focus on spirituality, broadly defined, more than religion per se, and to perform spiritual assessments and address spiritual distress.

Currently, around 60% of hospitals have chaplains.[24] Today, these spiritual care professionals have various religious and religious backgrounds and draw on insights from psychology, theology and other fields. They do not preach, but rather aid patients in confronting spiritual issues more broadly. Of U.S. chaplains, 30.3% are mainline Protestants, 24.6% Catholic, 16.7% Evangelical Protestants, and 9.3% Jewish; the rest are other, including 0.15% Muslim.[25] Roughly equal numbers are male and female; 63.8% are Caucasian, 9.0% African American, 2.6% Latino, and the rest are other.[24] Increasingly, many, but not all, healthcare chaplains are certified by the Association of Professional Chaplains, which requires that they: (1) have a master's degree in a religious discipline (such as divinity or a related field); (2) are ordained, supported, or endorsed by a religious or spiritual organization (such as a church); (3) have completed several units of training in a clinical pastoral education program; and (4) have worked at least 2,000 hours in the field.[27] Yet numerous chaplains are in the midst of this process and not yet certified. Organizations have also started for Catholic, Baptist, Jewish, Muslim, and other denominations of chaplains, providing ongoing education and support. In recent years, the field has increasingly emphasized nondenominational approaches as well.

Several scholars have begun to study several key aspects of spirituality and religion among patients, doctors, nurses, and chaplains. In her book *Paging God: Religion in the Halls of Medicine*, the sociologist Wendy Cadge has, for example, shed valuable light on the history and growth of hospital chaplains, chaplaincy departments, and chapels in America,[28] observing chaplains and ICU staff closely at a hospital and interviewing others, examining their daily work. Research has also begun to probe how often chaplains engage in various kinds of activities, such as prayer.[29,30]

Yet most people know little, if anything, about this field. In addition, many questions remain about who these spiritual care providers in varied institutions are; what exactly they do for patients of increasingly varied beliefs, and how and why; what challenges they face and how they address these; how they interact with doctors, hospitals, and other staff; and what insights they have about spiritual, religious, and existential issues more broadly.

Given the growing importance of these issues, *and the fact that religion and spirituality have become increasingly both polarized and pluralistic, I began to wonder what patients today believe, how they respond to threats of death and dying, and how chaplains help.* I therefore started to interview hospital chaplains. I initially talked with hospital chaplains informally, contacting them through word of mouth, and then soon launched a formal, systematic in-depth study of them, which I largely draw on here.

My approach was influenced to a considerable extent by one of my former professors, the anthropologist Clifford Geertz, who argued that to comprehend any social situation, we should try to obtain a "thick description,"[31] not by imposing preconceptions or theoretical structures on it, but by trying to grasp the views and perceptions of the individuals involved in their own words. This approach can elucidate not only what these individuals are doing, but also what they think they are doing and how they understand their lives and the challenges they confront.

This book focuses on the insights of the 21 board-certified chaplains I formally interviewed in depth by phone. As described more fully in Appendix A and B, these individuals came from across the United States and from different religious backgrounds—Protestant, Catholic, Jewish, Muslim, Buddhist, and secular humanist. Twelve were men and nine were women. They ranged in age from 42 to 75 years, with an average of 63. Ten were from the Northeast, and the others were from the Midwest, Southeast, Southwest, and West. They had practiced as chaplains for an average of 18 years (with a range between three and 30 years). Eight had master's degrees, and five held doctorates. (Appendix A and B provide further methodological details.)

I draw here, too, on interviews I have conducted as part of several research studies with doctors and patients confronting various diseases, including cancer[2] and HIV[32] and genetic testing results for various conditions.[3] All interviewees gave informed consent. I have changed the names and identifying details of all the individuals quoted here to protect their confidentiality. I have been influenced, too, by decades of participant-observation; conversations I've had as a doctor and psychiatrist with a wide range of patients and their families; and my own personal experiences.

I saw how chaplains have developed valuable and impressive methods for helping people in confronting the threats and terrors of serious disease and death, offering unique and essential lenses into how people face these issues today. These pastoral care providers each presented extraordinary stories of experiences and, at times, frustrations and challenges, working with patients and families, as well as with doctors and nurses, within complex, fragmented hospital systems that generally ignored patients' existential and spiritual concerns. Chaplains routinely witness courage and anguish, and help patients find meaning and fortitude. Like canaries in a coal mine, they convey to us vital insights on the current state of religious and spiritual beliefs among individuals facing life's ultimate crises.

I argue here that patients with serious disease and their families today often wrestle with profound existential, spiritual, and religious quandaries that physicians are generally uncomfortable with and/or lack the time and skills to discuss, and that, consequently, chaplains play ever more crucial roles, filling these gaps, assisting patients of differing beliefs in finding and constructing meaning, hope, and connections to broader moral principles or "higher powers." In so doing, these spiritual care providers have developed flexible approaches, and reveal insights and challenges that can aid all of us in navigating these troubled seas. I have reported a few of these findings in the scholarly literature,[33-45] but they are of wider interest and importance as well—reflecting human nature as well as our broader culture and attitudes.

Importantly, though public discourse on religion and spirituality is increasingly polarized between atheists and the religious right, patients commonly struggle in the middle, striving to cope and to find meaning and hope.

Unfortunately, in our ever more fractured healthcare system, doctors and nurses are stressed and lack time to address these existential and psychological strains. Hospitals usually have insufficient psychiatrists, psychologists, social workers, and other professionals to explore these realms.

Chaplains have thus come to provide, too, de facto psychotherapy, as well as fresh eyes, strikingly uncovering vital information about patients that abet diagnosis and treatment and overcome biases that hospital staff may have. These spiritual care providers also assist doctors and nurses with burnout and grief.

But chaplains face challenges. Communication about spiritual, religious, and existential quandaries is inherently subjective, ineffable, and potentially divisive, and thus difficult. Chaplains work in vital but highly amorphous spaces, and are often marginalized and under-resourced, able to see only a fraction of the patients in a hospital.[46] Regulations do not require that hospitals hire chaplains, and many hospitals rely not on board-certified chaplains, but on local community clergy without specific training to serve as volunteers. Most chaplaincy departments are relatively small, and hence cannot realistically include chaplains of every possible faith. Hospitals that are smaller or rural are less likely to even have chaplains.[33]

Yet, I contend here that *these spiritual care providers are unsung heroes*, and that hospitals, doctors, healthcare systems, insurers, and policymakers, as well as patients and families, need to recognize and appreciate these critical professionals far more. I suggest here how doctors and chaplains can also better address these topics.

Simple questionnaires, used to try to quantify the benefits offered by chaplains, have faced limitations and had mixed results. However, in-depth narratives of what these individuals actually do, with examples of how they help patients and families, illustrate the value of their work and insights in ways that statistics cannot. I have therefore sought to provide such descriptions here.

As a brief overview, this book divides these issues into six sections. Part I shows how patients encounter fundamental questions that physicians commonly do not discuss and that chaplains do. Part II sheds light on the range of specific types of beliefs about religion and spirituality that patients and their families draw on when facing medical crises and that chaplains work to address—from traditional faiths to being "spiritual but not religious," atheist or agnostic. Many religious patients, for instance, wonder if they are being punished by God. Pastoral care also aids individuals who are "spiritual but not religious" in finding their own sources of meaning. Part III probes how chaplains confront cross-cutting themes regardless of patients' particular beliefs, helping to reset priorities, creating prayers, and addressing patients' vulnerabilities related to disabilities, mental health, or other stigmatized characteristics. Part IV explores specific end-of-life dilemmas that chaplains help adults and children confront, concerning, for instance, questions about grief and the afterlife. Part V examines how these professionals can face hurdles with not only patients and families, but also other medical staff, especially doctors and nurses, who experience moral and physical distress. Yet physicians, in particular, are often wary of religion and spirituality. Part VI probes directions for the future for doctors, chaplains, and ultimately us all. I have chosen quotes to exemplify the major themes that emerge. (I have also highlighted some of the words for emphasis.)

These chapters present cross-cutting issues in organized ways to convey a sense of these topics as a whole, rather than offering merely a series of separated, individual portraits of each chaplain with whom I spoke. My goal is to paint a group portrait, a collage, similar to a documentary film, in which interviews with different people are intercut, with each individual discussing one particular issue at a time, and then reappearing later to talk about other subjects.

But this approach poses challenges. Documentaries have an advantage over written texts, letting viewers literally see each interviewee, and remember what he or she looks like. For several reasons, including needs to protect confidentiality, I cannot do that, and instead refer to each interviewee through brief descriptions. The relatively large number of speakers could, however, potentially confuse some readers, trying to keep all these individuals in mind. I could have left out some of these chaplains and included only a handful, but each one shared valuable experiences and insights. Their stories deepen and enrich the picture as a whole and, by the end, I think the reader will have a sense of each interviewee as a person, along with the field's approaches and insights as a whole. To aid readers, Appendix A also includes a list of the names (all pseudonyms) and brief descriptions of the chaplains who frequently appear. I beg for the reader's patience through these pages, in becoming familiar with each of these people.

I focus here on the United States, but pastoral care exists in countries throughout the world, with similar goals, benefits, and challenges.[47]

Several different groups of readers may benefit from this book—from general readers to professionals, including healthcare providers and trainees in medicine (including oncology, intensive care, palliative care, family medicine and psychiatry), nurses, chaplains, social workers and psychotherapists, lawyers (in estate planning and other areas), clergy who are currently practicing or in training, social scientists (e.g., psychologists, sociologists, anthropologists), and others.

The insights here can especially aid countless patients and families who often wrestle with these challenges, but may be unaware of the existence and potential benefits of chaplains. The vast majority of us (80%) will die not in our own beds, but in hospitals or nursing homes, and will face existential and spiritual quandaries. Many of our prior beliefs will fall short, and chaplains will be the ones to assist us and our loved ones to make sense of the existential and spiritual crises we then face. Heightened awareness and understanding of these amazing providers can aid us as we face these ultimate moments in our lives.

My goal is not to convince readers whether God exists or not. Various authors have attempted that, and readers have undoubtedly already considered that question at length. Rather, this book reveals *how*, in the context of ever-rising religious, cultural, and social polarization in our nation and world, people today grapple with these quandaries and forge new paths, and how spiritual care frequently assists us in better understanding these realms, and communicating about them with each other, while pointing ways forward for us. The individuals here have deeply moved and inspired me and can, I think, help countless others as well.

2

Asking "why me?" and second-guessing God

"What did I do to deserve this?" Jane Mayes, a 38-year-old woman who couldn't get pregnant, asked me. I met her as part of a study I was conducting on assisted reproductive technologies.[1] She had undergone multiple intrauterine inseminations and in vitro fertilization without success. "I don't have a relationship with my mother, so I wondered if karma came back to bite me. My husband has had a lot of health problems, so I thought maybe *that* was the reason." Jane knew that "logically," these were not the main causes. "But *emotionally, there's a whole process*—I wanted something, someone, some reason to *blame*. What brought this upon me?" Some days, she figured that maybe God did not want her to have a child. "I was definitely ticked off at God and thought: 'Just let it happen, it would be easier on both of us.' . . . I prayed, begged, pleaded, tried not praying—the whole spectrum. Mostly I kept it all in perspective: Maybe my body was just not able to. But I started thinking: 'Maybe it wasn't *meant* to happen. Maybe my body isn't *meant* to have a child.'"

Patients and families often ponder and ask, "Why me?" Among parents who lost a child in a motor vehicle accident, for instance, 91% asked this question and 59% said they were unable to answer it.[2]

I know personally how strongly these questions can arise, even if irrational. After 9/11, I, too, found myself wondering why my family had been one of the unlucky ones. No one else I knew had lost a family member on that horrific day. In the weeks after the attack, everyone I knew asked repeatedly how my family and I were faring. I appreciated their concern but didn't want to keep talking about it all the time. The questions kept reopening psychic wounds. I knew her death was random, but it still didn't seem at all fair to me. We had done nothing wrong. Why did my family have to deal with this grief, and personal and public ordeal? Why had we been singled out? Why did it have to be *us*? I knew these questions were irrational, but they still plagued me.

Doctor, Will You Pray for Me?. Robert L. Klitzman, Oxford University Press. © Oxford University Press 2024.
DOI: 10.1093/oso/9780197750841.003.0002

Jane Mayes, confronting trouble getting pregnant, and others search their own lives for causes of bad news, and seek more than physical, biochemical processes as reasons, wanting instead an explanation that emotionally makes sense.

One of the most compelling and discussed books in the Bible is the story of Job. His friends argue that he must have done something wrong to incur God's disfavor. Job disagrees. When he asks God why he suffers, God does not answer directly, but instead explains how God is vastly older and more powerful than Job, stating, "Where were you when I made the Heavens?"[3]

These questions of "Why me?" inherently pose larger metaphysical conclusions about whether some larger power or order in the universe exists.

"There are no atheists in a foxhole," a common adage says. The immediate threat of one's own death forces one to suddenly confront one's own mortality. As Samuel Johnson, the eighteenth-century writer and critic, similarly quipped, "When a man knows he is to be hanged in a fortnight, it concentrates his mind wonderfully."[4]

Patients with life-threatening disease, I have found, wrestle daily with dreadful threats to their own annihilation. Many are uncertain if they will ever leave the hospital alive, or again feel happy or see their parents, siblings, children, or friends.

One of the most difficult questions patients confront is why their particular fate has befallen them. Instinctively, we ponder why bad events are occurring to us. We evolved to seek causes and possible solutions to these questions. Through human evolution, these impulses have helped us. Desires to ask why and to want answers, to find underlying roots of problems and potentially ways of fixing them, instead of simply accepting helplessness and pure randomness and chaos, have been adaptive.

Yet definitive answers do not always exist. Though ever advancing, scientific knowledge frequently remains murky and incomplete. Medicine strives to predict future outcomes—whether and for how long we will each survive—but these forecasts are invariably cloudy. Cures are far rarer than we would like. Patients thus commonly wonder, "Why me?" and seek not only physical but also metaphysical explanations.

Connie Clark is a Wisconsin Catholic chaplain who works at a secular academic medical center. During the COVID-19 pandemic, she became burned out, took time off, started practicing yoga, and, on returning to work, began assisting hospital staff with their moral distress. "All patients in the hospital, particularly an intensive care unit, have concerns about survival," she told me. "Even if their prognosis is good, they face existential questions about 'Why am I here? Where am I going? What's the meaning of all of this?'" The threat of imminent death poses ambiguities regarding what to do about the disease and one's remaining time on Earth, however long it may be, and in turn, the purpose of life, how to keep going, and what is most important. She knew these feelings from her own personal experiences during COVID.

Even when a clear physical cause can be found, people also look for larger moral frameworks. When patients ask, "Why me?" they usually don't mean the question scientifically—what virus caused their life-threatening disease—but rather existentially. Even if a genetic mutation is involved, many people still wonder why they have the mutation while others do not.

Yet the seemingly simple two-word query "Why me?" in fact represents multiple different questions and concerns, the emotional valences of which vary across patients, seeking to better comprehend the roles of chance in a random universe. These simple two words involve profound and troubling existential and spiritual dilemmas and trigger a wide range of reactions, reflecting not just despair but epistemological unknowns, too.

This short phrase can in fact represent several different questions:

1. Why am I singled out? (Why *me* vs. someone else?)
2. What did I *do* to cause this, and what if I had acted differently?
3. Is this punishment?
4. Does this fate reflect some kind of order, rather than mere randomness?

This statement can also reflect anger and depression.

Many patients wonder if they somehow *deserve* bad outcomes, and at times feel that they do, related to guilt, anger, fear, desires to avoid blame, or other psychological factors, even if they recognize intellectually that such feelings are unhelpful. Disease can reanimate and reignite past lingering regrets.

Many people, like me after 9/11, realize there is no clear answer, but ask anyway. They recognize the irrationality, but wonder nonetheless. These questions spring up from deep wells in the human psyche. Patients may also disagree with friends or family members about the answers. Psychotherapeutic perspectives can help, but these quandaries can nonetheless linger.

Over the years, I have met a few patients who, when confronting disease, accept solely scientific answers and appear to reject broader existential questions. Yet these individuals tend to be rare and have had scientific training. For instance, Sandra Jones, a science major in college, worked for a technology company for several years, and then had a son who had a congenital heart deficit at birth. Her scientific background shaped her views. Her friends discussed religious perspectives, which she strongly dismissed: "They told me, 'God doesn't give you any more than you can handle,' which I think is *bullshit*. I don't believe God has anything to do with it. I think something happened, and this is what I got. It is what it is. I did not ask, 'Why me?' because that's not really productive. I'm a science person, so I kind of got the whole picture, and was interested in it from the scientific perspective as well as 'What does it mean for me personally?'"

Yet in sticking to a strictly scientific approach, given her education, Sandra is an exception. Jane Mayes, the woman with infertility, and most other patients I have met, especially if they face the threat of their own death, struggle at some point with larger, existential questions about why they are being singled out, and whether they may have done something to deserve this fate. *Physical explanations do not feel fully satisfying, prompting larger metaphysical queries.*

Many struggle, unsure, and conclude that "no one" or "only God" knows why they got sick. People generally don't want to believe that God would want them to suffer, and they feel that a larger plan, even if unfathomable, somehow exists. They feel that mixes of not only genes and environment, but also larger mysteries and unknowns, can be involved.

Psychotherapy can assist in coping with these questions but not necessarily eliminate them. "I don't believe that God wanted this," said Roberta Sinclair, a woman who, like Jane, grappled with infertility. Roberta had undergone eight years of unsuccessful treatments, and was now 38 years old and worked in marketing. "There is no reason for it. It's definitely unfair and stinks. Why does it happen to certain people? I don't know. I don't think *anyone* does." Nonetheless, "I went through all of those emotions. When I look online or go to the doctor and see all those other women there, I know I'm not the only one going through this. But I felt, 'Why is this happening to *me*? Why am *I* going through this? No one else I know is going through exactly the same thing.'"

"When you asked, 'Why me?'" I queried Roberta, "What did you tell yourself?"

"I don't know. I didn't really have an answer. That's what was so frustrating . . . I'm a good person. I haven't really done anything terribly wrong. A counselor put those feelings in perspective for me: They're normal, but not helpful. It's better to think, 'What am I going to do?' Have a game plan, think positively. If you want to have a child, one way or another you will." Roberta highlighted how existential and spiritual unease can fuel desires for "positive" reframing and thinking.

Ongoing psychotherapy over months or years can potentially help, but unfortunately not everyone who would benefit from it receives it. Many cannot afford it. Generally in the hospital, patients and families receive no kind of formal psychotherapy.

Since these questions have no answers, patients' views often fluctuate as new crises surface through the course of a disease. Amy Thompson, a suburban secretary whom I also met as part of research on genetics,[5] had two sons who died of a severe congenital disease. She underwent genetic testing herself, seeking a cause, but didn't find one. She now wondered, "Why would God allow this to happen—two children in a row? I was certain there must be some major wrong. When you've had such tragedy, you have a different perspective on life—that you're *unlucky*, that if something bad is going to happen, it's going to happen to *you*." Her sons' deaths anguished, angered, and grieved her and forced her to grapple with the religious tenets with which she had been raised, to try to make sense of these events.

On the one hand, her religion ostensibly gave her an answer. "Our faith plays a huge role. As Catholics, we believe that God doesn't make those decisions. We are free beings and make *our own* decisions. God is there more to give us strength and support—whatever life brings to us. Other people may believe God *does* look down and make these decisions, and if you pray hard enough or live your life a certain way, He's going to decide whether your child lives or dies."

When her genetic tests failed to explain her sons' deaths, she "felt tremendous relief to find out I was at least 'normal.'" Yet these questions continue to haunt her. Once she "got beyond" the bitterness, she "was able to say, 'OK, God *didn't* do this to me' or 'I don't fully grasp why it happened. I'm not going to understand. I just have to accept.'"

Still, even now, she fluctuates: "It's human nature to ask, '*Why?*' Every now and then it still creeps up on me, and I have to talk myself down from 'Why?' There's no answer. *It's an ongoing battle. I haven't completely overcome it. It's a journey* . . . a constant battle of 'Let it go.' *It just eats you up!*"

"You can live in a constant state of anger and frustration," she confessed, "and see your life wither away. *Or* you can decide, 'I'm going to keep working on accepting this, and do my best with what life has given me.'" Her beliefs evolved, partly due to external events such as test results, which offered some relief but did not wholly erase her perplexity. She keeps trying to accept strictly medical answers, yet still wrestles with these questions and emotions over time, torn between theological answers and her own internal emotional turmoil. Ultimately, of course, no real "evidence" can resolve these conundrums. Given our limited abilities to fathom Nature, many patients grapple with such quandaries, Job-like. The notion that events occur because of pure randomness threatens faith in human agency and hope, and can instead foster sadness and resignation.

We are hard-wired to construct stories with a beginning, a middle, and an end, to seek and create tales—even distorted, inaccurate, or false—that place painful events in narrative structures, to try to avoid despair and painful regrets, expand our larger sense of meaning, and calm us. As Joan Didion wrote, "We tell ourselves stories in order to live."[6] We evolved to construct such accounts as mental frameworks to organize social interactions and relationships, and make sense of other people and their motives. We are meaning-making machines.

Yet people, yearning for coherence and meaning, tend to have difficulty fitting their disease into their prior stories of their lives, to provide a sense of wholeness. On our ever-unfolding journeys battling disease, we strive to write and rewrite these narratives as we go, shaped by medical and psychological factors, wrestling to understand and find meaning, causes, and blame—from biology and physics to luck and metaphysics. Patients generally try to fall back on their pre-existing beliefs, which can help to a certain degree, but often now fall short and no longer feel wholly sufficient. In the terror of hospitalizations, countless people struggle to find a framework that works for them, and they frequently benefit from assistance.

3

"Doctor, do you believe in God?"

Physicians facing spiritual and religious questions

When on call as a hospital intern, I slept on a tiny cot in a barren, windowless, closet-sized room. On the white bare wall, a colleague had scribbled, "70% of patients get better on their own."

"God saves the other 30%," another intern had penned.

One more wrote, "10% will die anyway." This nihilism, though tinged with cynicism, spoke some truth—even if the percentages didn't add up to 100.

Over the doors of my hospital, words from Ecclesiasticus 38:2 are engraved in stone: "From the most high cometh healing." At parties, fellow medical trainees, getting drunk or high on marijuana, would laugh: "I guess we're the most high now!"

Only rarely, if ever, even to each other, do physicians acknowledge these domains or the limits of science. When we do so, it is only fleetingly and tacitly, around the edges, often through black humor.

Both of these ancient professions, medicine and religion, help us combat the horror and finitude of death, but they have had a long and complicated marriage. Physicians and clergy seek to heal patients' bodies and souls, respectively, and require extensive training and selflessness, but they differ and conflict. Medicine today aims to focus on scientific facts; religious and spiritual concepts all appear utterly subjective. Yet, religion and spirituality do influence doctors and other medical providers. Among OB/GYNs, for instance, 45% said that their religious and spiritual beliefs at least sometimes affected the medical options they offered patients.[1] Physicians who are more religious are more likely to suggest chemotherapy, and less likely to recommend hospice for cancer patients or to engage in medical aid-in-dying.[2] In one British study, 50% of nonreligious doctors, compared to only 32.3% of very or extremely religious doctors, had made a decision that involved an expectation or intent to hasten a patient's death.[3]

Religion and spirituality affect patients, too, both directly and indirectly—in terms of whether they consult clergy, pray, or use

Doctor, Will You Pray for Me?. Robert L. Klitzman, Oxford University Press. © Oxford University Press 2024.
DOI: 10.1093/oso/9780197750841.003.0003

complementary and alternative medicine; how they cope with stress and uncertainty; and how they handle decisional regret, end-of-life care, and advance care plans.[4]

But though religion clearly affects healthcare, and patients routinely ask, "Why me?" most doctors feel awkward discussing or mentioning these topics at work.

Patients want these conversations. A 2011 study showed that among inpatients, 41% wished to discuss religious or spiritual concerns with someone while in the hospital, but only half of them ended up having such conversations.[5] Among patients who initially indicated that they did not desire to discuss religious and spiritual topics with staff, 20% ended up having such a discussion anyway—and they were later more satisfied with their overall care than were respondents who did not see a chaplain.[6]

These days, hospitalized patients are typically treated by medical staff—doctors, assisted by nurses, physician assistants, and nurse practitioners—all of whom focus on diagnosing and treating disease. Social workers tend to concentrate on the logistics of discharge (such as to rehabilitation or long-term-care facilities). Chaplains address spiritual, religious, and existential issues that patients and their families confront. Doctors and other medical staff could potentially have these conversations as well, but commonly lack time, and hence do so only briefly, in passing, if at all.

Most physicians feel that their professional role includes engaging patients spiritually, that these issues are important personally, and that patients want such discussions.[6] Being aware of patients' spiritual concerns is vital and need not take more than a few moments. Yet doctors rarely broach these topics.[7] Among ICU attendings (or fully trained doctors), for instance, 79% thought that it was their responsibility to address patients' religious or spiritual needs, but only 14% and 7% say they frequently ask patients and families, respectively, about these topics.[6] Sixty percent report they would like to provide spiritual care to terminally ill patients, yet 41% do so less than they would like,[8] and about 18% of physicians say they never discuss these issues, even if the patient asks, even at the end of life.[7] Only around 15% of doctors ask about these issues, according to patients, and at most 19% do so at the end of life.[7] Similarly, religion is important to 88% of advanced cancer patients, but 72% say that the medical system supports their spiritual needs minimally or not at all.[9]

Forty-seven percent of physicians are personally uncomfortable with the topic.[10] Most doctors still say their training about these realms is nonexistent or inadequate. Over half of doctors report that they have received no education in this area, and 62% feel that what they got was insufficient.[10]

Patients tend to almost always initiate these conversations,[7,11] and physicians currently fail to support or facilitate the patients' religiosity.[12,13,15] Moreover, most physicians at times attempt to change the topic.[7]

But while physicians say that, especially in hospitals, lack of time and lack of private office space limit these discussions most, research shows that these two factors are not in fact significantly involved. Instead, major barriers are physicians' inadequate training and discomfort, especially with a patient whose beliefs differ from their own, feelings that patients do not want these conversations, and worries about patients feeling uncomfortable.[9] Physicians' perceptions concerning patient discomfort are thus not always accurate. Male doctors with lower spirituality are also less interested in obtaining more training in these areas than are their female colleagues.[10]

The pendulum has begun to swing back a bit. In recent years, JCAHO, which accredits hospitals, has begun to state that hospitals should assess patients' spiritual beliefs. Partly as a result, many medical schools began to include these topics in their curricula, but often inadequately, only for a few minutes at most, in passing. Initially, JCAHO stipulated that students learn the value but not the means of assessment. More recently, the organization has added that medical staff have "sensitivity" toward these topics. But the Commission has not addressed who should perform these assessments, what to do with the information once gathered, and how to incorporate it into communicating, interacting, or making decisions with patients.[14,15]

Only 7% of medical schools report that their curriculum includes electives or required material on spirituality and health.[16] Most medical school deans resist giving these topics more attention: Only 43% think that more material in the curriculum is needed, and only 40% think that it is important. Though 53% said teaching on the topic should be increased, most reported that they did not have faculty trained to teach it. Only 25% thought they would increase the amount of time on the topic in the curriculum, even if they were provided funding and training assistance. Only 32% feel that the Association of American Medical Colleges, the major organization addressing medical education,[17] should encourage more material in the curriculum.

Around the country, a few trainees and junior faculty have initiated their own small-scale lectures and demonstrations to address these realms, but deans have generally declined to support or continue these grassroots efforts after these altruistic individuals move on in their careers.

In society more generally, religion and spirituality remain largely taboo topics. "Never talk about religion or politics at dinner or the workplace," the old adage warns. Individuals who agree on other matters may clash, and fear seeming irrational.

Yet, awkwardness about these issues significantly impedes providers' and patients' communication and relationships. "In my training," a fellow psychiatrist told me, "a professor even told me, 'Don't say "good luck" to patients when discharging them from the ward, because it suggests they need luck— that they don't have the agency to do what they want.' We can't even with our patients good luck!"

Physicians face other barriers, too. Understandably, medicine concentrates on objective data, facts and evidence that treatments work, while religion and spirituality do not. As one chaplain told me, "I can't prove that there's a God, or that prayer is going to change a person's life. It may. Yet there are things that science can't explain. Our technology tries to figure problems out and crack the code to get the answer. With religion, you've got no code." Doctors tend to feel that science, not religion, has the solutions and can offer the most benefit and hope.

Yet doctors, geared toward curing disease, also generally see death as a failure rather than an ultimate inevitability, and commonly avoid discussing death and spiritualty altogether. As Ernest Becker, in his Pulitzer Prize-winning *Denial of Death*, and Jessica Mitford, in her classic *The American Way of Death*, described, our nation is youth-oriented and has difficulty accepting the harsh realities of human mortality.[18,19]

"In our death-phobic culture," Brenda Pierson, a pediatric chaplain in the Bible Belt, noted, "we can't even say 'dead.' We say, 'passed away' or 'passed on.' Even our hospital's electronic medical records system [EMR] recently switched its language. It used to say, 'You are opening the chart of a deceased patient.' The EMR company said they had had a complaint that 'deceased' was too harsh!"

Even in hospitals, death gets hidden, moved as far out of sight as possible. Jack Stone, a Buddhist, entered chaplaincy due to multiple losses in his life. When Jack was a child, his father died. His mother and his spouse both died young. He decided to pursue chaplaincy after seeing his mother perish in an ICU, "where machines outnumbered human beings. I finally found my calling—in the hospital, in these antiseptic realms of hell. If I can make someone, in the darkest, saddest time in their life, feel a little bit better or less traumatized, or at least realize that their loved one died with dignity and love, surrounded with a sense of humanity, then I have done my job. My own losses have put me in hard places that have opened my heart."

He sees how scientific medicine ignores the existential and even biological fact of death. "People aren't supposed to die in hospitals. Usually, the morgue itself is in the basement. When a body is moved in the hall, it's moved to a service, not a passenger, elevator. The room doors shut. It's slipped under the rug. People don't die in a hospital! Most people in fact, will die in a hospital. But some doctors feel that death is a failure, and that they've somehow failed their patient. So, they don't see death as a natural process. It's taboo." Patients or families may want, for instance, to discontinue additional chemotherapy, when it is harming more than helping, "but they don't want to disappoint the doctor who's been working on them for so long."

Physicians also face increasing pressures from insurance companies and hospitals to treat as many patients as possible each day. Senior physicians, rotating through wards, tend to have much shorter relationships with patients (note that my comments about patients generally apply to their families as well). A former journalist, Linda Porter now works as a pediatric chaplain at a large academic hospital in Maryland where attendings rotate weekly. When she asks families who their primary oncologist is, "They sometimes respond, 'Maybe the one who has the short brown hair,' " which Linda finds "not at all surprising. Our physicians are also doing academic research. So, if they're on service for a week here, they're not going deep into their patients' lives."

These limitations intensify needs for chaplains who have more time than doctors do to explore these topics with patients. "If I'm an attending," Linda continued, "I have to see 17 people on the transplant service every day. But, as a chaplain, I can spend a couple of hours with a family in crisis. So, it's very different." She sees her role as helping to fill this gap.

Especially at major academic medical centers, doctors can be superb researchers, but otherwise wholly miss such information, busy and focused on other realms. As Linda said, "There are some utterly brilliant doctors who do not have the best bedside manner, but I would still want them to save my child's life. There are many shades of gray."

Linda marveled that, as a result, "People tell me things that they don't tell the doctor. Sometimes I share it with a physician, if I think the physician would really care or need to know. Knowing who your patients are is so important." Yet senior doctors "often don't know the story or necessarily care. One father had a daughter with medulloblastoma," a common cancerous brain tumor in children. "He and his wife had trouble dealing with it. They just tried to switch it off. He was a Marine, and had done two tours in Iraq. He told me, 'Nothing I did there was as hard as this.' I told the doctors," who found it helpful, reminding them of parents' points of view.

The notion that doctors should ideally at least be aware of a patient's existential concerns has even become controversial. Critics have lambasted the possibility of doctors "prescribing" religion[20]—which they should not do. Yet occasionally, doctors themselves value religion and spirituality and see these as important to be aware of as factors in understanding patients' and families' medical decisions, responses, and abilities to cope with the stress of disease and death.

To be sure, a few physicians recognize the importance of spirituality, broadly defined, and try to draw on these realms professionally, leveraging potential spiritual supports for patients. Physicians vary somewhat, often related to their specialty. For example, 52% of internists and surgeons, yet only 29% of psychiatrists, describe themselves as religious. Most internists and surgeons, but not psychiatrists, pray at least daily (61% and 53% vs. 40%, respectively). Psychiatrists are more likely than internists and surgeons to be agnostic (24% vs. 13% and 11%). Internists and surgeons, but not psychiatrists, occasionally prayed with patients (29% and 27% vs. 0%, respectively).[21]

When they themselves become seriously ill, many, physicians, though not all, turn toward faith. Some were always religious. Roxanne Cuartas, a 48-year-old gastroenterologist from Brazil, had developed abdominal cancer and was undergoing chemotherapy. I met her in her spartan office at a major research medical center, as she sat before a large computer screen, a white plastic keyboard, and small and neat piles of recent pristine glossy scientific journals. Neatly dressed in an ivory cardigan sweater and black slacks with her brown hair closely cropped, she seemed smart, studious, rational, and down to earth, but dignified and calm. Born and raised in Brazil, where Catholicism deeply imbues the culture, her Catholicism has always been important to her and aided her now. "When on call," she explained with a slight accent, "I'd go to a priest and say, 'Father, I'm on call,' and he would bless me. I'd say, 'God help me not to make a decision when I don't know what to do.'"

But her faith also evolved. After her diagnosis, she "started to become grateful for whatever I have. I traveled as much as I could—to Rome and to Lourdes. Then, my abdomen expanded. My spleen crossed the midline. For three months, I stayed home."

Her spiritual life shifted. "One day, something happened—something expressed itself that had not before. I was a big fan of Caravaggio, and had seen all the Caravaggios in Rome; I started painting. I had always wanted to paint, but said I couldn't." She viewed this activity in spiritual terms. "I wondered if his spirit helped me paint, because I couldn't before. I now started painting portraits—of my father, grandfather, sister, and my dreams, and a nude self-portrait of my abdomen. I stood in the bathroom and looked right back at the mirror. Painting is going back to Mother Earth, to the mother of energy and life." Her faith and its new expressions strengthened and sustained her.

She also now seeks to integrate her medical work with her faith. "I use the word 'God' a lot in my practice. Some doctors may be offended by that. But I tell patients that I work with the help of God—that I'm an instrument of God." The strength of her religiosity, given her scientific training, was unusual.

I asked her where she felt such beliefs come from. "Spirituality is a gift," she replied. "You can't teach it. Either you feel it, or you don't. How come people don't have the feeling? I don't know. I give it all to God." I sensed, too, that her strong Catholic upbringing contributed.

Many doctors who have come to appreciate these issues have done so only after they themselves became older and/or ill and more fully faced their own mortality, gaining more experience and seeing the limits of medical knowledge. Hubris then falters. Jason Cooper, a Connecticut psychiatrist, is unusual in openly discussing with patients their spiritual and religious views and practices as potential sources of support. "As I've gotten older and closer to the end of my life," he explained, "I've paid more attention to these issues. Having a sense that there is something greater than myself has been comforting—even though I don't think that when I die, I'm going to be any more than chemicals going back into the universe. But the longer I've been practicing, the more I feel, as a therapist, when I'm really honed in the moment, that I'm channeling some larger force. It's through me, not of me. That's my spiritual side."

Yet while a few physicians, like Roxanne and Jason, are open to certain degrees to spirituality and religion, and feel comfortable discussing these topics, most doctors remain ill at ease. When asked by patients about their own beliefs, countless doctors are caught off guard. "How should I respond," a fellow physician recently asked me, "when dying patients say to me, 'I'm going to die and go to Heaven, right?' I don't believe in Heaven, but I don't want to take away their hope."

"You could say," I replied, "that many people have strongly felt that way for thousands of years."

He was surprised by the answer's simplicity, and very appreciative. I was struck that he was unsure, on his own, how to respond.

Physicians face challenges, especially, in communicating with a patient whose views differ from their own. "Patients have asked me if I believe in God," a young female colleague told me. "I don't know how to respond. I say, 'I was raised Catholic, but am now not sure. I think there may be a higher power' . . . I try to explain what an agnostic is—that people have different ways of conceiving God. I just sort of ramble. Sometimes I've lied. I'm Catholic, so I can 'talk the talk' and say the right things. But I don't believe it, and that doesn't feel good to me, either."

I replied, "I think just saying, 'I was raised Catholic, and now think there may be a higher power' could be effective." She looked at me, amazed that she could utter such a simple and straightforward statement. She had never thought it through.

Many doctors also fumble when patients ask them to pray with or for them. "Patients sometimes ask me: 'Will you pray for me?'" Jim Adams, a Philadelphia oncologist, similarly told me. He is usually surprised by these requests and uncertain, not fully sure how to respond. Wary of organized religion, he describes himself as "a lapsed Catholic. I suppose I'm now an agnostic, not an atheist—I still hold out hope. But I was an altar boy for three years, and see the Church basically as a way to control large groups of people."

"What do you tell patients when they ask you to pray?" I inquired.

"I say: 'Uhh . . .'" He stretched out his hand and the syllable, wavering, unsure. "OK . . .'" he finally mutters, still hesitant, the word lingering in the air with uncertainty. He shrugged, as if to say, "I guess so. Why not? It's no skin off my back. I do worse things every day"—giving patients potent chemotherapies in desperate attempts to extend lives by a few months, though these drugs have severe side effects and will probably fail. He thinks medical education needs to address these realms far better.

Unfortunately, these and many other doctors have received little, if any, education on how to respond to such patient queries.

As these brief examples suggest, patients often make small gambits, dropping tiny hints or suggestions about their fears, hopes, and beliefs that hover just on or below the surface. Doctors commonly miss or dismiss these cues. Physicians regularly ask, for instance, "How are you doing?" and patients answer, "I hope God is on my side" or "God won't let me down, will He?" Some doctors immediately reply medically, saying, "Did you make your follow-up appointment?" or "Have you been taking your medications?"—ignoring the potential implications of the patient's remark.

Clearly, doctors need to be prepared and have ready answers to these questions in some way, but frequently don't. Though uncomfortably avoided by doctors, these topics nonetheless preoccupy and vex countless patients and families.

4

Amazing graces

How chaplains enter the room

Given that doctors commonly eschew these existential, spiritual, and religious issues, hospital chaplains have come to fill critical voids. "Chaplains are better than Prozac," a fellow psychiatrist, who has treated hospitalized patients for decades, told me. "They make patients feel better in all kinds of ways."

Chaplains vary widely in their particular religious, personal, and professional backgrounds. One of the first chaplains I met when beginning to explore this area was a nun, Sister Francine. I had never before spoken to a nun at length. Based on tales from friends who had attended parochial school, I imagined nuns in black habits, formal, stiff, and doctrinaire. But Sister Francine wore a bright red turtleneck shirt and a white cardigan sweater with bright shiny red plastic buttons. Her blue eyes sparkled. She smiled warmly. A halo of soft curly white hair emanated from around her head. She lived in a convent, but worked as a hospital chaplain, and seemed very down to earth.

"I always carry around little prayers from different faiths," she told me, pulling out and unfolding two or three well-fingered pages of small, typed prayers from the back of the plastic pouch that hung around her neck and displayed her ID card. The paper's worn edges flopped down. "I see Jews, Christians, Muslims, Buddhists, Catholics, and everyone else. I say: 'You have a choice. I can say a prayer for you, or give you good wishes.' But I basically say the same thing to everyone.

"Yesterday, I 'knocked' on a patient's curtain, introduced myself, and said: 'I'm from the chaplaincy department.' An older gentleman was lying in bed, staring at the ceiling. 'No, thank you,' he said. 'We don't need you.' But his wife said to him, 'Come on, Joe. Why not? What's the harm?' Reluctantly, he agreed.

"I said, 'I give you good wishes: "Oh God, please give the anesthesiologist, surgeon, and recovery room nurses the guidance, good skill, and judgment

Doctor, Will You Pray for Me?. Robert L. Klitzman, Oxford University Press. © Oxford University Press 2024.
DOI: 10.1093/oso/9780197750841.003.0004

today. Especially if they face difficult issues, give them all the skill and good judgment You can so that they help Joe get better. We hope that he gets the best possible care, which he deserves. Let today be a new beginning for him, filled with hope and joy." ' He grabbed my hand. 'YES, Sister! I was just thinking about that this morning. Thank you for coming today!' He looked me in the eye and said, 'THANK YOU,' emphasizing each syllable, giving it added weight. 'YES!! YES!! God bless you.'"

"That's beautiful," I said.

"Really?" she responded. To my surprise, she seemed genuinely unsure. Her unassuming modesty and humility were striking.

"Essentially," she continued, "I end up saying the same thing to everyone: 'God, give us strength. Give the surgeon the skill, strength, and good judgment he needs.' Patients are almost always grateful."

She radiated a wise and deeply spiritual presence. "The nurses and doctors talk loudly: I have only a soft voice," she told me quietly. "But patients say to me, 'You make me feel so calm.'" She exuded a genuine, heartfelt compassion and sincerity that, I sensed, would surely soothe patients. Meeting her helped inspire me to write this book.

Becoming chaplains

Chaplains start their journeys from widely ranging points. Unlike Sister Francine, many of these professionals first entered other, far different fields. Several had worked as teachers, clergy, business people, or arts administrators and/or raised a family, and then wondered what to do next. Frequently, they had helped several family members and friends deal with disease, death, and dying, and found these interactions deeply rewarding. Hence, they entered a seminary and/or a pastoral care training program and became chaplains.

Often, they have faced significant losses, trauma, or abuse themselves, which helped propel them into this field. Indeed, the psychoanalyst Carl Jung and others have argued that clinicians should be "wounded healers"—to have endured trauma themselves in order to make them as sensitive as possible to patients' plights.[1] As we saw with Jack Stone, the Buddhist chaplain, many enter this field due to painful personal crises (such as a loved one's death). They find that this work constitutes a "calling" and can even be "redemptive," and that, in this field, "maturity is an advantage."

Given past experiences of the painful demise of loved ones, chaplains find their work deeply and uniquely gratifying. Hospice work in particular, seeing all of one's patients die, can devastate many people but attracts chaplains such as Jack Stone, who had witnessed a family member suffer a horrible demise that they now strive to avoid for others. Cathy Murray, for instance, a hospice chaplain at a Virginia Catholic hospital, had been a candy striper as a teenager. In high school, she had begun dating a guy "and was supposed to go to the homecoming game with him the next weekend. But an hour after he had left my house after coming to see me, the highway patrol phoned that he had been killed in an accident on his way home.

"I was so angry with God, but did not express that, even to myself, and especially not to anyone else. Two or three months later, I was sitting on the sofa with my mother, crying, saying, 'I'm so angry.' She said, 'With who?' I couldn't even say 'God' out loud, so I pointed up. She knew immediately what I meant, and was horrified. Her face told me that what I felt was wrong. So, I quickly straightened up, and was no longer angry at God. Immediately, I was 'just fine' and jumped back into dating another guy. We got engaged and married in a year, when I was 19—which should be illegal.

"After seven years, he wanted a divorce and that anger came back; I discovered that it had never gone away, I had just swallowed it. I had 'accepted Jesus into my heart' and done my best to 'live for Jesus,' and these things still happened! I'd been told God would take care of me, and He didn't. I was furious at God and thought, 'Screw this! I'm done! Stay out of my life! This isn't fair!' For the first time, I recognized I was angry with God, and frankly, didn't give a rat's ass if anybody didn't like that.

"After my divorce, my mother invited me to move back home. But I knew I then would never leave again, and nothing would ever change. I had gone to one year of college but was not interested. Now, I was ready to go back to school and seminary."

Cathy volunteered at a nursing home and enjoyed it but "didn't think that I necessarily wanted to be a chaplain. I thought I would be in the nonprofit world, working on hunger or other social justice issues." But then her grandmother "had a really terrible experience at death, and I did not want anyone else to have to go through that. They didn't know how much chemo to give her. She was a big personality, and could speak Italian, French, and English, but at the end, wasn't talking at all. I was her favorite grandchild, but she wouldn't even talk to me! People often work in hospice because a loved one's death went either really well with hospice, or really poorly without hospice."

Facilitating discussions about meaningful topics—the ultimate questions—proves profoundly satisfying. "I found it incredibly rewarding," Cathy continued, "because the level of conversation that you have as a chaplain in hospice is very different than what you normally would when you're first meeting people. It's a real gift."

In her work, she draws on lessons from her own personal experiences. Her past "helped form my pastoral care. It's weird that I'm a chaplain, since I told God to 'take a hike.' But in seminary, I realized that God 'taking care of us' doesn't mean that bad stuff isn't going to happen. Many conservative churches say, 'Accept Jesus into your heart. If you do that, you're saved: *Live with Jesus, and He will care for you.*' Preachers and Sunday school teachers never go beyond that. In some Christian traditions, especially the Baptists, it's literal. There's no ambiguity. But what does it mean that 'God will take care of you?' Crap happens in everybody's life!

"Preachers say we're not supposed to question God," Cathy continued, "But I now say to patients, 'It's OK to be angry with God. Job was angry with God.' Preachers don't talk about that. They say that Job's wife told him to 'curse God and die.' But they don't talk about how angry Job later got. Job said, 'The Lord giveth, and the Lord taketh away. Blessed be the name of the Lord'—setting up an impossible scenario that we're supposed to follow when hard stuff happens. But in seminary, I discovered that that is *not* what Job said."

Though patients often feel that challenging God is taboo, she instead encourages them to recognize and accept these emotions. "When patients say, 'I know I'm not supposed to question God,' I say, 'Let's talk about that. Let's talk about Job.' I live in the Baptist-heavy South. One of the last things Jesus said was, 'Why, God, have you forsaken me?' Sounds to me like Job was questioning God! People don't think of it that way because many churches discourage you to do so. Patients cock their heads at me as if to say, 'Huh?' When I say, 'That's not where Job stopped,' one nurse looked at me and said, 'Well, that's not what *I* was taught.' I said, 'Go read it!' She didn't say anything else, but I don't think she was going to read it."

These experiences also taught her the value of silence. After her boyfriend's death in high school, friends aided her just through their quiet and mere presence, rather than their words. "My best friend invited me to spend the night with her. I didn't want to go, but my mother thought it would be good.

My friend and I sat on opposite sides of the living room, just looking at each other. I couldn't talk. She just sat with me. Only later did I realize that that was such a gift. I probably made her uncomfortable, but she just sat with me in silence. To this day, 50 years later, I can't believe it. *That* has informed my pastoral care. People need someone to sit with them in silence. That's one of the lessons of Job: sitting in silence with somebody who's suffering. *There's nothing you can say to make it better. Anything you want to say, just keep to yourself."*

Conversely, she recalled, "For several months after my divorce, I talked to only one person. I was so angry, but she couldn't listen to me. She had to defend God. I was sorry I opened up to her." Chaplains learn the delicate art of when to speak and when not to.

What chaplains do

The field has developed several effective nondenominational approaches for talking with a wide range of patients about their deep and ultimate concerns. Generally, these professionals strive to help patients find hope, meaning, purpose, and spiritual ties. Given that the spectrum of patients runs from staunchly evangelical to vehemently atheist, these limber and nimble approaches are generally effective.

Broadly, these professionals visit, talk, and pray with patients and at times distribute Bibles, Qurans, or rosary beads. Several studies have sought to enumerate quantitatively the activities in which chaplains engage, such as "saying a prayer" or "performing a ritual."[2,3,4,5] Much of what chaplains do involves communication. In palliative care, chaplains report that their major activities are relationship building (76%), care at death (69%), and assisting with existential concerns or spiritual distress (49%).[5] The main chaplaincy interventions in palliative care in ICUs include active listening, demonstrating care and concern, providing pastoral presence, preserving dignity and respect, providing emotional support, demonstrating acceptance, collaborating with the team, and building rapport and connectedness.[6] Overall, chaplains address broad quality-of-life concerns more than religion and spirituality per se, and are most satisfied when engaging in activities such as prayer and touch, as well as active listening and discussions of both seemingly practical matters and ultimate concerns.[7]

Yet I found that chaplains in fact also use several broader cross-cutting methods to address specific challenges faced by patients of particular beliefs (from devoutly religious to atheist) as well as shared dilemmas across these varied groups, gaining trust and establishing relationships. In recent years, chaplains have increasingly embraced multifaith approaches, seeing themselves, professionally, as nondenominational and engaging with people of different faiths in innumerable ways.

A critic may object to this model of interfaith nondenominational chaplains, contending that Muslims or Orthodox Jews may not want to meet a Catholic or Hindu chaplain or vice versa. A devoutly Catholic patient may want a Latin Mass, Eucharist, or the sacrament of anointing the sick. Yet, chaplains assess patients, if patients are interested, and either assist directly or refer the patient to a colleague of a particular belief. Few chaplains, however, report ever actually needing to offer to make such a referral, though occasionally, late at night (when only one chaplain is on call in a hospital), preemptively suggesting the possibility for the morning if the patient wishes. These days, "telechaplaincy" can also allow involvement, if needed, of chaplains from faiths that a particular hospital lacks.

In certain ways, spiritual care resembles psychotherapy. Chaplains commonly see their work as "a *blend* of spirituality and mental health." As Jack Stone, the Buddhist chaplain, observed, "In a way, we are *spiritual therapists*." Other chaplains similarly see themselves as "in an indirect counseling mode."

But chaplains also differ from mental health providers in having a more open-ended agenda, giving them flexibility. In addition, less defined by boundaries of time or topic, their roles are more amorphous. Generally, psychotherapists have other priorities, eliminating symptoms of anxiety and depression that impede patients' functioning, and aiming less at helping patients to find meaning in and of itself. Not all psychotherapy patients focus on spiritual and existential questions and finding ultimate purpose, though many do. Chaplains and psychotherapists tend to differ, too, in the length of time of their relationships with patients. As Connie Clark, a Wisconsin Catholic chaplain who got burned out during COVID and needed to take a break, observed, "The difference between what I do and what a therapist does is that I stay with patients in that moment, helping them get through *that moment*. If patients are stuck, and need help going from point A to point B, I refer them to a psychotherapist."

These two fields can therefore complement and bolster each other, and chaplains try to collaborate closely with mental health providers who may be available.

"I'm from spiritual care": Entering the room

Usually, chaplains start by entering a patient's room and introducing themselves. But even this initial step can involve a complex choreography. Patients and/or their families may be open or wary or misunderstand. These spiritual care providers seek to establish trust through both the form and content of these interactions, and proceed accordingly based on the responses they receive. As Jack Stone said, "I wear a black uniform that Buddhist monks use called a Kāṣāya. It kind of looks like scrubs. Because of the color, when I walk into a patient's room and introduce myself, patients sometimes say, 'Oh, the Grim Reaper!' or wonder why I'm coming into their room: 'What are the doctors not telling me?' So, I alleviate that fear with humor, or by saying, 'I'm the specialist in listening to people. My job is to take care of your spirit, your mind, your soul—whatever that is. Whatever faith tradition you do or don't have, I am a good listening ear. How are you doing?'

"Sometimes, it's a cold call," Jack continued. "Staff refer patients to me to help with loss, bereavement, or grief. I'll knock on the door and say, 'I'm from pastoral care; do you have a minute or two? I'd like to introduce myself.'" They mostly agree. "Then I say, 'The doctors are interested in your physical condition, the social workers in your family and social connections. I'm interested in your mind, spirit, and soul. How are you doing in that realm?' Sometimes that visit's very short. I just leave a card and say, 'If you'd like, we can meet again.' Or if they're very interested, we can extend the visit five or 10 more minutes."

In trying to cover key topics, chaplains often use various memory devices, each denoted by an acronym. "I do a quick, generalized spiritual assessment using a mnemonic called a FICA," Jack explained—"faith, importance or influence, community, and address."[8] Jack asks, "Do you have a *faith*? What spirituality or religion is *important* to you? Do you have a *community*? Is your family important in your life? How can I *address* that in your care?' Within five minutes, I know if this is a sustainable visit. I can tell by their words and body language if they are going through spiritual distress or anxiety. Having been a chaplain for over 10 years, I've got the skills to see when I can help, or not. Maybe they're fine, and I won't visit them again. I always ask, 'Would you be open to another visit at another time?' Clergy can be very heavy and serious, so I love humor and just being real with them—just human to human."

Physical aspects of the interaction matter, too. Spiritual care providers try, for instance, to sit down, to be literally on the same level with patients. "I try not to stand above them, or physically look down on them," Jack explained. "I try to meet their level, and attune myself to their body language." As another pastoral care provider similarly told me, chaplains try to "focus directly eye to eye on the patient. Patients trust that. I don't just sit down. I ask, 'May I sit down?' Sometimes they're lying down. I try to get low enough where they can see eye to eye with me. I pull up a chair."

Unfortunately, the COVID-19 pandemic, especially initially, significantly impeded these physical aspects of conversations. Protective masks and gloves hampered communication. "It is challenging to read people's expressions and body language when they are covered in gowns, gloves, face shields, and masks in every encounter," Brenda Pierson, the pediatric chaplain, noted. "Previously, we would have pulled a chair up close to a child's bed and spent time talking, and playing cards or other games or drawing with crayons and markers. Now we couldn't touch anything or anybody. Human touch is so basic—an exchange of humanity that was now missing from every encounter."

Verbally, chaplains generally ask open-ended questions and actively listen, but doing so can involve complexities as well. Such active listening may sound passive but is not; in fact, it constitutes a skill and an art, requiring learning, adjustment and refinement of techniques over time, and knowing when to stop listening and to speak. "Most people want to be heard," Jack added. "So, we are listeners, but with *a different set of ears*. If we think more is going on, we ask, 'Say more about that.' Sometimes I'll just say, 'Can I challenge you about something? You're saying *this*, but also *that*. How do you reconcile that?' So, hearing, questioning, and gently being present with the person."

The process of reflecting back what patients say lets them see themselves more clearly. Jack strives to "walk alongside the patient or their family, and be a *mirror* to their thoughts and feelings, and replay it back to them: 'This is what I'm hearing. Help me if I got anything wrong, but it sounds to me that you have a lot of fear of the future and what might happen. You're frustrated that you're not getting the answers you want, and there are a lot of unknowns, and this is probably the most vulnerable time of your life. Help me to understand: Is that what's going on with you?' It opens up that therapeutic relationship."

For patients and families who have difficulty articulating their feelings, chaplains at times use poetry and pictures to find common ground and trigger conversations. "Rather than directly asking, 'How are you feeling today?'" Jack elaborated, "I might bring up a poem: 'Listen, this is a poem that I have in my pocket today; can I read it to you?' Or, I'll bring two or three photographs of nature or a painting by Picasso or Chagall and say, 'Tell me a story when you see this image.' I love working with images, poems, and music that come at it from different points of view, and aren't prayer bells and smells, which some people could find threatening."

Nurses and doctors also ask him to visit particular dying patients because he offers meditation and mindfulness techniques. "Not all chaplains include meditation in their work, but as a Buddhist, I've found ways to bring it into working with patients to help them sleep and relax, and undo some of their anxiety or stress."

He incorporates music, too, into his approaches. "Sometimes I get a referral at the end of life because they want to create an atmospheric condition where the dying person needs sound. I play a beautiful harp that helps patients relax, and enter the dying process less anxiously."

Other chaplains use different combinations of structured and unstructured approaches. For instance, Marvin Beck, a Protestant chaplain in New Hampshire, works at a small community hospital whose CEO strongly supports chaplaincy. Marvin has even arranged, for example, to read prayers over the loudspeaker. As a mnemonic, Marvin uses HOPES: "The H is for what does the person *hope* for—to get out of the hospital in a week to play golf or see their kid get married. The O stands for *organized* religion: 'Do you participate in an organized religion?' The P stands for what are the *practices*: 'Do you listen to meditation music, read the Bible, pray, go to church?' The E is the *emotion*: What is the person expressing? S is for what are the *supports*. That's what I listen for."

Yet patients also range considerably in what they need and desire, and chaplains thus adjust what they offer. "My first meeting is really goodwill, introductory," Marvin reported. "Some patients just want somebody to come and say, 'Good morning' or to have daily prayer. I'm there three or four minutes. That's all they want. Sometimes I'll ask, 'Now that you're recovering, who's going to be home with you?'—just to find out and see what kind of connections that person has. I might then say to the nurse, 'Maybe we need to have a social work consult because this person just had a knee operation and has stairs at home.' The social worker deals with the discharge, but sometimes just doesn't know."

Most importantly, chaplains seek to align with patients, finding each patient's sources of meaning—the specific forms and terms. "It could be their sports team, pets, or gardening," Marvin added, "something that helps them get through these next days in the hospital. We offer Bibles, rosary beads, spiritual readings, and just companionship. We might spend five to 10 minutes, unless they really want to discuss heavy-duty issues troubling them. Today, a few guys spoke about how our football team got screwed twice yesterday—two terrible calls! Then we leave our pamphlet. It's about making a connection with them, and finding out: *Do they have a spiritual resource in the broadest sense?*" Though people may see chaplaincy as discussing either ultimate concerns and mysteries or quotidian, mundane topics, the borders between these two realms commonly blur. Seemingly practical matters can reflect deeper concerns about life and death.

Through these interactions, these spiritual care providers aim to be highly receptive and responsive to the patient's needs. As Marvin tells trainees, "You know the expression: 'Don't just stand there, do something?' Well, ours is the opposite: 'Stand there and *don't* do anything. *Just listen.'*"

Chaplains tend to see varying religions as different roads to the same place. "As Muslims, Jews, and Christians, we are all praying to the same God," Marvin said. "If I drive to my state capital, I can take the interstate, but other people may want to take back roads. We're all going to get there, but in different ways." When meeting a patient of a different faith, chaplains commonly therefore inquire about it, which, Marvin observed, "patients like. With Muslims, I say '*as-salamu alaykum* (peace be with you),' and they respond, '*wa-alaikum-salaam* (peace be upon you also).' All of a sudden, they're relaxed. They fear that we think they're all terrorists. They're not!"

I have been struck by how open patients can be to such interfaith experiences, valuing a chaplain's ability to connect more than his or her particular religious faith. As Marvin, though a Protestant, continued, "One 93-year-old Jewish woman comes into the hospital all the time, and calls me her 'deacon.' She always says, 'I want *my deacon* to come in.' I told her, 'If you come in one more time, I'm going to have to baptize you and make you Catholic!' We laughed. The next time she came in, I said, 'I've come here to baptize you.' Her daughter, whom I had never met, happened to be there and asked me, startled and upset, 'What are you doing?' I said, 'I'm only kidding!'"

When asking open-ended questions and actively listening, chaplains, like psychotherapists, vary in terms of their individual styles, approaches, and techniques. As one chaplain said, "You can't force beliefs on people but can help them appreciate things beyond themselves. Asking patients simply, for instance, 'How do you find meaning in what's happening to you, and in what's in your heart?'" Chaplains then follow up as appropriate. "I hear the person's feelings. Maybe I'll ask another open-ended question, showing them that I've heard them—not necessarily to directly spur them to deeper thinking, but for that person to feel heard, and to summarize, paraphrase, and distill the heart of what they have said. My practice is much less about asking questions. I ask my students as a training exercise to make a visit without asking a single question."

Such open-ended inquiries and active hearing allows for wide flexibility and benefits, reflecting views about their own and other's beliefs. "There's a lot of *magic* to it," William Gibson, a chaplain in Vermont, said. He considers himself to be a humanist and atheist, "basically *secular*. That's just how I was raised to think." His mother was Jewish, and his father was Christian but "secular." As an undergraduate, he studied religious studies and loved it. "My parents are lawyers and I was going to go to law school, but at the last minute went to divinity school, where I heard that chaplaincy was a great field for somebody who could speak multiple faith languages. I thought, 'That's kind of what I've been doing!'"

He is now a member of an "atheistic, naturalist—as opposed to supernaturalist—organization. Sometimes, we call ourselves 'atheologians.' We try to do theology, and think about what could be sacred, and address religiousness and questions." This background shapes his approach with patients. "We seldom meet anyone in life who does not have an agenda, who hasn't already made up their mind on who we should be and what we should do. For my own spiritual life, I draw on certain poets. Poetry and its ways of 'being' and peacemaking are important to my personal life and politics." His wide stance helps him engage with all patients regardless of their beliefs.

He also draws on baseball. "I love the game and use it as a metaphor for life. When I enter a difficult clinical situation, I take a deep breath, as I did on the mound. In baseball, you're always thinking about what's happening. Being a good teammate means knowing what's going on in your teammates' lives. You never really lose. You either win or learn. As a child, I went to South America and didn't speak Spanish, but played baseball, and was therefore able to form a community. In college, teammates differed from me in race and class, but the game brought us together. It's a source of community—kind of like baptism."

Knowledgeable patients may request a chaplain for related reasons—to receive nonjudgmental, nonstigmatized psychological support. William Gibson recalled a patient's spouse who was "totally atheist" but requested a chaplain. "We didn't talk about religion, atheism, or spirituality, just about his wife, and how he was feeling about that. At some point, I asked, 'Why did you ask for the chaplain?' . . . He said that he was in the military and that 'everybody in the military knows that the chaplain is the one person you can really confide in.' . . . It's almost like an *on-call therapist*." Unfortunately, in the military there is stigma about seeking psychological care. In hospitals today, chaplains similarly often provide the only de facto psychotherapy available to patients.

Outsiders commonly miscomprehend and underestimate the active listening involved in chaplains' interactions. "Folks think of us as just this lovely, empathetic listening presence," another chaplain told me. "But many of us are a lot more directive. We assess, intervene, and check outcomes, just like doses of medicine. We're not *just* nice, friendly visitors. Some of us are—and that's a problem."

Active listening therefore entails being exquisitely sensitive to patients' and families' language—the feelings underlying statements or questions—and responding appropriately, appreciating the subtleties of language, and not saying the wrong thing. But in the hurly-burly of spontaneous interactions with diverse patients, reacting optimally and avoiding inadvertently callous comments is not always easy. Seemingly small, innocuous comments can come across as insensitive.

Even seasoned chaplains occasionally say the wrong thing rather than acting more carefully and professionally. "At times, I've totally messed up," William, the humanist, admitted. "I've learned the hard way that showing up as the chaplain in the ICU waiting room can scare families badly—if I just say, 'Hi, are you the family of so-and-so?' I've learned to say quickly, 'I'm a chaplain but *there's no news*! Nothing's wrong.' Once, I told a patient before surgery, 'We'll see you on *the other side*'—in other words, 'See you later.' But that doesn't sound good coming from the chaplain. The patient in the next bed ended up laughing, and it broke the ice. Sometimes we're only human and mess up."

Even small, seemingly innocent words and gestures can unintentionally upset patients and families. Chaplains thus adjust their practices over time.

Even Adam Quincy, who pays close attention to language, has at times erred in his comments. Once at 3 a.m. on call and in bed, for instance, he got paged to see a woman who had just lost her husband of 64 years. He walked into the room and said, "It's going to be all right." "She said, 'It's *not* going to be all right! And you can leave!' Obviously, I should have said, 'I'm so sorry for your loss,' and been much more subtle. I never made that mistake again." Chaplains, doctors, nurses, families, and friends may make such ostensibly well-intentioned comments, hoping to help, not thinking how the suffering patient or family may respond. Chaplains strive to learn from these errors and self-correct. Here, too, they reveal important, broadly applicable life lessons.

Being nondenominational

The fluid, nondenominational approaches that chaplains have developed meet broad human needs. As William Gibson suggested, chaplains each have their own tradition but are interfaith. In working with patients from across a host of beliefs other than their own, these professionals' specific faith matters far less than their interpersonal skills. These flexible approaches differ from those of clergy, who are tied to a particular established institution. Chaplains "meet people where they are," and, as William indicated, do not all even consider themselves to be part of a faith tradition.

Pastoral care providers in fact provide a new model—of a "*post-religious profession*" for a "*post-religious*" world, in which countless people feel that traditional religious institutions no longer meet their needs. Instead, they now recognize and embrace more varied and supple forms of belief. Margaret Dixon, a Pennsylvania chaplain, began her career in arts management, raised a family, and, after her children went to college, attended seminary. She sees the field as reflecting the country's shifting religious landscape: "Familiarity with the Bible, the Quran, I Ching, or the Bhagavad Gita is important, but only slim slices of the pie. They're just runway lights, pointers. Yet that's hard for people to understand."

Traditional religious institutions fail to respond to the needs of mounting numbers of people. "Churches and synagogues feel stuck in the twentieth century," she continued. "How do they respond to the twenty-first century—getting people not to be afraid to say, 'I have doubts'—just calling out the logical inconsistencies in religious doctrines? Christ dying for our sins on the cross is weird. I've read about it 14 different ways, but still don't get it! Am I the only person who's not understanding? Nobody likes to talk about that. It's OK if people can't figure out the Resurrection. But there's such fear. Everybody's scared that the whole house of cards is going to tumble down. It's not. We need to start talking about what holds up, and what doesn't. If we don't, we're going to keep losing members."

She and others see contemporary chaplaincy as providing a useful, wide-encompassing model, distinct from what clergy offer. "In the twenty-first century, we have to be doing *secular* chaplaincy. Our training gives us inter-faith grounding. Catholic priests come into a patient's room with their Last Rites sacraments to perform and little wafers. I appreciate that. But many people have had spiritual injury and are suspicious of clergy or have been silenced by them." More pluralistic models are essential.

Chaplains must gauge as well how much to be a neutral blank slate in each encounter, including whether, for instance, to wear visible uniforms or other symbols revealing their particular faith. Many chaplains seek instead to be a *tabula rasa* onto which patients can project whatever aids them most. Margaret Dixon, for instance, remains unsure about how she will dress after her ordination. "I'm not sure I'll wear my collar, just like I don't now wear a cross or a rainbow flag. I don't want somebody to look at me and feel they have to modulate themselves in any way." Still, she wavers. "I go back and forth. A nun I work with wears her cross in front. It's her identity, who she is. But for patients who are not Catholic or Christian, to have a chaplain come in with a collar and giant crucifix around her neck can be complicating, especially if they've had some spiritual injury in their life. Plenty of great chaplains wear collars and see all patients, but I would be concerned that it *puts a third element* in the room, as opposed to me being an empty vessel. I'd be coming in with a giant symbol!"

Relatedly, chaplains face questions of whether to divulge their own beliefs. While some observers argue that chaplains need to declare their own faith to a patient, others disagree. "Some people say, 'You've got to disclose your faith and say whether you believe or don't,'" another chaplain told me. "But that doesn't feel right to me. Patients want to talk about what *they're* experiencing—what *they* need. The chaplain's own personal religious beliefs are irrelevant." Patients require a listening ear and don't care about the chaplain's own views, as long as the interaction is comfortable.

Choosing topics

In picking what to discuss, chaplains select topics based on their perceptions of specific patients' challenges or struggles. The topics need not always be explicitly religious or necessarily even spiritual, but rather reflect the patient's existential concerns. Chaplains regularly try to engage patients in such broader issues, rather than religion per se, and avoid explicit, specific religious jargon. Adam Quincy, a Catholic North Carolina hospice chaplain, reads widely about other religions of the world, which has shaped his approach. He advises trainees: "Don't come across with a lot of religious dogma. That turns people off."

Overly complicated, rather than simpler, more straightforward, language can unnecessarily hamper interactions. As Adam continued, "It's important to avoid so-called 'seminary terms'—$50 terms—when a $2 one will do. I once said to a patient, 'That is really *sacerdotalism*'—the idea that the priest is a sacrament of the Church, so that when the priest blesses you, it's effective because of the priest's position. The patient looked at me as if to say, 'Why are you using those huge words? What are you doing here?' We need to make sure we put it in terms they understand."

Instead, Adam argues, focus on broader issues. "Walk in and tap into what people find interesting about religion—that life is a paradox, that we're all going to die someday so that we are *living to die*. Religion is relevant in giving us *perspectives on how to live our lives*, bringing courage, joy, peace, and intrinsic rewards and satisfactions that we wouldn't want to live without. *You're selling interest in religion*, which is more interesting to people. People are tired of political rhetoric and fighting, and want to be shown something wonderful and marvelous. If you can use religion to do that, it can be very positive." As our world becomes ever more politically and religiously polarized, these insights can benefit all of us.

He and his colleagues strive to be supportive: "A key principle is to *do no harm*," Adam continued. "You don't ever want to piss the patient off, or say, 'The reason you're in the hospital is because you screwed up your life.' I've seen chaplains do that! Every chaplain visit needs to be positive and affirming."

Patients can have vehement but incorrect religious views, and responding to these is not always easy. Chaplains try to avoid contradicting patients' inaccurate remarks about religion. "Patients make wrong or insulting statements about the Bible," Adam added. "That's OK. I avoid whacking people with the Bible. I don't say, 'The Catholic Church never said anything like that.'"

Still, theological arguments can unfortunately erupt. "One chaplain I was supervising," Adam added, "got into a debate with a fundamentalist Protestant patient who said, 'Martin Luther was the one responsible for getting the Book of James and the Book of Hebrews taken out of the New Testament.' The chaplain said, 'That's not true. You're wrong.' You never want to say that, but instead say something like: 'Wow, that's interesting. You have a lot of background in church history. I was not aware of that.' But chaplains can be very 'teachy,' because their training is. Yet it gets the patient mad. The family will call and complain, which can jeopardize the whole chaplaincy program."

At times, Adam, too, relies just on silence, instead of words. "Staff have to know when *not* to speak," Adam noted. He not only avoids religious jargon but also values wordlessness. "When somebody has been through a devastating event, silence sometimes speaks much louder. I once sat in the ER with a woman for four hours. Her husband had broken his neck in a motorcycle accident. She was so upset, she couldn't talk. She needed someone to sit there with her—not watch TV, but sit there with her and say nothing. No words. Nothing. She had tears in her eyes. I thought, 'This is not a time to talk. Just be present.'

"At the end, she said, 'Thanks for talking with me. This means so much to me.' I thought, 'I haven't said a word for four hours!' But it was the *not* saying something—that was what needed to be said. That's 'ministry of presence.' You validate people emotionally and psychologically: They can tell you're there and aren't thinking about something else or watching TV, but are really there in the moment. If you have an opinion, say nothing or as little as possible. That's where chaplains make the most mistakes: saying something inappropriate, and projecting their own self-image onto the patient or family, who don't care about *us*. We are just there to support *them*."

Creating narratives

Chaplains benefit patients, too, in constructing narratives of experiences that help organize new, unwanted, and seemingly chaotic events. As patients and families tell their story, they come to understand and forge new identities.

Psychological research has described a therapeutic technique of cognitive "reframing," to help patients view their situations differently in order to change their perceptions of stresses they confront from negative to positive, to enhance their well-being or alter their behavior.[9] As we will see, chaplains regularly employ this method as well. "People create some of their understanding of their identity through story," explained Cathy Murray, the chaplain at a Virginia Catholic hospital who had been a candy striper and whose boyfriend had been killed in high school. "How they tell and understand their story, and see it in the context of other peoples' stories, and a larger faith story. We hear and validate the story as important—and reframe that the patient is a good person."

Pastoral care affirms and validates patients' experience by "bearing witness" to the patients' suffering and plight. For Cathy, this means "bringing graciousness, gentleness, compassion, and respect to the story. Patients don't always have reliable, nonjudgmental witnesses to their story. Other people are so busy, it's hard to hear one's whole story."

Additionally, a chaplain can convey these stories to doctors, helping these providers to feel more emphatic.

Building therapeutic relationships

The strength of the ties they build can astonish even chaplains—how meaningful these relationships become to patients and families, who frequently seek to maintain these bonds even after hospitalization. While chaplains themselves may feel they are not doing much, a patient or family may see them as nonetheless embodying or representing the imprimatur and gravitas of religion and spirituality. "Thirty years ago," Nancy Cutler, a South Carolina pediatric chaplain, recalled, "my supervisor told me that if I went into a room and somebody there was raised religious, even tangentially, and had some exposure, and I introduce myself as a chaplain, *'in their eyes, you are God. You are God's representative!'*" When one family asked her to officiate at their deceased child's funeral, Nancy was surprised. "An awesome little four-year-old girl had a brain tumor and died. I was with her parents through her death. I didn't feel I did anything for the mother, so I was shocked when she called me a couple of days afterwards and asked about the *funeral*. I said, 'But I never really did anything for you.' She said, '*You knew my little girl!* I don't want somebody who doesn't know her do her funeral.' They didn't attend church and approached a relative's Baptist church, but the pastor there said that because I'm a woman, I could not do the service. When the mother told me, I steeled myself to hear, 'I'm sorry, you can't do the service after all.' But she said, 'We're finding another church.' That blew me away."

In emotional crises, such support can be not just verbal, but also physical. A hug can communicate more than words. Cathy, whose boyfriend had died in high school, described how she met the family of an elderly man who had just died in the ICU. "His teenage granddaughter was crying and upset. The family were saying, 'He's in a better place. God has a plan and never makes mistakes,' attempting to comfort her and shut her up. She didn't say anything, but opened the stairwell door and ran down the stairs, slamming the door behind her.

"They started going after her. I said, 'I'll go.' I went down the stairs and just held her. She threw her arms around me and we just stood there like that while she sobbed. She just wanted everybody to shut up, and let her grieve. When she was ready, we walked back upstairs. I was instinctively able to tell what she needed, or at least I hoped I did and tried."

Generally, physical contact between providers and patients or families is taboo, but here it seemed appropriate. Female chaplains may face obstacles but also have certain advantages, more readily able to hug patients and family. "There are downsides to being a woman in pastoral care," Cathy explained. "But one upside is that female chaplains can touch patients and families, which can be important. We're less likely to be questioned with teenagers than a male chaplain would be. He would be told, 'Get your hands off her! That's inappropriate!' This granddaughter was young enough to be my daughter. But hugging her just felt right. It was just automatic."

Drawing on a patient's own terms: Using metaphors

In communicating about these ineffable realms, chaplains regularly use metaphors that may reflect a patient's frames of reference and can help in probing concerns. Just as William Gibson, the secular chaplain, drew in part on baseball images, pastoral care providers use various analogies to convey deep but elusive concepts. "Metaphors go to nonverbal parts of our brains," Kristine Baker, a rural Texan chaplain, said. "When patients talk, I look for metaphors. Anytime I can reframe a metaphor that is familiar to them is powerful because it's concrete, and goes into the body." She and other chaplains strive to use a patient's own language, not theoretical or abstract terms. "I want to figure out if I can get in their worldview and use the images *they* use. When I can access these, I can play with the edges of what is verbal."

"Metaphors convey visual images better than words alone," Kristine continued. "The verbal is not robust enough. I listen for metaphors, whether about God, house cleaning, bowling, or birds. If somebody's using a metaphor of golf or engineering, I'll use *that*. I'll see if I can fold the metaphor into what I'm talking about.

"I live in a rural area, so I use farming metaphors. In a clinical trial, one farmer responded extremely well to a particular treatment, while other patients did not. The doctor realized that it was because this patient believed in it so much. When other patients found out it was placebo, it didn't work. But this farmer said, 'I didn't take so seriously the fact that they said it might not work, because the state agricultural department said corn wouldn't grow on my farm. But I planted it and it grows. So, people who think they know everything, don't always!'"

Chaplains use their own tropes, too, to help convey these ethereal topics. Kristine, for instance, also uses the metaphor of ballroom dancing. "In college, I took a dance class, and there weren't enough guys, so my best friend was my partner. I had to learn how to lead as well as follow. Being a chaplain is a little like being the female partner in ballroom dancing. You go in trying not to be stable, happy, or sad, but *neutral*."

Yet, especially in highly fraught emotional situations, providers may at times be unaware of the metaphorical implications of the words they utter, and the ways a listener may misinterpret comments. Kristine described, for example, how a mother was barred, because of COVID-19, from going to the morgue to see a daughter who had just died. This distraught mother asked a junior chaplain, "Is my daughter in a *box*?" This chaplain answered, "No, she's in a *bag!*" The mother exclaimed, upset, "Oh my God!" As Kristine astutely observed, "Just because someone asks you a question, you do not have to answer it. *Almost every question is actually a statement, not a question.*" This insight applies far more generally in life, too. The mother really wanted to know that "the body is respected and safe. The trainee knew his response had been offensive, but didn't know how to respond better. I told him, 'If you get that question again, what you want to say is that the daughter is on a bed and covered up.'"

Kristine tries to understand, rather than automatically assume, what patients mean by the terms they employ. She and other chaplains strive to understand patients' perspectives without rushing to conclusions. Many trainees and others want, for instance, to swiftly cheer up distressed patients. But Kristine teaches medical and chaplaincy students to "not so quickly provide reassurance before hearing the whole story. When patients say, 'I'm pregnant,' I do not answer, 'Congratulations!' or 'I'm sorry.' Rather, I say, 'Well, what's that like for you?' I want to find out whether this pregnancy was planned or unplanned. Is she happy about it or sad and in an abusive relationship? Students often go in and have decided that they're going to opt for sadness or happiness. But I don't yet know what that patient needs. I have to go in a little off-balance. Yet none of us like to be off-balance. We want to go in and have our minds made up where this visit is going to go.

"Patients can't have any sense of confessing or being forgiven until they have told the whole story. So, trainees should bear witness not just to the surface story, but to the complexity of the *whole* story. They could say simply, 'Tell me some more about that,' or 'What makes you feel guilty about that?'"

These efforts require patience—pausing, giving time, and creating stillness to allow deeper and wider exploration and reflection. As Kristine continued, "W. B. Yeats summed up my approach to being a chaplain: to 'make our minds, so like still water, that beings gather about us that they may see their own images.'[10] That's my approach: to try to create that still space where people can reflect for themselves. And I can help reflect that back to them.

"People don't do that for themselves much," Kristine went on, "but instead quickly decide that they're wrong or at fault, instead of thinking, 'I did the best I could.' We should bear witness to the complexity of our stories."

Chaplains detect and explore metaphors to help patients articulate and understand underlying feelings. Marvin Beck, the New Hampshire chaplain at a small community hospital, similarly described a patient who had fought in World War II and was now struggling to make sense of cancer: "I told him, 'It looks like you're fighting another battle here with this cancer.' He said, 'I am. It's another battle!' So, we talked about the war. But we were really talking about his cancer." The patient felt better after this conversation, having found points of reference and strength.

In particular, patients who do not draw on a traditional religious framework can suggest, through metaphors, glimmerings of how they organize and view key aspects of their lives, even if just symbolically and imperceptibly. Margaret Dixon, for instance, the Pennsylvania chaplain who wondered whether to wear a collar after her ordination, described a young atheist artist with bad edema. "Her art form was textiles. She made enormous clothes that she would put in various shapes. She loved her work and lit up when talking about it. I said, 'I wonder what it would be like for you to think about putting on those clothes?' She just burst into tears: 'I never thought of that.' She was palliating herself with art she made from her heart."

Such comments on images and metaphors can tap into half-hidden emotions. As Margaret added, "One patient showed me little fragile sculptures she made from twigs. The sculptures could barely stand up. I said, 'When I see your sculptures, I think of *you*.' She began crying."

With patients of wide varieties of belief, these spiritual care professionals thus employ careful methods, introducing themselves to patients and families, asking open-minded questions, actively listening, avoiding a rush to conclusions, drawing on metaphors, and at times remaining silent. Chaplains' insights and sensitivities can also help doctors, nurses, families, and friends—in short, all of us—in being as attuned as possible to such nuanced aspects of interpersonal communication. Yet, as we will see, these approaches, although they seem simple and straightforward, can nonetheless pose challenges, depending on particular patients' and families' prior beliefs and current crises.

PART II
"COMING IN WITH THE RELIGION THEY HAVE"

Aiding patients with particular beliefs

5

"Why has God let me down?"

Helping religious patients

Specific aspects of patients' or families' longstanding religious or spiritual beliefs can pose particular unique complications. Before they confront serious disease and the prospect of death, most people have had beliefs of some kind—whether religious, spiritual, agnostic, or atheistic—but now face novel conundrums. Patients differ in their responses, based partly on whether they are devoutly religious, atheist, agnostic, or spiritual but not religious.

Frequently, patients try to draw on the religious tradition with which they were raised, but now find that it comes up short, and that they must pick and choose which particular behaviors, identities, or organizational affiliations to embrace. At first, they commonly struggle on their own, trying to rely on these past perspectives. Some consult with their longstanding clergy from outside the hospital and do not require much input from hospital chaplains. But countless others end up needing or benefiting from pastoral care.

Past views can provide some sustenance, but frequently now shift. For Roxanne Cuartas, for example, the Brazilian-born gastroenterologist battling abdominal cancer, religion has always been important. Yet after her diagnosis, her beliefs evolved as well as she began to paint.

Prior religious convictions, while helping many patients to various degrees, also frequently falter or flounder before the horrific new uncertainties of severe disease and threats of death. When experiencing trauma, numerous members of evangelical or other conservative Christian churches can struggle deeply with these questions. As Margaret Dixon, who debated whether to wear a collar, said, "When patients say, 'Jesus is my Savior. God will take care of it. God's got me covered. It's all good.' I think, 'OK, but when the pain is bad or a miserable experience is compromising you, some of that crumbles. It just does.' That's when I can come in, and begin to reframe what that means. One patient said, 'It's been tough, but God doesn't give you more than you can handle.' This patient seemed reluctant to admit that he was wrestling with this idea. What do I say in response?

Doctor, Will You Pray for Me?. Robert L. Klitzman, Oxford University Press. © Oxford University Press 2024.
DOI: 10.1093/oso/9780197750841.003.0005

That I don't believe that? I think God gives people a lot *more* than they can handle. Patients break. But, if that is what he believes, I'm not going to dissuade him. I say, 'That's cool,' and not dwell on it. We talk and keep exploring. You don't lose your faith but, because you are alive, are in *conversation* with it. It is dynamic and real."

Religious patients and families often come to feel disappointed and incensed at God. Chaplains can normalize such feelings. Connie Clark, the chaplain who got burned out during COVID and took time off, said, "Patients are irate at God or wonder, 'Why me?' I'll say, 'How could you *not* be angry? *I* would be angry if I were you.' That is very reassuring to patients, because *many grew up thinking that they can't question or second-guess God.* I say, 'Do you love your husband?' 'Yes.' 'Do you ever get angry at him?' 'Yes.' 'Well, it's sort of the same with God. It's a relationship: God understands.' Once I remove the guilt about that, I can help them process it."

Even "unwaveringly devout" patients can still struggle spiritually and religiously with anger, at times almost instinctively. Juan Rodriquez, a chaplain who developed cancer, found that his experiences as a patient and chaplain affected each other. His diagnosis strengthened his sense of what patients endure, and he then had profounder encounters with them. "I've been dying for two years, but have continued working." He helped, for instance, "a fervent devout Catholic patient who had done everything right and never deviated. She felt, 'God is going to get me through this. I am going to be fine.' Unfortunately, she got worse and was furious, angry at everything. One day I said, 'You seem a little upset today.' She's said, 'I'm *so angry!*' She felt God did not hold up the promise that she believed was hers. 'Sometimes I wish I could hit something,' she said. I said, 'I'm here. Hit me.'" Juan put up his hand, palm facing her. "She started laughing, but was then able to open up more. A lot of her pent-up anger was released. She realized that God did not give her cancer. Her God had not changed. It was the same God. That interaction was a profound prayer for her and for me. I felt so present. Two weeks later, she passed." Sadly, Juan, too, died the month after he spoke with me.

Many religious patients struggle to retain their faith, wrestling with doubt and questions of whether God has forsaken them. Chaplains respond in several ways, partly by giving prayers of lamentation. William Gibson, the Vermont humanist chaplain, for instance, described a patient whose toes had been amputated due to very advanced diabetes, and was now enduring enormous post-amputation pain. "He was Christian, and trying to keep God on his side and be grateful for what there is to be grateful about. But he was having doubts, and feeling, 'God, what else do I have to do?'

"My prayer with him was of lamentation," William explained. " 'God, why have you forsaken me? Why do you turn your face away from me? We don't understand your ways. But we're grateful to you.' The prayer was petitionary, not 'God, why are you doing this?' but 'God, please help.' "

Yet angry patients also pose difficulties for chaplains, raising complex emotions. "I once supervised a younger chaplain working at a nursing home with older Holocaust survivors," another chaplain told me. "This younger chaplain emphasized forgiveness. The Holocaust survivors all told him, 'I'm *never* going to forgive the Nazis!' This trainee didn't know what to do. I told him, 'Let them be angry about that. Anger can be energizing.' "

Patients can also clash about these issues with their family and friends. Tina Edwards, a nurse I interviewed for a study on genetic testing, had had breast cancer, as did her sister, and explained how they each perceived their risks differently. "My sister said her cancer is God's will," Tina told me. "She thinks that cancer is part of *God's plan for her*, and that He is not punishing her, and that God spared me because I prayed." For Tina's sister, religion provided a complete explanatory system. Tina disagreed: "Many people say, 'So-and-so was in a car wreck, but God spared them.' But is that the same God who makes bad things happen?"

Numerous patients thus argue with their families or others regarding religious beliefs, in ways with which chaplains can potentially assist. These feelings are not wholly rational but rather spring from deep emotional wells in the human psyche. Such ruminations are related to questions of "why me?" but differ as well, at times forming a subset of secondary contemplations. Though not all patients ponder if they are now facing retribution, many do so, and vary in their responses.

When patients or families feel they have somehow done something wrong, guilt increases. Humans evolved with this deep instinctual feeling, which promotes moral behavior, motivating us to avoid harming and instead trying to help other people. But at other times, this emotion can balloon too large relative to the imagined offense, causing stress. The presumed offense may not in fact have contributed to the problem faced.

Though strongly religious patients experience these qualms most poignantly, countless others, who have moved away from the faith with which they were raised, nonetheless experience these emotions, too. "Patients just have a sense of, 'I feel I'm being punished,' " explained Connie Clark, who got burned out during COVID. "Even if they're *not* religious, they can feel 'the universe is punishing me.' It doesn't have to be from a God with a long white beard."

Chaplains differ in their specific language and, methods depending partly on the patient's or family member's particular views, but generally encourage these individuals to stand back and reevaluate such feelings. "People use negative images of God to cope," Connie continued. "When they feel they're being punished. I say, 'Wow, so you feel like you *caused* this?' Some say, 'Well, no. I didn't.' That frees them to piece these thoughts together. Others think, 'Well, yes, I think I do deserve it.' That's a different conversation, helping them verbalize their deepest fears and concerns. *Just being able to say that out loud, and be heard, can be very healing in and of itself.* If you can say something out loud, it loses its power: 'Do you think you caused this? Really?' I carry them through to those logical conclusions." A chaplain can thus reflect back to patients their own words or thoughts to challenge them and lead them to shift their focus.

At times, patients also ask chaplains for direct assistance with forgiveness and expiation of sins. Not all chaplains feel comfortable potentially offering such redemption, though it doubtlessly aids many patients, illustrating how individual chaplains vary, based partly on their own beliefs and those of the particular patient. "Forgiveness comes up," Connie continued. "Patients want to make deathbed confessions. They just want to be heard. So, I'll hear them. Sometimes, they will want to be absolved of their sins. That's not really my thing, but I think, alright: 'In the name of Jesus Christ,' or whatever deity they believe in, 'you are forgiven.' I wouldn't say 'absolve.' Generally, they had a Catholic upbringing, and that's important for them to hear. For all I know, they *are* forgiven. I look at it as pastoral care: This person needs to hear these words. It's like baptizing a dead baby: Theologically, I'm not supposed to do it because it's not a live person, but if the family wants it, I'm not going to refuse."

Patients who may have injured others, whether intentionally or not, can confront guilt and feelings of punishment with particular force. Combat veterans regularly struggle with these quandaries, particularly if they themselves had been seriously hurt growing up. Victor Simmons, a chaplain at a midwestern Veterans Affairs hospital, for instance, described a patient who was on a Navy fighter ship in the Persian Gulf in the 1990s, fighting 15 Iranian boats. "The Navy ship was called to engage, and sank five of them. The crew was excited, pumped up. The patient was one of the radar techs and got a call that a jet was heading their direction, and that they needed to engage it. His job was to help decide if each radar blip was an enemy, unknown or friend. If they delayed, the plane could attack. They said it was an enemy. He had some questions about it, but they were only in the back of his mind. So, his ship shot the plane down. Then, they realized that it was a civilian airliner, containing 290 souls, including 60 children heading to their Disneyland. The Navy pulled the dead bodies out of the sea with hooks and piled them up.

"Since then, this patient has suffered all kinds of guilt, and subsequently addiction. He came into our ward saying, 'I'm going to Hell. I'm just trying to figure out how to make life livable before then.' He killed not just people, but *innocents*. 'We ended their lives. We stopped a generation of lives.' Those dead children's faces woke him up at night: 'I believe in God, but I feel His judgment on me is already done and final. There's nothing I can do about that.'

"My role was to find out where his beliefs were coming from," Victor continued. "So, I was curious about his religious upbringing. He was raised Presbyterian with a staunch Presbyterian mother. Where did his hope stop or slow down? Did it stop in the Persian Gulf or was he already feeling guilty because of some adverse childhood event that the military magnified?

"The patient said, 'I think I know that salvation is possible, but I don't know how to access it, because mine feels too much.'"

Victor helped this patient, conveying that forgiveness is possible. "If a person's moral injury comes from a religious upbringing," Victor explained, "we do them a disservice by not going back to that. A chaplain doesn't proselytize or tell patients what to believe, but explores how they were raised, so that they can understand how their hopelessness comes from their religious upbringing. Childhood traumas magnify combat ones.

"Another patient was an interrogator in Iraq and Afghanistan," Victor continued. "He interrogated guys like Saddam Hussein, and told me, 'I was surrounded by evil. I felt like *I* was evil.' He was raised Catholic and had a strong sense of guilt, and had started to investigate a Protestant evangelical approach, which resonated with him more. His mother was also very manipulative. Parents teach kids about God for good or bad, and choose churches that match the parents' various traits, embedding their view of God into their kids. I did it with *my* children. It's a function of parenthood. Kids get the good and the bad." Chaplains thus try to learn from their own past personal experience as well.

In addressing feelings of punishment, a chaplain may therefore try to get patients to grasp the sources of these attitudes. Victor wants them "to recognize where that voice is coming from. It's usually a parent's voice.

"With the vet who shot down kids," Victor continued, "we read the Bible together, and I asked, 'What did you hear?' He told me. I said, 'The voice of God has your mother's face on it. What if we read the Bible from the perspective of your dad, who was much more giving, gracious, and fun?' The patient felt he was 'totally relearning God here. I perceived God as my mom. Apparently He's not.'

"This patient is still struggling, and resorts to alcohol because of his guilt. He was in the hospital again this week. He's now got fourth-stage pancreatic cancer. The guilt still gets to him: 'I've got everything I want, but just can't enjoy it.' I'm working with him, but that trauma might just be too much."

"This sounds like psychotherapy," I said.

"I work with his psychotherapist as a team," Victor explained. "Chaplains seek to connect the domains of body, mind, and spirit, which often get separated in the hospital, but are complementary. I'm in the 'spirituality' lane. But the best treatment is when all three of these are working together. Patients come in for detox and feel shame. The doctors rebalance the chemistry, then send the patient home. I'll ask a patient, 'What's going to happen now?' and he'll respond, 'Relapse.' Why? Because we didn't deal with the mind and the spirit. That's part of my job."

These perspectives can be especially critical in treating PTSD and other mental health problems. As Victor explained, "Moral injury occurs when people get into war or life events happen, and they don't live up to their own moral, spiritual, or religious expectations. They enlisted in the military to defend their country, but ended up shooting innocent women or children. They confront their own guilt, shame, and sources of forgiveness.

"We deal with the problem of evil," Victor continued. He asks patients, "'Where do your thoughts about it come from? How is that based on your religious beliefs? How do you find forgiveness?'—not just the redemption of guilt, but hopefully its elimination. We help patients identify how their childhood affects their moral compass and religious beliefs. Ultimately, to overcome the problem of evil in any relationship, we need to have a choice—an ability to walk away. Love, too, is a choice."

He and other chaplains who have felt disillusioned with the faith with which they were raised draw on various specific aspects of their own personal journeys. Victor's earlier conservative religious background, for instance, aids him with patients who struggle to leave their own strict dogmatic upbringing when it causes problems. "Some of my views and approaches come from my *own* childhood experiences," he explained. "I was born in the South. My dad became a Christian in the Southern Baptist Revival and was very conservative, racist, evangelical, and right-wing. He was distant, very judgmental and rule-focused. So, we went to very judgmental churches. They talked about grace and forgiveness, but the reality was, 'If you do *that*, I wouldn't want to be in *your* shoes! If you walk away from home, you'll go to Hell!' *Patients find a religious organization that fits their dysfunction.* They defend and fight for it, because otherwise there is a dysfunction in *them*, and thus with God."

Victor attended "an extremely conservative college that lost its tax-free status because they wouldn't allow whites to date Blacks. My seminary interpreted the Bible literally. So, I grew up with a pretty narrow view of who's in and who's out. I had that same perception of God, even though I knew better. I still don't pray very well, because my conversations with my dad were very short. I could preach a great sermon and be passionate about the need for compassion, because I felt I was missing it."

His own emotional distress and shame compelled him to enter chaplaincy, but have also humbled him. The later collapse of his marriage led him to switch from being a pastor to being a chaplain. "I went through my own trauma, going through a divorce. Pastors aren't supposed to do that. My congregation was pretty good about it, but I didn't have the energy to give them. So, I stumbled around for a while. I felt guilt, unqualified. I had talked about grace, but didn't know what to do about it for myself. I started asking the hard questions. A friend talked to me about chaplaincy—how going through recovery or grief work makes you a 'natural' for helping other people in trauma, grief or life adjustment.

"I thought chaplaincy was what retired pastors do to keep getting salary and benefits. I didn't respect it much, but thought, 'I really need to start addressing these issues. I'll do that part, and figure out the chaplaincy part later.' Once I did that, I realized I could be with people in their pain. So, it became a *calling*. It's deeper work than pastoral ministry."

Victor's own path, pain, and uncertainties have made him more sensitive to patients: "Before, I thought, 'I have to fix that.' *But I can't even fix myself!* So, I've taken off some of the pressure to have to fix people. I also don't judge patients if they pose questions they're not supposed to ask."

His past experiences also prompt him to scrutinize his daily practice. "In raising difficult issues with patients, I know I'm creating the potential for hopelessness. I wonder, 'Am I doing more harm than good? Is some of my-self coming up too much?' Patients know it's going to get worse before it gets better, but when I'm the one causing that harm, can I make it better? For some patients it's too much. My prayer is: 'God, do something that I can't do. Take what I've got and multiply it,' because I want to heal, not harm." He also readily refers patients to psychotherapists when he needs to: "I stay in my lane."

Even nonreligious patients can at times feel intense guilt that affects both their mind and body and that chaplains can help ameliorate. Many people experience remorse even if they are not in fact responsible for a bad event. As Cathy Murray, the Catholic hospital chaplain whose boyfriend was killed in a car accident, described, "One patient phoned the on-call nurse every night at 2 a.m., complaining of pain. The nurse tried everything, changing pain medicines. Finally, I said, 'Perhaps it isn't just physical pain, but an aspect of spiritual pain. What if I spoke with him?' The patient turned out to be car-rying massive guilt from his mother's suicide when he was 18. He felt it was his fault. I arranged for his older siblings to talk about it. They were aghast. They had no idea he'd been carrying this regret all these years. They reminded him that their mother had mental health issues: 'Don't you remember?' It was like a 50-pound weight had been lifted. After that, he never again called the nurses at night."

Parents of ill children also frequently feel guilty that they are somehow re-sponsible for their offspring's disease, when that is not the case. "I hear a lot of guilt," said Linda Porter, the Maryland pediatric chaplain and former jour-nalist. "One mother had a daughter with Down's syndrome who eventually died. For four months while the child was hospitalized, I saw the family every day. The family cherished the daughter. She was the star of the family, but now had leukemia. They were devout Catholics. One day while her daughter was sleeping, the mother said to me, just apropos of nothing, '*Do you think God gave my daughter leukemia because when she was born with Down's, I prayed for her to die?*'

"The mother had been pregnant at 40 and didn't know she was carrying a child with Down's, and at birth, found that her daughter had trisomy 21 and serious cardiac problems. Overwhelmed and afraid her child might suffer, the mother said, 'Please, God, take her.' That was an utterly human feeling. She didn't say that to anyone, but carried that *in her heart*. That was her question to God, her 'quiet prayer.' At some deep level in her psyche, she then carried guilt about merely having *thought* that. Surgery corrected the daughter's cardiac problems, but the doctors weren't sure how severe the ongoing problems would be. Then, this daughter developed leukemia.

"On the ward, her daughter was cheerful and happy—a great kid who sailed through treatment. But she then collapsed from a respiratory virus. She was in the pediatric intensive care unit [PICU] for a month. Ultimately, the family had to remove her from life support. The end was pure anguish. It was a terrible tragedy because the leukemia treatment was successful, but she died from something else."

Here and elsewhere, a chaplain can help patients and families reconceive their views of God, even if holding different personal perspectives. "I come from a liberal, progressive tradition," Linda continued. "I don't believe in a punitive God who gives children dreadful diseases to teach parents. I never say that bluntly. But I hear many religious parents feeling guilty and ashamed and feeling they're being punished.

"I asked this mother: 'Do you think of God as a loving God?' She said, 'Yes, of course.' 'Do you see the love that your daughter has brought into the world? Could you pray to a loving God if He was hurting your child?' 'Well, no . . .,' she replied. 'I really don't think *that* . . .'

"*People come into the hospital with the faith they have, and sometimes it comes up short,*" Linda observed. "Some people believe that God doesn't make mistakes, or that everything happens for a reason or because God must be trying to teach them something. I never tell such patients what I feel: 'You've got to be fucking kidding me! This is so fucked up! How can you possibly believe that?' I just say, 'I hear what you're saying, but tell me about your image of God.' 'Well, God is love. God loves us and wants the best for us.' I say, 'You talk about Jesus as loving children, so how could anyone hurt a child in the name of God?' I try to shine a light into their narrow view of God."

As Linda noted, the mother of the girl with Down's syndrome had a "quiet prayer" that this mother kept "in her heart" and uttered to no one. Yet doctors generally don't think of "things kept in the heart." Medicine ignores things metaphorically "in the heart"—if anything, biomedicine sees all thoughts as encoded in the brain—underscoring the importance of chaplains' discourse.

Religious patients can worry about not just past but also future punishment. Linda described, for instance, another mother who "had a twin pregnancy, in which one twin was draining off nutrition from the other. The mother could terminate one and have a 90% chance of having a healthy baby, or continue the pregnancy and possibly lose *both* or have a severely damaged child. Before the procedure, she asked me, 'Will God punish me for killing my baby?'"

Linda and other chaplains generally feel that we cannot know the answers to these ultimate questions, but nonetheless ask. As Linda continued, "I hear ad nauseam, 'Everything happens for a reason' and 'God never gives you more than you can handle'—all those platitudes. That's what people have been taught. I'm not judging that. I listen and try to expand their thinking: There are two ways of thinking about that. Some people believe that God causes everything to happen—COVID-19, tsunamis, or children dying of cancer. But other people believe Jesus' statement: I am with you always. You can never separate yourself from the love of God."

In helping patients examine and recast such questions and feelings, Linda and other chaplains judge whether, how, and when to draw on their own views. "I believe that God is with you through everything," Linda said, "but does *not* cause everything to happen. There's a certain *randomness* in the world. Yet within that, people have alternatives. I try to engage patients, and make their world a little larger. Inside, I feel judgmental, but I never dismiss what someone says."

Pastoral care helps patients overcome assumptions about God causing disease, and accept the realities of our chaotic cosmos. "People are very self-punishing, and feel relieved knowing that their problem is *not* their fault," Linda continued. "Parents whose child gets a bad diagnosis immediately ransack their life to figure out what they did: 'I should have gone to the pediatrician two weeks earlier,' even though the doctors assured them that they didn't miss anything. Our human psyches need to control and understand. It's much easier to blame ourselves than to think the world is an utterly random, freakish place."

By probing patients' views in detail, chaplains assist. "When parents say, 'My mother said that if I had gone to church, this wouldn't have happened, and that it's my fault,'" Linda continued. "I say, 'How do you feel about it? . . . I don't think God is judging you. I feel the depth of your love for this child. A loving God is not going to hurt your child to teach you something. Don't you think, if you believe God created the universe, that He'd have some other way to get your attention without hurting your baby?'"

Feelings of being punished seep out from deep roots and religious school precepts, underscoring how powerful early indoctrination of children can be—no doubt why religious institutions strongly pursue it. Brenda Pierson, a pediatric chaplain in the Bible Belt, trained in a faith-affiliated hospital where pictures of Jesus and quotes from Scripture hung on the walls. She explained how mothers frequently ask, "Is my baby sick because I smoked marijuana in high school? Is God mad at me because I was living with my boyfriend? Am I in trouble because I had sex before getting married, or had sex with three people or seven people—that God is somehow now judging my behavior, and my baby is now being punished?" "I say, 'Tell me what makes you think that.' They will pull out a dire sermon they heard in middle school. If the Bible is authoritative for them, I suggest verses about forgiveness, love, kindness, and children being valuable to God. If the Bible is not authoritative, I go back to a time when they experienced God as loving, gracious, or kind, or when someone whom they thought was connected to God showed them those feelings, behaviors, or examples. Sometimes this journey lasts one to three months while their child is in the NICU or getting a bone marrow transplant. Nobody's neutral about their child."

Yet clergy from outside the hospital may instead inculcate and promulgate such punitive doctrines. As Brenda continued, "Televangelists say, 'If you pray *this* way, God will answer you with riches, blessing, and good health.' If you put the right prayer in the vending machine of God, and push the right button, the biggest Hershey bar with almonds comes out!" Brenda added sarcastically. "It takes a lot of energy to question and deconstruct one's theology. In a lot of communities, that is unwelcome, unhealthy, and unheard of."

In various ways, chaplains thus aid religious patients who feel let down, angry at God, guilty, or punished for their behavior. Chaplains range in their tactics and language, drawing on their own past experiences, travails, and training, but ultimately manage to succor patients and families with wide arrays of beliefs.

6

"I just look at sunsets and stars"

Aiding patients who are spiritual but not religious

After my sister died on 9/11, Nature uniquely comforted me, reminding me of the far greater universe that extends beyond us, existing for billions of years before humans evolved, and surely fated to persist for billions more after we're gone.

Choral music by Bach, Mozart, Beethoven, Vaughan Williams, and others similarly transports me, elevating my spirits—the clear voices of sopranos, tenors, violins, horns, and trumpets, each rising in crescendos above the other into the pure air, sweeping like birds, gliding forward together, then separately, then swooping upwards together again. The sounds wash over each other like waves. In religious services, inspired song and moments of silence have uplifted and cleansed me, separate from any explicit religious content per se. But other parts of religious services feel to me long and rote. I understand why many people increasingly dislike these rituals and do not attend.

Chaplains assist not only religious patients but also those who are "spiritual but not religious." Many patients are wary of religion per se yet still value connections, which chaplains can help strengthen if patients wish.

When asked on surveys whether they follow a major religion, increasing proportions of people describe themselves as "none of the above," and are hence dubbed "Nones." Wariness of religious practices dates back to the beginning of recorded time. Socrates questioned the ancient Greek gods' authority and existence. Moses complained of Jews' idolatry in the desert. Corrupt popes fill Dante's Inferno.

But in recent decades, given scientific advances and church scandals, criticism of organized religions has been growing. "Nones" include individuals who are atheist, agnostic, or nothing in particular, and reflect the fastest-rising category of beliefs in America. In a 2016 study of U.S. adults, 80% had a religious affiliation, 11% had no religious preference, 6.3% were agnostics, and 2.8% were atheists,[1] and 36% of young Millennials say they are religiously

Doctor, Will You Pray for Me?. Robert L. Klitzman, Oxford University Press. © Oxford University Press 2024.
DOI: 10.1093/oso/9780197750841.003.0006

unaffiliated.[2] I found, though, that when they face serious disease, unaffiliated patients and families commonly grapple with quandaries with which chaplains can help.

Many studies of religion focus on relatively rigid binary categories, such as whether or not a person is affiliated with a religious institution or believes in God. These forced choices fail, however, to capture the vast ranges of people's beliefs.

Leeriness toward religion takes widely varying forms. Given the ever-mounting mobility of people and ideas, I have seen how patients in fact fall across broad and fluid continuums, mixing and matching beliefs from multiple faiths, adopting New Age views and practices, and rejecting traditional frameworks altogether and/or formulating their own. Even within the standard broad categories, patients start out and end up in differing places. While my own beliefs have fluctuated but remained overall within the broad, loose framework of Judaism, many people have dramatically moved between markedly contrasting faiths. *The boundaries between these creeds appear far more permeable than in the past.*

The terms "religion" and "spirituality" themselves have very wide spectrums of meanings in varying academic disciplines. "Religion" derives from the Latin *religio* (meaning "obligation, bond"[3]). The ancient Greeks had no word for "religion" per se. Julius Caesar developed the term to refer to captured soldiers taking an oath to their captors.[4] In the 1200s, the term came to refer in English to a life bound to monastic orders.[5] Only in the 1500s did the word begin to refer to the realm of the Church as opposed to worldly things.[6] Various scholars have defined "religion" differently. Anthropologists, for instance, have defined the term as "human interaction with a culturally postulated non-falsifiable reality."[7,8]

In contrast, *The Oxford English Dictionary* defines "spirit," from the Latin *spiritus* (meaning "breathing"), as "the animating or vital principle in humans and animals; that which gives life to the body, in contrast to its purely material being; the life force, the breath of life."[9] Some sociologists have said that a community is needed—but people who are spiritual but not religious are often parts of various communities as well, from book clubs to yoga classes, consisting of like-minded individuals.

In practice, Jack Stone, the Buddhist chaplain, perceives religion and spirituality as "two sides of the same hand. Look at the front of your hand: a palm. Then, look at the back side of your hand. Which is more important? Neither! They're both important. Both the front and the back make up your hand. The spiritual aspect might be the palm, and the religious aspect the back of the hand. Religion would be the dogma, belief systems, and specific nature of how we human beings meet the sacred—the words, the language, the stories we tell, the belief systems. Spirituality is much more broad. It's how we connect with the sacred. You can be spiritual but not religious."

Sociologists have described three different aspects of religion or the "three B's"—religious *belonging* (to institutions), *behavior*, and *belief*.[10] But I have found that, among and within these three broad categories, patients range widely, and can fluctuate over time and in which aspects of the "three B's" they follow, and how. For example, about a third of Americans today who "don't know" if they believe in God nonetheless attend religious services at least once a week. Most agnostics (55%) feel a sense of wonder about the universe at least once a week, 68% feel a sense of spiritual peace and well-being at least several times a year, 20% pray at least monthly, 14% believe in Heaven, and 9% believe in Hell.[1]

In his book *What We Talk About When We Talk About God*,[11] Rob Bell suggests that what we discuss when we talk about God is a "unitary" phenomenon. But people vary widely in how they define "God," "religion," "spirituality," "agnosticism," "atheism," "doubt," "prayer," and "grace," influenced by their parents, upbringing, personalities, stresses, spouses, medical diagnoses, and other factors. "God is any number of things that we want God to be," explained Margaret Dixon, who debated whether to wear a collar after her ordination. "That's not necessarily bad. It can be very helpful, an anodyne to suffering." *The simple three-letter word "God" can reflect myriad existential and spiritual views.*

Observers commonly see "Nones" as a single distinct, relatively well-defined group,[12] and view this category in essentialist ways—lumping together various individuals, including those who are "nothing in particular," "spiritual but not religious," and at times atheists and agnostics. Many observers are also highly critical of these groups. But "Nones" is a large catch-all phrase that in fact squeezes together highly diverse sets of people, defining and uniting them merely by a single question about what they are *not* (i.e., "none of the above") and ignoring major distinctions. This one term by itself is not especially useful. Within this broad category, patients vary widely, constructing their beliefs in diverse ways. To try to clump this broad spectrum of people into one fixed category does them a disservice.

While some researchers have attempted to subdivide Nones, numerous questions persist about how best to do so. Most religiously "unaffiliated" individuals (68%) believe in God, as do 97% of those who are "affiliated" and 80% of the U.S. population as a whole. Among unaffiliated people, 41% pray at least monthly (vs. 88% of the affiliated and 79% of the general population), 18% think of themselves as "religious," 37% as "spiritual but not religious" (vs. 75% and 15%, respectively, of affiliated individuals), and 42% as "neither spiritual nor religious" (vs. 8% of those who are affiliated and 15% of the general population).[13] The meanings of these terms therefore blur. Individuals may check "none of the above" because they fit the other boxes only partially, or fit more than one. Atheists and agnostics are also more likely than others to be male, younger, better educated and white, from the western United States, and less obese, and to have fewer medical problems, but also to have lower happiness, self-esteem, and optimism, and more anxiety.[14] As Brian Post, a Michigan chaplain department administrator, said, "The label of 'None' isn't helpful, and doesn't tell you much. Some Nones are more spiritual than 're-ligious' individuals! Just because somebody identifies as a None, Catholic, Orthodox Jew, or another label doesn't begin to tell me about this person's individual spirituality. Within any of these labels, some people have relatively developed and mature personal spirituality. Others don't.

"The hospital admission process asks patients their religious preference and it's somewhere in the chart," Brian continued, "but I never thought it was particularly important to look up. If I saw it, I might make note of it. *But the label doesn't communicate how the person will cope with the existential challenges they face.*

"Some Nones," Brian observed, "have much more spiritual maturity than people wearing a particular religious label, and are able to face their impending death in the next hours or days with a settled peace, and form healthy relationships and express gratitude, joy and meaning. Those are characteristics of 'mature spirituality,' regardless of religion."

Chaplains can often uniquely assist patients with such beliefs when serious diseases threaten lives. "Some Nones are very *anti-religious,*" Brian noted, "and don't believe in religion and just hate it, seeing it as all merely wish ful-fillment and fantasy. But they might still appreciate somebody listening to them when they are facing death and dying. We are better suited to care for Nones than are most congregational-based clergy. Nones usually don't have a pre-existing relationship with a clergyperson, spiritual advisor, or leader. So, that increases our value."

An increasing group of Nones, in fact, want to become chaplains. "Larger numbers of young people are Nones, interested in ministry as a career, and feel drawn to this kind of work," Brian continued, "but would rather not do it in a church, synagogue, or mosque, and prefer an institutional setting like chaplaincy."

Spirituality appears relatively ubiquitous. As Brenda Pierson, the pediatric chaplain from the Bible Belt, said, "I think we are created to have a spiritual self that longs for something more than simply a physical life."

Yet the wide range of beliefs of patients who are spiritual but not religious has astonished me. These broad spectrums of beliefs are important to note, since to grasp what chaplains do, it is essential to understand the breadth and depth of the beliefs of patients whom they encounter and attempt to help. Spiritual care providers must learn how to address each such stance, and they therefore develop and hone wide and flexible approaches to adapt to each patient.

Many people, for instance, say "none of the above" partly because they amalgamate their own unique combination of concepts from several traditions, not ascribing solely to any one of them. "I have a Quaker background, my mother is Pennsylvania Dutch and Lutheran, and my father was Methodist," Roy Gifford, a retired salesman with a chronic disease whom I interviewed as part of a study, told me. "I used to joke that I'll be married Jewish and buried Druid. I just lump them all together as 'the God fetish.'" A tall, thin man with wavy light brown hair, he had moved around the country from the East Coast to California, and now to the Southwest, and seemed to have a bit of wanderlust geographically as well as spiritually.

Countless patients were raised in one religion, but then marry spouses from another tradition, subsequently join a third faith or avoid churches altogether for a while, and afterwards seek another, feeling that no single religious institution entirely meets all their needs. Since 1960, the rate of interfaith marriages, for example, has roughly doubled, from 19% to 39%. Among unmarried couples living together, 49% are of different faiths.[15]

In certain ways, such mixing and matching and constructing one's own religion are very American traits. Ralph Waldo Emerson, for example, preached spirituality but was wary of organized religion and other institutions. "That which shows God in me, fortifies me,"[16] he wrote, but also quipped, "Whoso would be a man, must be a nonconformist. . . .I am ashamed to think how easily we capitulate . . . [to] dead institutions."[17] As the late literary critic Harold Bloom wrote, "American religion consists of individuals drawing on their own experiences to forge their own way."[18]

"I've done a lot of reading," one ill surgeon told me. "The Quran, Hindu literature, Mary Baker Eddy and Christian Science, and Bible stuff. I found the old parable of the elephant helpful. One man feels his leg, one his trunk, etc. They've all got a little piece." He and numerous other patients draw on whatever feels nurturing to them at the moment, with less ongoing allegiance to any one single faith.

"I tried different religions, even Hinduism, and finally *made up my own religion,*" a colleague recently told me. "Just as some creatures live on flat surfaces and only experience two dimensions, I think a fourth dimension exists that we just don't know about."

God as Nature

Poets have long celebrated Nature itself as representing the hand of the Divine, however we may define it—the source and mystery of life, connecting the smallest creatures with the largest organizing principles of the universe—and reminding us to appreciate these details. In the face of chaos, Nature, ever able to renew itself, can grant a sense of order, connection, and escape to something beyond. From Henry David Thoreau, Walt Whitman, Emily Dickinson, and Ralph Waldo Emerson, through today, Nature can resplendently solace us.

The psychiatrist Robert Jay Lifton detected that survivors of the atomic bombs at Hiroshima and Nagasaki, facing widespread death, sought sources of "symbolic immortality"—ways of symbolically living on—and do so through five means: through religion, children, creative work, experiential transcendence ("sex, drugs, and rock and roll!"), or Nature.[19] Many patients, I have observed, follow similar patterns. Some patients, on their own, come to see Nature as divine. But for others, chaplains can help instill this sense.

Nature can serve several functions. Appreciation of the larger universe beyond ourselves—physical evidence of something far vaster, outside us—can calm us, helping us to place stressors in a much broader context and thereby reducing their relative weight. "If a nuclear bomb wiped out all human beings," Nora, a 39-year-old physician with metastatic breast cancer, told me, "there'd still be some little cockroach. And after eons of time, there'd be a whole new population of things. A process is moving forward in some way— some mysterious force . . . That by itself is the meaning of life: We don't understand it. It's great that we don't. Maybe we would be sad if we did."

Her spiritual beliefs are unconnected to a religion per se but have succored her. She has come to see change as the only constant, and suffering as ever-present—principal tenets of Buddhism, though she does not note this commonality. "In the beginning, I thought I had a bad prognosis but maybe skimmed by—maybe I'd be lucky, and the cancer wouldn't come back. Then, it came back. So now, I try to stop thinking about the future, because just when you think you see how it's going to go, something changes. That's traumatic. I have some trips scheduled until June, but not beyond. When things happen, they will be dealt with. We'll all be on top of it—do as much as we can. Hopefully, I won't suffer much."

"My oncologist immediately tried to medicate away my distress with Valium," she continued, but Nora refused. Physicians commonly respond to a patient's existential despair by prescribing medication—often because of their own discomfort with these challenges. But Nora bravely wanted to confront the fact that she was dying.

She located spirituality in biology and science, and integrated her spiritual beliefs with her medical training. Her hobby was gardening, which for her exemplified and reaffirmed the ever-changing cosmos: "The tree or shrub I love this year is already too big next year. Things are always changing. Nothing stays the same."

Chaplains and other providers can assist patients, if interested, in forging such ties. A psychiatrist I admire now routinely asks all his patients if they are religious or spiritual. If they answer no, he asks, " 'Do you believe in a higher power?' Some say, 'No, not really.' I then inquire, 'Do you ever feel awe?' Some ask, 'What do you mean?' I say, 'Do you ever look at the sunset or a forest and feel one with nature?' 'Sure.' 'Well, that can be a form of spirituality.' 'I guess you're right,' they say, relieved. It gives them a way of feeling part of something larger than themselves. Pointing this out to them feels like a helpful gift. They feel soothed, less alone. Some patients say they drink alcohol or use drugs to feel that way."

Patients from a wide range of cultural and economic backgrounds come to see nature—the extraordinary beauty of multi-hued trees, leaves, birds, and stars—as reflecting a larger force or order. "Yesterday evening I looked at the sky," Olana Ramirez, a Latina patient from the Bronx whom I had interviewed for a study, told me. She had injected heroin and was now sober but had HIV. "It was a beautiful sunset: orange and purple. When I look at something like that, I know there's *got* to be something greater to create so much beauty. Man can't create that. So, I have a lot of faith in a higher power. It's blind faith, but it beats no faith at all."

Faith in nature transcends social and economic divides. Olana never finished high school but appreciated the deep intricacies of biology: "What fascinates me is how the body is built. I've seen videos about the immune system fighting, and it's beautiful. I feel joy when I see it. God made us perfect: He made one little cell send a message to another cell to go fight. They communicate with one another. Our eyes see. The liver filters. When I think of that, I'm grateful we have the ability to fight." For her and others, disease and suffering are a means through which to heighten appreciation of God as embodied in nature, and to feel more grateful.

"Would God create something so magnificent just to live a little while and die and be buried and that's it?" Olana asked. "There *has* to be something else. Nobody builds anything so beautiful, so intricate, and just throws it away. That's ridiculous!" For her, the very complexity of human biology suggests the presence of a force beyond it. Still, she remains unclear as to the specifics, and is unconcerned about that lack of clarity: "I don't believe I'll come back as a bird or something. I'm put here for a purpose. God has something else planned for me. I don't know what." She sees evidence of God but accepts inherent mysteries, ambiguities, and unknowns. God can serve as a stand-in for the randomness and vast unknowns of the universe.

"I pray every night," Olana continued. "I say, 'God . . .' The first part I say in Spanish because that's the way I learned it when I was in church. I'll start as if I'm talking to a person. Sometimes, I ask Him to forgive me for being weak."

Nature can spark spiritual and religious sentiments, yet individuals may not explicitly recognize the role of illness itself in triggering these thoughts. Wanda, an HIV-infected African American woman, for instance, felt she didn't deserve to contract HIV, but then listed all of her sexual partners and felt embarrassed and regretful about her past behavior. A profound religious experience now sustained her: "I was standing up on a mountaintop at an upstate retreat overlooking the Hudson River when all of a sudden I heard God's voice," she said. "I feel like I just cleansed my soul out and have a new one now." Still, of note, she feels that this experience occurred because of God directly, not her illness, and that this connection came from outside, not inside, herself. The Bible, too, presents numerous stories of Divine Recognition emanating from outside oneself. Moses saw the Burning Bush and received the Ten Commandments, and Abraham heard God telling him to sacrifice and then spare Isaac—all seen as signs of God's existence.

Others actively seek these experiences of nature in and of itself, without an explicit link to religion per se. "In the past, when I had a car, I would drive to certain places, like up a hill, and just sit and look at the river," said Roy Gifford, the retired salesman who had a Quaker background and now mixed and matched beliefs. "Or I'd go to a spring. I had favorite places. I still take walks . . . wherever the spirit goes. I forget about what upsets me, leave it behind or work it through." Nature itself can thus offer order, escape, and evidence of forces greater than oneself—more implicit than explicit, but nonetheless stabilizing and grounding.

The threat of death can fuel these quests. "When a person knows they're going to die, they appreciate nature," a patient who lived in the inner-city Bronx and now had a chronic disease told me. Before her diagnosis, she didn't even think about death. "Now, I look at the clouds and hear the birds once more. I go sit out on the porch at night and look at the stars, and think, 'This is beautiful—the human body, the stars, and the leaves.' Nothing dies in this world. A tree loses its leaves, but they go on to become something else. Everything is part of a cycle. A Supreme Being definitely put all of this together. I look up and see the sky and feel I want to be there one day.

"Sometimes I just walk down by the river," she continued, "and simply keep walking. Wherever, whatever, it doesn't matter. The water comforts and calms me. I look at the sky, just to put my mind in a state that I forget everything until I have to go back home." She seeks such comfort not all the time, but only at particular points. "At home, I turn on the faucet and just sit and let the water go through my hand, listening, like when it rains."

Spirituality in science

Science, probing great cosmic complexities and mysteries beyond our ken, inspires many Nones. Individuals trained in biology or physics often see these disciplines as reflecting or embodying a sense of spirituality. Jack Stone, the Buddhist chaplain, views the awe that he has encountered among some scientists as spiritual. He assists such patients in discovering their own answers to the riddles of the cosmos. "One astronomer with cancer was not religious, but told me, 'You're a Buddhist, and the Buddhists have the closest affinity to scientists. If I had a religion or spirituality, I would be more

Buddhist than anyone!' When I first met him, he was not dying per se, and was trying to find all the chemo available to him. But he was having an existential crisis, trying to find meaning in what was happening to him. He was sick and vulnerable—the cancer could kill him—and was asking, 'What is this all about?'"

Jack asked him, "What brings you a sense of awe? Tell me about a time in your life when you felt spiritual, for lack of a better word, or felt that the world or universe was larger than you." He told Jack "about a turning point in his life, as a teenager, that got him into astronomy. He was watching the Milky Way and thought about the stars, the planets, the enormity of the universe, and all of its mysteries, complexities, and unknowns. That opened something with him, which led him into his life's path—to science, and studying the planets and stars. It was a spiritual experience for him. For him, *that* was spirituality. He wouldn't name it that, but I told him *I* would. 'That opening that you experienced—many saints, monks, and religious people throughout the ages would call it different things, but you had an *opening* of some kind.' Patients say, 'I'm not a religious person.' I say, 'OK, but have you had an experience in your life, at some point, that made you open yourself up to something perhaps larger, though you might not know what it is?' How does the space of the sacred touch a person's life—even though he or she might not define it that way? Most people are open to it: 'I might not believe in all the deities of Hinduism, or in an old man sitting in a chair governing over what's happening in my life, like a chessboard, but there's something maybe helping, awakening, guiding, and supporting us. I don't know what that is.' I don't have the answers, but *help patients find their own answers* that they need in this moment."

A hospital chaplain can aid such patients, appreciating their views, at times more than even family or friends do. William Gibson, the humanist Vermont chaplain who draws on poetry, described a patient who "felt the hugeness of the universe, suggesting God, but he didn't feel cared for by Him. The patient wasn't particularly religious, but had a strong sense of God as the Creator of the Universe. He was raised nominally Protestant, but other family members were very religious. He developed very serious lung disease and was on life support, and found himself watching YouTube videos about the universe, showing how unbelievably tiny Earth is compared to Jupiter and other celestial objects. He had me watch with him. It helped him sense the 'hugeness' of God, and that there *is* a God. But he had no sense that that God would care about him. And he wanted to feel cared for. I joined him in prayer, and said I hoped that the Creator of the Universe cared about him and would help him.

"When it was clear he was going to die, he asked me to speak at his memorial service, to share his spiritual thoughts with his family and friends—his view from his foxhole. He wanted people to know that even though he wasn't particularly religious, he really did believe that there was something bigger, and that he was a part of it. He wanted his wife and daughter to know he loved them—his final thoughts from his deathbed." This patient feared that his immediate family might not understand or appreciate his beliefs, so private can these be.

God as love

Other Nones see *love* as the essence and source of spirituality and God. The idea of "God as love" may seem diffuse, trite, or abstract, but chaplains often draw on it effectively. Connie Clark, the chaplain who took time off during COVID, applies what she calls an "ethics of love: There are four principles for making bioethical decisions," she said, referring to the basic tenets of patient autonomy, beneficence, justice, and avoidance of harm.[20] "I also apply an *ethics of love*. I say, 'If you're making a decision out of love, in love, or for love, even if it's imperfect, it will be blessed by God, because God is *love*. Your intent matters.' That seems to comfort a lot of people. The 'love ethic' is the overarching ethic to all of this."

These various forms of spirituality without religion—seeing God in love, nature, or science—are not mutually exclusive and can blend. Margaret Dixon, who had debated whether to wear a collar after her ordination, described, for instance, a cancer patient with "a lot of angst, rancor, and edginess in his relationships with his children from several marriages. Yesterday, he told me he had a 'moment of awareness' about the world. He was standing on the porch, looking at his backyard, seeing nature, and able to watch it and stay with it for longer periods than ever before. He realized, 'There's so much we can't control.' We can't control much of anything— except how we interact with each other in relationships, ethically. God is an *ethics* between people: how we love people, and are in awe of something, and stop and are stunned by something beautiful. The sense of awe and the ways we treat each other are almost like a horizontal and a vertical—a cross," she said, smiling.

Spirituality despite oneself

Chaplains can aid patients in getting in touch, too, with inchoate beliefs that prove helpful. The degrees to which varied beliefs are not always self-willed have repeatedly surprised me. When confronting disease, these spiritual notions can seem to emerge from outside one's conscious awareness. Many people become more attuned to these feelings despite themselves, and struggle to grasp these ideas. "I certainly don't have any relationship to any kind of deism or God," Walter Cunningham, an internist with lymphoma, for instance, told me. "At some points when I've been really sick, I remember thinking it would be really good to find serenity in believing that an all-powerful figure was going to look after me during and after death. But I could never quite bring myself to believe that." Science encourages searches for facts and *skepticism* of assumptions, and strongly attracts individuals with these predilections.

Still, once facing death, Walter Cunningham and many others trained in science become more open to spirituality. "Human beings can share something with each other—through touch or caring," Walter said, though adding, "I'm not sure where that falls in any *spirituality* range." He remains unclear how to define or conceptualize these notions, sensing possible connections but also ineffable ambiguity. "In college, I became more politically active," he continued. He started reading Karl Marx and Vladimir Lenin. "Marx was a Positivist, reflecting the philosophy of the Enlightenment: You could understand the world . . . If you could just understand the world enough, then you could figure out how to make it better." He became an activist, working as a physician with poor, marginalized populations all over the world.

Then he developed lymphoma. "My doctor looked at the CT scan and said, 'There's nothing we can do.' I was devastated. He said, 'You'll never be able to eat. You have tumors everywhere. If we operate and get into your abdomen and there's tumor everywhere, what do you want us to do? It will hurt and won't change the outcome. You'll be dead.' He didn't mean it to be devastating, but it was . . . I was convinced I would die." This treating physician may have felt he was merely conveying the facts of the case, but was oblivious to his words' emotional impacts.

Though believing in Marx, a fierce critic of religion, Walter felt, in the hospital, a strength from outside himself, aiding him. "One really strange story that probably was a result of delirium: I had already been in septic shock, and was going downhill. For a couple of days, I had a very strong sensation that

(1) I was strongly rooted to the ground . . . I had almost a tree root from my back through the bed, into the ground, and that it was rooting me, and giving me strength; and (2) I was getting strength from outside myself.

"I was quite surprised. I didn't know how to process it. There was nothing I could do about it, but it was a strong sensation. It lasted a couple of days and never came back. I was not delirious. Sounds like some of my more psychotic patients: I felt like there *were vibrations coming from outside* . . . and they did good things inside me."

He did not know how to understand and integrate these spiritual experiences with his prior atheism. At first, he mused that the experience was "probably" because of "delirium," but he later stated emphatically that he had *not* been delirious. His feelings about faith clashed—he wanted to believe in a hereafter (to provide a sense of comfort) but was unable to embrace this notion fully. The seeming irrationality embarrassed him. He felt unable to comprehend the experience fully, or to integrate it within his existing beliefs, highlighting the broader conflicts between spirituality and reason. His scientific training cautioned him about irrational beliefs that lacked evidence.

He and many others do not seek these beliefs, but feel that these notions are somehow thrust upon them. Despite their conscious attitudes, they feel these ideas emerge in their minds, unsought and surprising. Countless people end up having certain beliefs without undergoing a process of rational choice. Clergy describe having a "calling" that they cannot and do not will. Similarly, many patients come to have certain beliefs, not attained through conscious logic alone.

After my sister's death on 9/11, when I sat in Central Park for hours, I, too, didn't "look for" the beliefs I now have. Somehow, it seemed they found me. While major theologians from St. Paul to St. Augustine have undergone major religious conversions, numerous patients today experience transformations unwittingly, unclear how to interpret or process these—not whole-heartedly embracing them, but unwilling to dismiss them either. Their views are not necessarily internally consistent, but rather amalgams of various faiths and feelings that may not wholly cohere.

Wanting *more* belief

Chaplains also help patients who have some faint, amorphous beliefs but want additional or stronger ones. People who are spiritual but not religious vary in not only types but also degrees of beliefs. The fact that religion and spirituality are not always self-willed leads some individuals to yearn for or seek more. Yet like love, these sentiments cannot be forced or easily described or defined. "I'm almost *envious*," a social worker with breast cancer and the gene for it, told me. "I've seen people have tremendous strength from believing in God, praying, worshipping, and going to church or temple—having something you can focus on, and really feeling that there is a Greater Being that can make it all OK. I don't have that. *I wish I did!*" Many patients want to believe in something, but struggle and can't bring themselves to do so.

"The first time I ever wished I were religious was when I had cancer," she continued. "I'm Jewish, but was not brought up in a religious house-hold. Jewish identity was always important to me, but *not* in terms of the religion—going to temple, believing in a God, or praying. I guess I'm too skeptical, for whatever reason." Her intellectual caution impeded her ability to draw emotionally on spirituality, and outweighed her desire to believe. Still, she does not wholly grasp her inner obstacles to faith, and feels she must simply accept them.

In having "some" spirituality, possessing certain extents of belief, but desiring additional amounts, patients highlight how degrees of belief fall across wide continua, and are not entirely self-willed. For instance, "I wish I was more spiritual," Steven, an endocrinologist with a chronic disease, told me. "I'm open to the idea—at least I *think* I am. It makes a big difference in most people's lives . . . Those who have some kind of centering around a spir-itual belief seem to do better. As a kid, I used to pray a lot—because you're *supposed* to. Even to this day, I find myself praying—that this blood result will be good, that You're going to let this be good news—without planning or thinking about it *consciously*." But, "the past few times, my prayer wasn't answered." He looked down, disappointed.

Still, he tries. "Once in a while, I'll pray at night, and it makes me feel a little better. I don't know why I don't do it more often. Perhaps I should." He paused and shook his head to himself. "But I don't know really what to pray *to*. I'm not very religious. I was brought up Methodist. After traveling in India and the Far East, I like Buddhism. I find Hinduism interesting, but don't be-lieve in all their multiplicity of gods. I've come to feel that Christ, Buddha, and Allah all actually represent the same horse. I pray to the Lord—if you can call it God—for strength to get me through this, and wisdom to help me make the right decisions."

Yet he isn't actually consistently involved with any religious institution. "I haven't been to church in years. I usually go when I'm home, visiting my parents. It seems to make them happy. A friend of mine is a therapist who incorporates religion into her therapy—the idea of a spiritual being, no matter what religion it is. I feel the need to be *more* spiritual, and to access that part of my being, which has been dormant a long time. I would do better if I had it in my life more. I just have this darn skepticism . . . On the one hand, I want it and need it. On the other, I feel it's what weak, simple people rely on: *a crutch*." He sees religion as something for people who are needy or dependent, which he vehemently does not want to be.

In seeing himself as "not very religious," he further underscores how differing degrees of religiousness exist in wanting to believe or believe more, but finding it hard. He and many others wrestle with conflicts and ambivalence that they cannot wholly overcome, but that chaplains can help address.

Confidence in science and opposition to the rigidity, hypocrisy, and corruption of many churches can make it hard to believe more fully in a higher power, despite desires to do so. Daniel, a psychiatrist with a chronic disease, said that outsiders would probably describe him as spiritual, though he himself did not think of himself as such. He in fact wants more belief in his life. He follows rituals but feels he lacks "true faith," viewing himself, if anything, as "religious but not spiritual. I'm looking for a spiritual component, but I tend to be kind of an agnostic. I wish I weren't. It would be more comforting. But I have such a scientific bent, and organized religion and most people who believe it, with their crystals, are such a turn-off. It's difficult for me to open up to it. I'm trying to be open to that. It seems like it's just a more successful way to live. But I don't know what to do about it."

Conflicted, Daniel feels that religion would help him but that his scientific rigor impedes his ability to believe. His negative views of other people's religiosity also taint his perceptions. In seeing himself as both "religious but not spiritual" and "kind of an agnostic," he underscores, too, how broad and complex people's definitions of these terms can be. People vary in not only whether they fit into each of the three B's (belonging, behavior, and belief) but also to what degrees.

Defining labels in one's own way

Pastoral care faces challenges because patients define, in their own ways, categories of religious and spiritual beliefs and may say they are "not religious" or "atheist" but nonetheless have practices and beliefs that observers might view otherwise. Patients' own definitions of these terms, as well as of "belief," "agnosticism," and "none of the above" point to underlying complexities. Individuals may reject the full tenets of any one stance, and in effect construct their own. Jeremy, a tall WASPy blond-haired California HIV-positive doctor, illustrates the diversity of patients' individual conceptions, saying, for instance, that he is "agnostic" about the existence of God as a Divine Being, but feels he is "doing God's work," pursuing broad humanistic and humanitarian values, as a physician. "I think of myself as a very religious person, *inwardly*, deeply," Jeremy explained. "But my religion is around philosophical, mathematical, and scientific concepts. I am religious in the deepest sense of the term: *I care about people!* I will fight for principles . . . sacrifice my own issues, my own needs, to get issues dealt with. But I don't go to any church."

He developed these views on his own, not from his family. "I was raised Presbyterian and was fairly active in my church—not because of the religious nature of it, but because the church had a pipe organ I could use," he continued, illustrating how a church can serve a variety of functions from which people can then choose.

"As an organist, I played in different kinds of churches, and got to see Catholics and Jews. My eyes opened." Though smart and well educated, he had known little about faiths other than his own. Most people are exposed only to their own tradition, and each faith claims that it uniquely possesses the truth.

"I think *I do God's work in my job*. But I don't see God as an anthropological being. I don't think it's God's work to put down gay people, for instance.

"In learning about religion," he continued, "I've tried to sort out the abiding *principles*—what to look at more closely, and what to totally dismiss. That's how I approach religion: *I'm doing God's work*, identifying principles that make humanistic sense and can be applied, pushing systems for the better. Being scientific and mathematical and being religious are not antithetical. Math is very clean. Mathematical principles apply in virtually every circumstance where they are tested. They are the most abiding principles. Chemistry is a very clean science. Physics is a very predictive science."

He searches for similar principles and behaviors. " 'Do unto others as you would have them do unto you' is a very clean principle—not as clean as 'One plus one equals two,' but simple. If everyone did it, we would live in a much better place. To me, they're all just another set of principles or tools to use to make the world better."

He thinks that many people interpret the orderliness of some things "to mean that some creative intelligence must have been involved. But the universe is *unfathomable*. I don't know that one has to conclude that an intelligent creature put these laws into practice. I'm willing just to say that part of it is unknown to me." Order in and of itself can fuel awe and respect, even in the absence of a divine creator per se. He occasionally spars with opponents, but concludes that we simply cannot know the ways of the cosmos. "I know how to use some of these principles, but just have to speculate about where they come from. I don't mind talking about it, but others are not going to convince me they have the answer."

For him and many others, science and medicine *embody but do not replace* the notion of an underlying order in the universe, answering some questions but not others. Helping humanity by advancing public health also gives him and other physicians a sense of purpose. As a researcher, he practices and values science, which for him includes acknowledging and embracing the mysteries that persist.

Jeremy constructs his own beliefs and might not score very high on surveys seeking to quantify spirituality. The fact that he and others may not feel themselves to be spiritual per se, but nevertheless engage in activities and hold beliefs that outsiders would probably see otherwise, underscores the difficulty of defining these concepts. He thus further illustrates the complexities of three B's suggested by sociologists.[21] Individuals may perhaps fit in a category in ways that they may not see themselves as doing. Torn between agnosticism, religiosity, and spirituality, innumerable people remain unsure. Self-reports depend on what definition, standards, and thresholds a person uses. Chaplains must work across all these perspectives.

Are people who are "just spiritual" missing anything?: Criticism of spirituality without religion

Theologians frequently chastise individuals who are "spiritual but not religious" as superficial or lacking key benefits that religion provides, but chaplains tend to defend such individuals. For instance, In her book *Choosing Our Religion: The Spiritual Lives of America's Nones*, Elizabeth Drescher, a Christian theologian, writes, "Noneness, by definition, does not connect one to any common philosophical, theological, spiritual, or ethical system that defines life purpose and shapes the formation of their children."[22] She sees

Nones as "worrisome" because they "seem to identify no specific, practical obligation" toward others who are "part of a spiritual community."[23]

But patients illustrate how Nones have wide-ranging beliefs and should not be collapsed into one of a few boxes (such as Protestant, Catholic, Jewish, other, or "none of the above").

Attacks on religiously-unaffiliated individuals can be surprisingly vehement. "People who are spiritual but not religious are fundamentally selfish!" a prominent Jewish theologian I know insists. "*They don't want to come and set up the chairs for others at temple or church!* There's no community. They think it's just about them and God. No one else! But you can't have meaningful beliefs without being part of a community. And there is no moral guidance. No specific moral precepts. No sense of caring about others or social justice. All these people who say they are 'spiritual but not religious' are kidding themselves. It's just their ego. Narcissism!"

"But," I replied, "many people who feel spiritual but not religious are in fact members of like-minded communities and groups. They engage with communities that share values and beliefs today, for example through Facebook."

"They just don't like someone telling them what to think or do. Religions embody important wisdom through the ages. For centuries, people have carefully thought about the issues."

"But these people *do* draw on philosophy and religion. They *have* beliefs. They see God in Nature, for instance."

"That's paganism!"

"But Spinoza saw God in Nature."

"Spinoza, was a pagan!"

"So, then, was Georgia O'Keeffe!" I replied. "A lot of people are."

"Belief needs a *practice*!" she said, ignoring my point.

"But sometimes they have practices—they pray and meditate! And they feel comforted by their spiritual beliefs," I argued. She brushed away my arguments in the air with the side of her hand. Her fervor astonished me.

Mandatory attendance at organized services at specific times of the week is not essential to leading a full and satisfying life. Yet the extent to which well-meaning people feel free to attack others' beliefs amazes me. Not everyone in a church folds chairs. Not all spiritual-only individuals are selfish, just as not all religious people are necessarily always altruistic.

Many patients have also felt spurned by religious institutions. Patients who have engaged in activities condemned by churches, such as homosexuality, drug use, contraception, abortion, or divorce, tend to be especially wary of religious institutions. "Churches didn't work for me," Yvette Bing, an HIV-infected African American woman in her 30s, told me. "The Catholic faith doesn't like condoms. The Church will help you die but won't help you stay alive. I couldn't understand that. The Episcopalians and Baptists don't like people who use drugs or have been in prison. They claim to love God, but they don't love *you*. The Muslim faith gives a Black person dignity. But if God made all people equal, why must the women sit behind the men?" She illustrates how individuals reason through the pros and cons of various faiths.

"Right now, I'm just a person who believes in something mightier than man," Yvette continued. She, too, has had beliefs seemingly despite herself. "I've always believed in a higher power. At the age of five, I remember knowing inside of me, without ever hearing it, that something made the trees and put the sun up there. I've had numerous spiritual awakenings throughout my life. I didn't know what they were, but they happened. I've prayed and felt that something put my body in a praying position. I believe there is a Supreme Being. If there weren't, I wouldn't still be here." Though rejected by churches, she and many others nonetheless still feel firmly connected to God, though grappling with certain religious institutions' hostility to certain behaviors.

Overall, chaplains feel that nonreligious individuals are not necessarily lacking meaningful social bonds or anything else. "If they are missing a community, that's bad," said Brian Post, the chaplaincy department administrator. "But I wouldn't assume that just because they are Nones, they *are* missing a community. Community can happen in your neighborhood bar, a 12-step program, or a pottery class. Having a community, a network of mature and healthy relationships, is an important part of spiritual health for any of us."

Though criticized by many religious leaders, patients who feel "spiritual but not religious" have valuable perspectives and experiences that aid them. "For those who are religious," Jack Stone observed, "a church, temple, or mosque provides a place to all come together and share a sense of love, compassion, companionship, and connection with others in a *formal* way. Yet, people can get that out of a Harry Potter meet-up group, a narrative writing group, a musical, art, dance, opera, quilting, humanities, or drinking group, or group therapy. Anywhere human beings bond together with a certain particular purpose can be healing, beneficial, and spiritual. It doesn't have to be, but it can be.

"Especially now, with COVID-19, relationships have broken down," Jack continued, "and we've had to find other ways to connect with each other. I don't think of it as missing or lacking. What are we talking about in that Harry Potter meet-up group? Love, good over evil, being human, the complexities of life. Anything that is going to be a mirror or bond to share, investigate, or explore together can be spiritual. People just don't define it in that way, though."

Some spiritual-but-not-religious patients may encounter added obstacles, yet criticism about them is largely moot because religious beliefs can hardly be imposed on people. "People who need a structure may look down at others who are 'spiritual but not religious,'" explained Jason Cooper, a Connecticut psychiatrist who asks his patients about their religious and spiritual beliefs to probe for possible sources of resilience. "Spirituality without religion can be sustaining, but less so. Nonetheless, you can't *make* people believe. People who feel 'spiritual but not religious' are not missing something, but it's easier to live if you believe. And the more organized or child-like your beliefs, the easier life is. It's just harder otherwise. Belief in a higher power isn't always as sustaining as a belief in Jesus, or Buddha, or Whomever."

Ultimately, spiritual-only patients tend to face similar core existential and spiritual questions to other patients. "We shouldn't treat them particularly different from any others," said William Gibson, the Vermont humanist chaplain. "They are not, in general, harder or easier to care for. Some chaplains sense that such patients are more atomistic and individualistic and don't have as much community. But they usually *do* have a community. They wouldn't say they have a 'spiritual or religious' community, but they get together with people and often feel part of a tradition—pulling from whatever indigenous spirituality or actual community. I basically assess them the same—to know what their spirituality's like, how it relates to what they're going through, and whether we can draw on that. I wouldn't presume any particular kind of themes or particular existential questions."

Chaplains, too, may themselves no longer attend or be affiliated with any organized religious institution. Connie Clark didn't think "people miss anything by not going to a church. I'm an ordained minister, but *I* don't now go to church. I consider myself more spiritual than religious. Every day, I meditate and pray. The yoga mat to me is a very sacred place. It's important to be able to tap into a sense of spirituality, and have an understanding of how the world works. But people have been *cobbling things together for themselves* for quite some time."

She, too, felt that Nones do not experience more difficulty than others. "Everybody has some kind of spiritual belief; even those who claim to have no spiritual or religious belief still believe in love, in goodness. A rose by any other name is still a rose."

In his research, the sociologist Robert Bellah[24] found one woman who made up her own religion. I found that many people, such as Connie, do so, in varying ways. These searches can constitute ongoing journeys.

In sum, whether inspired by science, nature, or religious traditions, numerous patients and families who are spiritual but not religious now confront harsh threats of death. Pastoral care helps them, heightening their appreciation and feelings of being part of the larger cosmos, and providing a sense of meaning, hope, and connection to something beyond them—however they define it.

7

"The thousand kinds of atheism"

Assisting atheist, agnostic, and uncertain patients

Before my mother died at the age of 92, she looked at me hard in the eye and said, "When you're dead, you're dead." I was stunned. Throughout her life, she had attended synagogue at least several times a year. Strongly dedicated to making the world a better place, she had regularly staffed a small gray metal folding table outside Zabar's on Manhattan's Upper West Side, even in the cold, collecting signatures for liberal Democratic candidates and political causes. She tried to see her children and grandchild weekly. In her small apartment, she devoted years to growing scores of potted avocado, lemon, and flowering tomato and green pepper plants. She believed in the inherent beauty and specialness of human beings, plants, animals, and our planet, but not that anything transcendent exists. She affirmed Reformed Judaism's tenet that "the deceased still live on through the good deeds they have done, and in the hearts of those who cherished them." Yet that was all.

She bravely faced her death. Two hours before she died, she called me to say that she loved me and goodbye. Yet only a month before had she told me her existential beliefs about the absolute definitude of death. I will never forget how matter of fact she was, and how little, I realized, we may know about others' views—even those to whom we are close. Perhaps, though, only by confronting death do patients crystallize their ideas.

Chaplains assist patients who are not just religious or only spiritual, but also atheist or agnostic. Such patients commonly value core moral ideals or principles, and also seek meaning, purpose, and hope, even if not wanting to label these as "spiritual." "One staunch atheist," Jack Stone related, "put her hands up in front of her in a cross, saying, 'Get out! I don't want you. You are anathema to me! My religion is watching CNN. That is my religion—politics and knowledge.' So, I said, 'OK, that's fine,' and left."

Yet he and other chaplains tend to return to such patients another day, usually to the patient's surprise, and often ultimately establish vital connections. The next afternoon, Jack "came back just to try it out. I said, 'Hi, remember

Doctor, Will You Pray for Me?. Robert L. Klitzman, Oxford University Press. © Oxford University Press 2024.
DOI: 10.1093/oso/9780197750841.003.0007

me?' She said, 'Yeah . . .?' I said, 'I know your religion is CNN, but what do you think about what's going on now?' At that point, Fox was making fun of Obama's beige suit. People were up in arms, saying it was the wrong color for a president to wear. (Things have so turned now!) But that was the start of our conversation.

"I sat down, and she talked to me about her life and family, her vacation house, why she was an atheist, and what's bad about religion. It became a wonderful visit. Very few times do I hear 'Get out,' but there's usually a story to it. It just may be a defense about something; so, I just try again and see. I've got nothing to lose, except my pride."

Chaplains address such situations in varying ways, following their own internal scripts. Marvin Beck, the New Hampshire chaplain at a small community hospital, described how "one patient told me, 'Just go away. I don't believe. Don't even leave your little pamphlet.' I said, 'OK, that's fine. God bless you; have a nice day'—that's sincere, but a little jab. But I always go back to the patient. The next day, he said, 'I told you: No.' I said, 'I know. I'm only going to take 30 seconds of your time to thank you so much for not wasting my time. That was perfect! You didn't waste my time, and I didn't waste your time. And I've got to tell you: I wish more people would be upfront and honest with me. OK, I'll see you later.'" Marvin started to walk away. "Then, all of a sudden, the patient said, 'No, wait, deacon, hold on. Let me just . . .' If you don't fight with them, and go with the flow, most times that's what happens— they want to sit and chat. It might be a goodwill conversation, a goodwill meeting. Sometimes when I'm talking with patients, I'm not even sure what I'm talking about. They'll talk about anything. When I'm training chaplains, they want to know what 'the cookbook structure' is: OK, you say this first, then this second, this third and fourth. I don't know. I like to speak with them in metaphors. This guy talked about our baseball team, and how they messed up." So Marvin discussed baseball with him.

Humans evolved with impulses to seek purpose, meaning, hope, and connection. Historically, we received these beliefs from our communities, through norms and religion. We evolved to want a sense of purpose: often to make our community or world better. Evolutionarily, this impulse has perpetuated our own and our relatives' or group's genes. Those bands of people with genes for cooperation have been stronger, all else being equal, and survived better than other groups that lacked these genes. We therefore carry these traits, among others.

Today, atheists and agnostics are rapidly rising in number, but clearly vary considerably in their views. Generally, though, they believe in firm moral principles and ideals. For instance, as one friend, a scientist, self-professed atheist, and "defunct Catholic," explained, "I have a strong moral core. My family were strong Catholics. But I see religion now as all just made-up stories, and people in churches worshipping the bones of saints."

"Do you believe in anything beyond the mere physical world?"

"No."

"Do you think science now explains everything or will at some point?" I asked.

"No—not for a long time, and maybe it never will."

"So, do we just live in a dog-eat-dog world?"

"No. I have high principles. I think we should work to save the planet, for instance."

"Why?"

"Because it's a wonderful thing. It supports life. It has been good to us, so should be good to others."

Such ideals give him a strong sense of moral guidance.

"*There are thousands of varieties of atheism!*" William Gibson, the Vermont humanist, added. Indeed, the term "atheism," like "Nones," defines people by what they are *not*. "Some atheists are more philosophical or thoughtful," he explained. "Others draw on sources of meaning that aren't about God per se, but music, poetry, or baseball—secular sources of community, meaning, and purpose." After illness, many atheists also question their beliefs. Chaplains have developed open-ended ways of assisting such patients. William attempts to translate what he learned in seminary "for patients on the 'atheism spectrum.' I try to distill the basic components of spirituality and religion and put them together in ways that make sense to patients who say they are atheists.

"Atheists are not part of a church community," he continued, "but I ask them, 'What group of people do you draw strength from?' You may not literally congregate with them, but you are just a part of this wider community—your sense of belonging. It could be online or about *Star Wars*. And I explore: What is a person's moral core? What would someone *die* for? I look for what helps—what's their version of mindfulness, being present and honest about their experience, what would they *pray* for?

"Very few people," William continued, "have nothing that they would die for, or find more important than their own superficial, material well-being. The poet William Stafford said, 'Everyone is a conscientious objector to something.' I promote these themes with my patients, even though we don't talk about 'prayer,' 'baptism,' or 'death.'"

Individuals who wholly lack belief in a "higher power"—to use a term employed by Alcoholics Anonymous—however they may define it, may encounter difficulties. "Nobody is deep in their bones an atheist," Jason Cooper, the psychiatrist, observed. "Culturally I'm Jewish, but religion is not relevant for me. Yet, I'm not atheist. A lot of people are like that. They just don't feel that's part of where they are.

"It's always nice to have an explanation for the meaning of existence," Jason explained. "Nonbelievers have a hard time with that. Some people find that spirituality gives them sustenance. It's just harder if you don't believe, which doesn't necessarily mean you're an atheist. Still, you can't make people believe."

Religious institutions have in fact hurt not only people who are "spiritual, but not religious," but also atheists and agnostics, whom chaplains therefore seek to understand and assist as well. "Some patients say they are atheists or agnostics because they have been abused in the name of God," Victor Simmons, the VA chaplain, said. "If they list 'atheist' or 'agnostic' as their religious preference, I visit them *first*, before other patients. *Nobody's born that way. They get that way.* So, I'll say, 'Can you tell me, how did you come to that conclusion?' One patient said, 'You don't want to mess with me. I'll argue you under the table.' I said, 'I'm not interested in the argument, but the *story*. What happened?' His parents were very religious and very hypocritical. They used religion as a cover for their dysfunction and sexual abuse, and nobody knew what was going on. But *he* did. They would go to church, and everything was great, just hunky-dory: good marriage, good family. Then, they'd come home, and the father would beat the hell out of him. My patient thought, 'I'll never be part of *that*, if *that's* the only use for God.' A lot of vets say, 'I've been to war. If that's what is going on, and God knows about it and doesn't do anything: No thanks.' This patient was struggling spiritually. He would call himself an agnostic, but thought, 'I wish God was what people said He was. I really do. But I can't separate God from my dad.' Atheists say, 'I've decided there is no God.' That's extreme. But agnostics are saying, 'I can't know.' That's almost a desperation."

Agnosticism

While atheists take a definitive, absolute view, agnostics remain unsure. Given our lack of definitive knowledge about whether God exists or not, agnosticism arguably follows most logically from the lack of available facts either way.

Various personal experiences have led me to appreciate this stance far more. I had always dreamt of visiting Egypt and the wonders of its ancient civilization—a birthplace of Western culture—and once voyaged there. After arriving in Cairo, I headed to the Great Pyramid at Giza, the grandest Egyptian monument, one of the only surviving original Great Wonders of the World, and the oldest, built around 2,600 BCE. More time had elapsed between the building of this magnificent structure and the birth of Jesus than between Jesus' birth and today.

Before boarding a bus there, I bought a bottle of water and a loaf of bread, and stuffed them into my knapsack in case I got hungry or thirsty. Slowly, the bus trundled across the bridge over the Nile. On the horizon, the pyramids shimmered in the desert heat like a mirage. By the time I arrived, it was probably late afternoon, but I didn't notice, too excited about finally being there.

I climbed up a small rickety stairway to a small door, once hidden, on the pyramid's side, and descended the long dark stairway, following an occasional bare lightbulb. Dazzling, painted walls and ceilings surrounded me. Images of bright blue birds with yellow wings appeared new, but had been preserved for thousands of years.

I descended further down the stairs. Near the bottom, I followed a narrow walkway past the ancient stones, and turned right, then left, then right. Finally, I arrived at the end—the burial chamber.

Here, deep inside the bottom of the pyramid, the Pharaoh had been interred around 4,600 years earlier. A bare yellow bulb dimly lit the tiny chamber. Paintings of hieroglyphics, white-robed servants, and gods with heads of jackals and birds surrounded me on pale yellow walls. In the small silent room, I was alone, transported into an ancient world.

Suddenly, a sharp thought pierced my mind. A voice in my head said, "If the lights go out, don't panic. You will be OK. You have a bottle of water and bread, and I can climb my way back out."

Then, just as suddenly, the lights went out.

I have never been in such utter darkness. But, somehow, because of the voice, I didn't panic. I started to grope and crawl my way out on my hands and knees. I had no flashlight. Smartphones did not yet exist. In the pitch darkness, I inched forward on my bare hands and knees, one cold rough ancient stone at a time, unsure how long it would take to get out. But because of the voice, I remained calm and unafraid. Otherwise, I would have freaked out, terrified. Finally, several hours later, I reached a small metal door. Would it be locked? I pushed. It opened, groaning on old creaky hinges.

The desert sunlight glared.

An Arab man in a white turban and long flowing robes squatted near the bottom of the external metal stairs and looked surprised. He spoke to me in Arabic, pointing to his watch and then raised his hand in the air, palms up, gesturing. I sensed he was saying that he didn't know anyone was still down there, and had assumed everyone had already left.

This experience still bewilders me. It was not a profound transcendent "religious experience," as if accompanied by soaring music. The voice seemed more matter of fact, isolated—out of nowhere. The blackout and the voice may have been mere coincidences. But the words had been very specific and distinct, and saved me from panic. It was uncanny.

I have had several other such experiences. They come out of the blue—I can never will them. They are not always about major events, sometimes just relatively minor occurrences.

Once, walking in Central Park, I heard a voice saying, "Sit on this rock!" It was very odd, but I sat down. A few minutes later, my sister, whom I hadn't seen in a few months, walked by with her new husband. They were going to the Boathouse Café to celebrate their one-year anniversary. I ended up joining them, which thrilled them.

In early 2001, I had a dream that I was in an elevator at Boston's Logan Airport that suddenly stopped midway between floors. Dark, dangerous-looking foreigners pushed to enter. I felt horror. I had trouble breathing, and finally managed to escape outside. In the wind, papers and debris swirled. On the ground lay a newspaper—the *New York Post*. The front page bore a headline, "Pol Pot," and a picture of one of my younger sisters. I woke up shaken and disturbed by this nightmare.

As a psychiatrist, I had read Freud's *The Interpretation of Dreams*,[1] undergone psychoanalysis, and trained to probe dreams for unconscious meanings. For a few days, I wondered what this dream meant and why I had it. Why Logan Airport? Why the *New York Post*? Why my sister? Why "Pol Pot"? Was it something political? It seemed odd—very different from other dreams.

Six months later, on September 11, 2001, terrorists boarded planes in Logan Airport and murdered my sister. A few days after her death, her name and picture appeared in the *New York Post*. Pol Pot was, I realized, a mass murderer.

Perhaps these are mere coincidences, but they seemed to have an odd distinctness and force. I have had other such experiences—about a dozen in all. They may certainly, of course, all be merely random, chance events, but I confess that I am not 100% sure.

I had never thought about the implications of these experiences very seriously, and have never written about these or mentioned them to more than a handful of people. I fear they may be seen as loony or worse. But they were my experiences—I am not making them up. Patients and others have told me of similar and other types of spiritual and metaphysical experiences and views.

The eighteenth-century Scottish philosopher David Hume argued that we lack evidence both for and against God. Wary of both positions, he insisted instead that it is necessary to maintain a skeptical but open mind. He believed in the existence of a God but was highly dubious about religious institutions, perceiving the benefits of spirituality to humans but also criticizing pure atheists. Hume believed in "Reasoning & Enquiry." As he wrote, "The worst speculative Sceptic I ever knew was a much better Man than the best superstitious Devotee & Bigot."[2] Yet he warned elsewhere, "[T]ake care; push not matters too far: allow not your zeal against false religion to undermine your veneration for the true.[3] . . . [M]en, when afflicted, find consolation in religion."[3] To me, this seems sensible.

Recently, I met Kip Thorne, the 2017 Nobel laureate in Physics, and asked him questions that have long perplexed me.

"What happened before the Big Bang?"

"We don't know," he said simply, unembarrassed by our ignorance.

"How does gravity work?"

"We don't know."

"What does dark matter do?"

"We don't know."

"What makes 'spooky forces at a distance' or 'entanglement' work?" (In these phenomena, particles separated by thousands of light years can nonetheless be "entangled," affecting each other simultaneously, as if somehow still connected.[4])

"We don't know." He didn't feel able to speculate—or the need to know. He seemed to embody Hume's skepticism.

I am therefore relatively agnostic about these experiences in Egypt and elsewhere, open to the possibility that something more exists, or at least that physical phenomena exist that we can hardly imagine and certainly not explain. Yet, that position is not easy to maintain. Physics may one day explain such phenomena, but cannot yet do so. No one can now definitely answer these quandaries.

Nevertheless, I feel fortunate and grateful for these incidents, since they have led me to appreciate how much we may not know about possible metaphysical phenomena, making me skeptical of the hubris of thinking that we understand or can readily comprehend everything and should hence immediately dismiss as nonsense patients' spiritual and religious notions, as numerous doctors and critics do. I remain wary of definitive "truths" in these realms, open to what we cannot fathom, and appreciate the mysteries and beauties of the universe and nature that we can't explain.

If you have not had such experiences, your logical conclusion would be to see them as ludicrous and to reject them. If I hadn't had these experiences, I would be far more leery. Nothing outside of these experiences supports the possibility of these beliefs having any grounding in experience.

Still, I make few claims for these uncanny experiences.

Every few blocks in New York City, palm readers and "psychics" fill storefronts, presuming to foresee the future. Once, after 9/11, I visited a psychic who said she could communicate with the dead. I was dubious, but went. She spoke to me for an hour. "I see you," she said, "going to Cap Ferrat," where I was about to visit on a vacation. But the rest of what she said had no connection to my life before or since. She said, "Your next book," she said, "will be about flowers." I left, unpersuaded.

But I concluded that it is vital at least to be open to other people's beliefs, and not just immediately denigrate them as pure rubbish. Maybe they *are* rubbish. But, I would argue, we cannot know for sure. Rather, a provider should consider seriously the significance *to patients* of their spiritual and religious beliefs.

A lot of nonsense is uttered about religion and spirituality. By no means do I support it all. I am skeptical of much that is said, but am open to the possibility that *something* may exist more than mere strict materialism as we understand it today.

For me, the Jewish tradition remains important, and I draw on it to a certain extent. I don't believe in literal interpretations of the Bible—Noah's Ark, Moses parting the Red Sea, or the burning bush. Historical evidence does not support that Noah's flood occurred as described in the Bible or even that the Jews wandered for 40 years in the desert. I am wary of various practices, such as women in Orthodox temples still having to sit in the back or balcony and shave their heads and wear wigs after marriage. I don't observe many Jewish holidays, but respect centuries of rabbis who pondered the Old Testament and the Talmud, and I sense that something incarnate may exist and go on. I see this notion, though, as consistent with, rather than inimical to, core Jewish beliefs, as well as with Christianity, Islam, Buddhism, and other faiths.

Atheism versus agnosticism

While many people, including scholars, sharply divide atheists from agnostics, individuals who describe themselves using these terms do so in varying ways. In people's lived lives, these categories blur. A person might disbelieve in a single intelligent being (and hence be "atheistic") but nonetheless be unsure about the existence of some kind of unfathomable forces beyond us (and thus be "agnostic"). Even scholars use these terms in widely different ways, too, ultimately limiting these words' utility. In certain respects, these terms are akin to words such as "good," "bad," "beauty," "virtue," "evil," "ugly," or "love"—employed in varying and frequently inconsistent manners.

Individuals commonly invoke these terms partly as ways of repudiating other people's beliefs. "I'm a devout atheist," a German friend recently told me.

"So, you believe that there is nothing out there?" I asked him. "That when you die, that's it?"

"Well, I'm really agnostic, but like to be contrarian and say, 'I'm an atheist.' I come from southern Germany where many bad things were done in the name of Catholicism. I like to let my family know that I reject all that. But certain events have happened in my life—bad things occur and then, out of the blue, something amazing happens. So, I think that there is *something* more, but I don't know what it is."

Other atheists at times adopt religious terms or practices, *even if unthinkingly.* "I am not religious or spiritual. I'm a rationalist," a lawyer who had breast cancer, along with her sisters, told me. "I would never ask '*Why me?*' I might, though, say it and *fall on my knees and pray to the God I don't believe in*, just because that's a natural reaction." She distinguishes between her emotional and cognitive reactions. Such prayers soothed her.

Others describe themselves as "atheist" but hold free-floating metaphysical beliefs about cosmic nature. "I'm an atheist but believe that *what goes around comes around*," a young medical school professor recently told me. "Over the years, I've helped many students, and feel that those acts will come back to me—that people will therefore help *me* in *my* career." He senses that his faith in cosmic justice contradicts his atheism, but he is unsure how to reconcile this conflict. Nor does he, however, feel the need to do so. Many people hold apparently clashing ideas, but little heed the tension until others point it out—and then, still, commonly don't feel particularly obligated to integrate the seeming inconsistencies.

Individuals vary in how much they tolerate the inherent murkiness of agnosticism, and prefer atheism as a more definitive answer. Other self-described atheists periodically question and have doubts about their beliefs. "I've always been an atheist," a humanities professor recently told me. "Maybe I wasn't for 30 minutes as a kid. I've only once been in a church for a service that wasn't a wedding, funeral, or concert. I wasn't raised with any religion. My mother was a psychiatrist. No psychiatrists are religious.

"But," he said, tilting his head and glancing off, perplexed, to one side, "then I think about the Big Bang! At one point, all was darkness. Then, BOOM!! 'Let there be light.'" He spread his arms out as wide, as far as they stretched. "And there was light. That's a lot to think about. It makes you wonder."

"What do you think about that?" I asked him.

"I say I am atheist, because I don't accept things just on faith, but I realize how much I *do*, in fact, accept just on faith, without evidence. I believe in hope and the value of love. Jesus preached, 'Love your enemy' and 'Turn the other cheek.' Does that work empirically? We don't know. There is a lack of clear empirical support either way."

Empirical evidence suggests, however, that love is beneficial, impelling people to enter and stay in relationships, which help them fare better than those who don't.

He and others observe, too, how the zeitgeist is shifting, leading them to reconsider their own beliefs. "Religion is coming back," this professor continued. "In the late Sixties, when I went to college, most people were atheists, or at least agnostics. But today, most of my students are Buddhists, into mindfulness, meditation, or yoga. It helps them. They think there is something greater than them.

"I suppose maybe I *am* an agnostic. But then . . ."—he shook his head back and forth to himself, and shifted in his chair as if cramped—"that feels uncomfortable and not right, so I feel I'm an atheist." He glanced around, as if looking for further justification for his conclusion. "Ultimately, religion becomes about power," he continued. "Even Buddhists tell me, 'My teacher says *he* is the teacher, and *I* am just a student.' I see how much killing goes on in the name of religion." He is torn: an atheist intellectually, but emotionally somewhat agnostic.

Though many individuals, when asked on questionnaires about their religion, check off "none," that single word fails to convey the rich breadth and variety of their feelings. This humanities professor and others are wary of the standard labels about beliefs ("religious," "atheist," or "agnostic") since these carry complex, loaded meanings in various people's minds.

These labels serve many functions but also cause confusion. Labeling theory argues that we create and reify certain terms as social constructs as forms of social control to categorize deviant behavior as stigmatized (e.g., in using terms such as "psychotic" or "whore").[5,6]

But in religion, labels may serve additional functions because of the lack of clear, shared definitions for these terms and perceived ambiguities. Countless people see themselves as neither "religious" nor "spiritual" but range in their self-views, grappling with these quandaries, often uncomfortable with labels. Chaplains have figured out ways of untangling such labels, identifying and tapping into individuals' underlying beliefs.

Atheists attacking others' views

Occasionally chaplains encounter atheists—such as the woman who said her religion was CNN—who attack all religion as delusion and dogma, reflecting the deep polarization from both sides in contemporary political, social, and religious debates. Since beliefs are private and lack any clear objective evidence for or against them, tolerance of each other's conclusions should prevail. Yet strikingly, many atheists, like religious diehards, fiercely berate others' views. As a psychiatrist colleague from Washington, DC, recently told me over dinner with his wife, "Religion is all nonsense! *None* of it is true! Scientifically, there is no evidence for it. When we die, we're just atoms!"

"But 96% of all matter is invisible 'dark matter' that we don't comprehend," I replied.

"But we *know* what it is: It's dark matter!" he retorted, as if that, in itself, explained it. "Human intelligence and science can explain everything!" Chemicals alone, he believed, account for all of human experience, or will do soon.

I cocked my head sideways, wondering how to respond. "Don't you believe that?" he suddenly asked, wondering if I were in fact sane.

"Maybe we *will* one day be able to explain all the mysteries of the universe," I replied. "But it could take hundreds or thousands of years. Our species may not even survive that long. Until then, we understand as little about the universe as an ant does about the planet—only relatively tiny bits. So, why not say we just don't know?"

"Because we *do* know: It's all just atoms!"

I told him about my experience in the Egyptian pyramid.

"But think of all the thousands of other experiences you've had," he said. "Why focus on this one?"

"In part, because of Pascal's Wager," I continued. "It is better to believe and be wrong than not to believe."

"The problem with Pascal's Wager is that there are hundreds of different beliefs you could have. It doesn't tell you which *one* belief to accept: Catholicism? Buddhism? Islam? They can't *all* be right. If one is right, then the others aren't."

"But they all share certain underlying tenets. These core principles can all be valid."

"But that's not what *they* say."

"That doesn't matter."

He sensed that we had reached an impasse. "I think, though," he said, backing down slightly, since we were, after all, at a casual, social occasion, "that my wife is agnostic." Interestingly, he wasn't fully certain of her beliefs.

"The choice," she explained, "is either you believe it all, or you don't believe it all."

"What about not being sure?" I replied. "Just not knowing?"

"Well, I guess . . .," she murmured, mostly out of politeness, unconvinced. "But the answer is either one or the other." Atheists, not only zealots, want definitive answers.

Yet, these friends' adult children have rejected their parents' atheism. "Our kids all center their lives around meditation," my friend confided a few minutes later. "One daughter lives in a Zen center. Our son is becoming an Orthodox Jew." As opposed to their parents' staunch atheism, they all felt needs for some form of greater meaning.

Generally, atheists aver that they are being scientific, citing a lack of evidence of God. Dawkins argues that the lack of clear evidence of God means that God doesn't exist. I once asked Dawkins about the fact that *the absence of evidence is not evidence of absence*. He blithely dismissed my concerns, undeterred. But evidence is absent either way. No randomized controlled trial shows that parachutes prevent death, because no placebo control group has ever been used. But, given the choice, no one without a parachute would ever leap from a plane. We commonly proceed in life without scientific proof.

Many atheists forcefully fight all religious and spiritual beliefs, due to the harms religions have perpetrated. Others cite scientific explanations of the universe. Those perceiving institutional harms could alternatively, as Hume suggests, accept the possibility of spirituality and reject religious institutions, but they frequently don't.

Atheists commonly argue that spiritual and religious beliefs are merely inventions from earlier, more tribal, less scientific eras. But larger forces of Nature outside of us certainly exist, and for innumerable people constitute a higher power.

Uncertainties and doubts

Still, uncertainties persist, and chaplains aid many patients who are unsure about beliefs, or previously held firm ideas, but now harbor doubts. "I don't really know *what* to believe," a South Asian physician raised in Hinduism told me, "somewhere between an actual God and an energy. It changes." She and countless others debate or fluctuate between forms of atheism and agnosticism.

"I am *undecided* whether things are predestined or not," she continued, delineating her reasoning: "Sometimes I think it's all just chaos. Other times I think we're given what we can deal with on purpose, and there are reasons." Her mother, aunt, and uncle had all died of metastatic breast cancer. Terrified, this physician has not yet had symptoms or undergone genetic testing for it, and wrestles with questions about her "fate." "With all the cancer in my family, I've always just sort of felt I'm going to get it. I almost became OK with that. My mother had it twice; it's been in my house four times now. I'm used to it.

"*I believe what I need to at the time.* In very difficult periods, I feel there *has* to be a bigger picture, and Someone actually looking out for me: that this is happening for a *reason*, and I'm going to learn a lesson from this, find inner strength. There's a purpose to all of this happening—there *has* to be. I can't just be randomly put through this for no reason. If you look at physics, we're all energy and just transform. We don't stop and start, but just change, become something else, some other form. So, there's *something*. Other times,

I think we just kind of stop being, but just can't accept that . . . When things are going OK, I think about it less, and don't have as strong a need to reach for something."

She and many others commonly look to science and its certainties or mysteries to support their beliefs. But, as she suggests, beliefs also shift, based on a person's altering needs over time. Patients often see themselves as wandering on ever-unfolding journeys, though much scholarship still views beliefs as fixed, unchanging entities.

Spiritual care providers assist patients, from very different religious traditions, who hesitate, stepping back and forth over bridges between beliefs and doubt. In part, science itself contains uncertainties and limitations, and can be seen as constituting a Rorschach test—as a glass either half-full or half-empty. Religion can be viewed as The Truth or as a psychological phenomenon, a set of social constraints, or a combination of these.

Many theologians argue that doubt constitutes an inherent part of faith. St. Augustine felt, "I doubt, therefore I am."[7] Yet, some people lack such self-questioning and humility, thinking that their views are *unequivocally correct* and that all others are simply wrong.

People without an established religious tradition often grapple to articulate larger sources of ultimate connection, but have difficulty doing so. A 65-year-old retired scientist and engineer with muscular dystrophy described these vagaries and tensions, which chaplains commonly help to address. "I don't know that I'm an atheist as much as an agnostic," he said. "I was in Protestant seminary for a year, but am not religious. I may be spiritual to some degree, but not in a particularly studied or organized way. I don't believe in fate, religions, or religiosity. Basically, I rely on a strong, well-thought-out *humanistic* base—a strong morality and belief system based in humanism." He highlights the fluidity and uncertainty about the personal definitions and boundaries of these terms.

Definitive answers provide psychological benefits, but not clear truth. "I tend to wrestle these things out with myself," he explained. "But assigning answers is more comfortable. For a lot of *big* questions, I just don't have answers. I sort of *live* with those. I see significant connections in nature and between people. They can be described molecularly, *but something else is there*. I don't know what, or who created it or how it evolved. Science gives some interesting clues—as valuable as anything I have—but there are 'things' that tie people together. I'm struggling to describe this." As a scientist with religious training, he accepts wrestling with these questions, not knowing the answers, and striving to tolerate the ambiguities. He admits, too, his difficulty even articulating these feelings, underscoring how these notions lie beyond words. This unfathomability bothers him, but he accepts it, since no clear evidence exists to persuade him otherwise. In the absence of evidence, patients commonly choose one of several conclusions—believing in God because of personal experience, taking Pascal's Wager, or remaining agnostic. Given that people frequently have trouble even verbalizing these vagaries, and waver in how well they tolerate such murkiness, chaplains can often help.

Nonbelief and depression

Patients who want to believe but find that doing so is difficult can be depressed. Belief in nothing can foster despair. Questions arise, though, of which came first: skepticism or gloom. Specifically, depression may impede confidence that something exists beyond oneself; and failure to believe in something larger can also fuel depression. Difficulty hoping or believing can be a symptom of depression. Many patients see the benefits of spirituality when facing illness, but nevertheless find belief hard and face existential despair, raising key questions of who is "touched by the light" or not, and why. The reasons appear manifold.

Questions of causality arise here. Depression and lack of religiosity can in fact exacerbate each other. Religiosity can protect against depression to a certain degree, but can also result from searches for solace and help in the face of disease.[8] Innumerable people feel emotionally connected to individuals in a church or other faith community, even if not knowing them well, because of a sense of shared values and belonging. As several of the patients here suggest, however, spirituality is not always fully voluntary, but rather can be partly unconscious. Despair and depression cannot be wholly untangled from lack of hope.

People have differing degrees of comfort or unease with religious quandaries. "I'm not even *prepared* to deal with the existence of God," an internist in her late 60s with leukemia told me. "I just put that aside," she laughed. "A few years ago, before I became ill, my husband died in a terrible automobile accident. I spent months crying myself to sleep every night. Even with all the wonderful support," his death "took enormous energy out of me."

She wanted to have faith in a higher entity but found it hard to achieve, and felt depressed. She thought that religion helps people "accept things that we can't rationally come to terms with," but she felt that religious institutions had historically abused these psychological needs. Still, she valued the existence of order and morality in the universe: "I guess that can be called 'God,' but it doesn't have to be." She remained unsure, fatalistic, and baffled by her predicament, continuing to work hard daily, though she was dying.

Her medical research was her "therapy" and provided the main source of meaning in her life. When hospitalized, she took her laptop and looked for articles about treatments for her particular disease, since her physician said he could not find any: "In the ICU, I did my literature search." Her doctors couldn't find any literature on her condition, but "it took me about five seconds." Even though cancer had spread through her body, she continued to work on her computer. Estranged from her family, she felt driven to succeed in her career and did not know "what else to do" with her life.

She contemplated these issues but remained uncertain. "Before my husband died and I got sick, I moved toward not knowing what I valued." Now, she reflected, "I have a need in that area, and am not coming to grips with how to do it."

She did not feel fully satisfied, or at peace with her decision to keep working. I admired her dedication, but sadly, several months after we spoke, she died. A psychotherapist or chaplain might have helped her make sense of these predicaments. As we will see, not all patients who might benefit from seeing a chaplain end up doing so.

PART III

"MEETING PATIENTS WHEREVER THEY ARE"

Helping patients regardless of their beliefs

8

"The most important moment in our lives"

Resetting priorities and appreciating the present

Now that I'm in my 60s, several friends my age are beginning to develop cancer, Parkinson's disease, and heart attacks, and in certain cases die, painfully reminding me of our mortality. Statistically, roughly two-thirds of my life is now probably gone—which sobers me. I have begun to think more about how I want to spend my remaining years, and how to make them as meaningful and satisfying as possible.

Regardless of our particular beliefs about the existence or nature of God, from evangelical to atheist, patients share certain mutual challenges, coping with aging, disease, pain, and threats of death, and therefore having to make tough medical decisions, and re-evaluate priorities and futures. Chaplains help patients and families with questions not only within each of the large categories above—being religious, spiritual, atheist, or agnostic—but also with dilemmas that cut across these broad classifications.

The threat of serious disease leads patients of varying beliefs to reassess their values and lives. While hospitalized individuals could potentially do so by themselves, chaplains often help by focusing on "the here and now." Frequently, when facing the imminent prospect of death, patients despair and benefit from exploring their feelings and fears, engaging in positive thinking, and finding or constructing meaning and purpose in their lives to overcome negative thoughts. "Thinking positively" may sound simple, but getting patients to do it can prove arduous. When patients ask, "Why me?" chaplains can assist by refocusing these quandaries. "People need help accepting that He or She is a little busy upstairs to pick you out individually for testing here," Jason Cooper, the Connecticut psychiatrist, said. "Shit happens. We could focus on why, but you can't make a better past. You've got to figure how to try *to live* with your cancer each day, as opposed to die with it."

Doctor, Will You Pray for Me?. Robert L. Klitzman, Oxford University Press. © Oxford University Press 2024.
DOI: 10.1093/oso/9780197750841.003.0008

Reassessing and revising priorities

A key component of re-envisioning a future is resetting priorities. We can't always foresee how we will react to serious disease. "We don't know how someone's going to process the reality of their dying," said Margaret Dixon, the Pennsylvania chaplain who was unsure whether to wear a collar after her ordination. "We may *think* we know, but we don't. Patients cut away the chaff. *Everything* cuts away. One patient said, 'I don't want to engage with anything that isn't to the bone. What do I care about? My son, my parents, friends, and being able to see another beautiful day.' *That* surfaces for everybody."

Disease prompts patients to re-evaluate and alter their values and goals and come to appreciate their lives far more. These transformations can, however, be complicated and occur only after perceived medical, social, or psychological defeats. While patients occasionally come to recalibrate their lives on their own, many others do so only with chaplains' input. Bruce, a 45-year-old physician, for instance, arrived at this point on his own, but only after multiple ordeals. He had planned to be a medical missionary, but instead, over several years, had become less religious. Unfortunately, as a doctor, he then acquired hepatitis C from a patient and became extremely sick, forcing him to reconsider and alter his views and behavior. "I'm stoical," he continued. "I said, 'OK, I've got hepatitis C. Big deal,' and really didn't think about it." But his viral load and liver enzymes then increased. He developed side effects to medications, including high fevers, shaking chills, nausea, vomiting, insomnia, anorexia, and weight loss.

"I became acting director of the department and was competing to become department director . . . wearing a lot of hats, taking on a lot of responsibility and working at least one overnight shift a week. Sometimes two. Some afternoons, I had difficulty concentrating, and fell asleep in my desk chair. So, the disease significantly impacted my performance. I wonder how I made it through."

He lost his bid to become director: "For all my work and effort I wasn't rewarded!" He was bitter, but spiritual and religious perspectives solaced him. In particular, he re-evaluated his life's larger meaning: "The illness actually brought me back to my prior religious training. I had become *less attentive*." Given the responsibilities of his many jobs, he had no longer "reserved special, quiet time for myself." But he now strove to do so.

His disease compelled him to "step back and say, '*I'm not going to kill myself for stuff that's basically temporary.*'" Faced with serious disease, he reviewed his values and priorities—what really is important, and what isn't. "I put my heart into work, but now, if I don't get it done, it's not going to get done. I'll do it tomorrow. I'll leave at five or six instead of eight."

Yet though he returned to his faith tradition, he did so *with a difference*. He is now "*religious in a sense*, but not pious. I'm spiritually oriented: I try to be quiet, and listen to myself." He and others now make their own such distinctions.

His condition also affected his medical practice and teaching. He now sees the need to pass his newly gained insights to the next generation. Now, for instance, he is more likely to check whether a trainee asks patients and families if they have any questions—"to make sure medical students and residents sit down and talk with pediatric patients' parents to really understand the parents' concerns. I've always done that, but am *more* attentive now. I ask my patients, 'Anything you don't understand?' . . . I'm more vigilant—talking about side effects and what to expect. I say, 'An hour before you get this, the nurse ought to be giving you a pill. Make sure you get it.'" He illustrates, too, how being more religious or spiritual can involve differences in *degrees*, not necessarily just *kinds* of commitments and activities.

But countless patients have difficulty realigning their values. Pastoral care thus commonly leads patients to these insights—to appreciate more fully the beauty of even small moments. Adam Quincy, for example, a Catholic North Carolina hospice chaplain who strove to avoid religious jargon, described a home hospice patient who "knew he was actively dying, and should be dead within six months." The patient asked him, "Why has God kept me alive? What for? I have no idea why I'm still alive. What benefit is there? I'm a burden to my kids. I'm not valuable. I don't contribute to society anymore."

Adam "picked up a piece of bread from the meal tray and said, 'Let's talk about bread for a moment. Bread is really amazing, isn't it? Just to enjoy the taste of a piece of bread! Christ is called the 'Bread of Life.' Maybe life is not meant to be lived according to external accomplishments, or measured based on the world's system of the monetary or other impact we have. What if it's OK just to enjoy the days you have?' That really knocked this patient backwards. He eventually said, 'I see I need to change my perspective. There are all kinds of wonderful things going on in the right here and now of my daily life that I'm missing because I'm not paying attention, because I'm so focused on thinking about the past.'

"The next time I visited, this patient's mood totally changed. He said, 'Hey, chaplain! How are you doing today? Let me tell you something I did . . .' He saw me as an enlightened person, *living* life instead of barely surviving it. That's what patients want—what resonates with them. He was more up-beat, positive, and a tad bit ashamed for having been dejected and forgetting that every day is a gift. A chaplain should use religion as a fulcrum to *move patients' perspectives*, to transition these into the transcendent instead of the imminent realm. I told him, 'Your story is something that I'm going to take with me to other people. They're going to be encouraged, strengthened, and motivated by it.'"

Patients facing serious disease mourn the loss of the future they had imagined, and must forge a new one. A chaplain or other provider can help them shift their goals and points of view—reframing, recreating, or reimagining a future. The psychological notion of "cognitive reframing" may suggest merely altering the outer edges of an idea, but clearly entails far more transformation, altering something deeper than merely the "frame," realigning one's very life.

In order to foster openness and trust, chaplains at times divulge their own experiences to patients. Adam, for example, described a 32-year-old woman who had "destroyed" her body with illegal drug use, and was resistant to talking to a chaplain, out of shame: "As a strategy, I shared events in my own life, to help her reframe her own. I said, 'I'm just a fellow struggler in this life, just like you. Let's talk. What's going on?' She said, 'There's no hope for me. I ruined my life with drugs. I'm probably not going to live a whole lot longer. The pain and sadness of that is terrible.'

"At that point, I empathized, and said, 'If I told you some of the disappointments in *my* life, we'd be here 10 or 12 hours. But let's talk about *hope* for a minute. None of us know what's going to happen next. But we need hope. What does hope mean to you?'"

A variety of approaches can, therefore, potentially inspire patients to appreciate the present far more. Adam aids patients, too, by encouraging them to segue from negative to other, more positive thoughts. "I tried moving her away from the idea that things are terrible, to the idea that life is actually a wonderful gift—that every day is a wonderful gift, and that you can find meaning, purpose, and significance in that. The only thing any of us ever really have is this very moment in our lives. Regardless of what we've done in the past, *this moment is the most important one in our lives.*"

He and other chaplains try to guide patients away from past self-reproaches, toward future aspirations. "Then I can start down the road of processing the guilt," Adam continued, "and say, 'We get into drugs for lots of reasons. Tell me *your* story. How did *you* get into this?' Once I build hope in her, I can talk about why she's feeling guilty, and about the importance of her life, regardless of her past."

A chaplain can thus assist patients by tapping into the specific details of their lives to rethink their perspectives on their lives. With this woman, for instance, Adam commended her honesty and courage, further helping her shift her focus: "I highlighted her humility of being willing to say, 'I wasted my life.' I said, 'Many people with drug problems have huge denial and narcissism. I appreciate your ability to be that self-aware, humble, self-reflective, and respectful even of life itself.' Even though such patients are deeply unhappy about their lives, these words make them feel *validated* and good, and move the conversation from how the world measures success, into a different context—of appreciation of the value of life. You can transform a patient's mood."

Adam and his colleagues hence strive to remind patients that the ultimate purpose of life may not be to achieve particular indices of "success," but rather simply to enjoy it. He emphasizes that "maybe there doesn't have to be purpose like accomplishing a financial or vocational goal. What if it's just to enjoy the beauty of life—a slice of bread, or the sunshine. What if that's really the ultimate purpose—to enjoy and be at peace with God's creation? *That* changes patients' perspectives. They stop thinking about how the world is set up, and start to hear the wonder of just being alive. That perspective reenergizes them and reinstitutes hope." Intellectually, we may know the importance of focusing on the present, but periodically we need to be reminded, especially when facing crises.

With such patients, chaplains and other providers must determine how best to foster hope, while remaining realistic and not denying the reality that death may hover closely. When confronting the prospect of their annihilation, patients commonly now select to spend more time with family and friends than with their career, and may not return to their prior religion per se, but increase their appreciation for life and nature more generally, reprioritizing their values and goals. "I've been more reflective," said Peter Haines, an HIV-positive medical student, "and learned to appreciate things—the ocean, the sky—to take time for people. Not just important people, but anybody. It's made me a lot more happy." It is striking that more people don't experience this before becoming sick.

Doctors and nurses can discuss these issues with patients as well, but generally have far less time and inclination to do so. Nonetheless, doing so need not take much time. "I've been a mean son of a bitch my whole life," an old grizzly patient I once treated for heart disease confessed to me late one night in the hospital. He was dying and depressed. "I left my wife and kids when they were young. They haven't talked to me in 10 years. I fucked up." He said he believed in nothing.

"Is there *anything* you believe in that helps you in any way?" He shook his head no.

"Anything you're looking forward to?"

"No."

I was surprised. "Nothing?"

He shrugged. "Well, I guess I could try to see my kids," he said.

"Why not try calling them?" I suggested. He eventually did, and felt glad.

Chaplains help countless patients in part by first seeking to understand how these individuals got to a point of existential pain and/or despair. "I've not met too many people who say, 'Nothing matters to me, and nothing ever has,'" William Gibson said. "At some point in their life, most people have felt some sense of spiritual crisis. I try to figure out what was meaningful to them and what changed. If you just help someone normalize their struggle, and give them options, they'll do the transformation on their own—when they're ready. A lot of people have felt, deep down, 'God has forsaken me.' There's usually a story to that. I don't feel stymied by that response. I just feel their pain. I have that in my own life, though I guess I've been fortunate: I haven't had that a lot lately."

Re-envisioning a future can be especially crucial for patients with chronic pain, who need to significantly alter their sense of their life going forward. Even if not explicitly tied to religious doctrine, guilt and remorse can exacerbate spiritual suffering and, in turn, chronic physical pain and distress. Kristine Baker, the Texas chaplain who draws on metaphors, including ballroom dancing, mentioned that long-term unrelenting chronic pain "is one of the hardest things I have ever had to work with, especially if patients blame themselves for it. One woman drove off the road, drunk, and killed her two children. She had disability from the accident and had chronic pain, and a sense of being unredeemable. I just sit and am witness to that kind of suffering. I ask, 'How long do you think you're going to need to punish yourself for this act? Will you ever not do so? Is there really such a thing as an *unforgivable sin*?"

These strains aggravate the emotional, physical and spiritual suffering that chaplains can help patients re-evaluate and thus cope with better. "More than anything, I am constantly reframing," Kristine continued. "Emotions amplify pain. Patients have pain and feel they're never going to get over it or work again. I say, 'Yes, you will have pain, debilitating at times. You may *always* have that pain. But people can live with that and still have meaningful lives. You have to make a decision *to be the type of person who makes it through this.*'

"One patient fell off his roof and has been in chronic physical pain ever since," she added. "He was angry when he went up there, and now thought he would never have joy in his life again. I worried he would either commit suicide or internalize an identity as a victim. I realized that *he had to grieve for the future he had constructed for himself*—that he would be doing various things. He had to talk though the loss of his future self. We create not only our *past* stories but our *future* ones. I asked him, 'What brings you joy? What did you do for fun as a child?' I helped him re-find a passion he had as a child—woodworking. A lot of people had a hobby as a child that they now don't pursue—because it doesn't make money.

"Most people, even those with quadriplegia," she continued, "come back to baseline if they can get through the first six months. But in those six months, some people kill themselves. Eventually, this patient found a life trajectory that contained some joy.

"I try to help patients dismantle and undo negative predictions about the future. I say, 'You are not God. You do not know the future. No one can know if you're always going to be in chronic pain. Nobody understands pain well or the autonomic nervous system. If somebody tells you they do: Run.' Yet society has also let some people down so badly that they feel they can't escape."

Here, too, chaplains' own experiences inform their approaches. Kristine's personal trauma exquisitely sensitizes her to these challenges: "I was abused as a child and still have to do a lot of self-care. I walk for over an hour every day. I paint, craft, and have a wonderful family. Sometimes, I spend more time with these activities than I feel I deserve. Sometimes I dissociate from it all, 'blocking it out.' But I say, 'It's OK to disassociate for a while.' "

A chaplain can motivate patients to modify their views about not only their past, present, and future, but also their larger place in the cosmos. As Kristine explained, "We reframe the patient's future story. Everybody has a past, but also a *future* story—an image of how their future should go. Yet, many people feel that if they don't get that future, their God has abandoned them. Reframing the identity of a person and of God are completely integrated. I can never tease apart how I see myself versus God and my community.

"I don't *give* people reframes," Kristine elaborated, "but explore and ex-pand their sense of how they could *reframe themselves*." Chaplains often see their roles as helping a patient to recast his or her own story, rather than as providing such altered perspectives themselves.

The only recasting Kristine at times offers is very broad and nonspecific—to "live in the present, rather than in the future or the past. I'm constantly saying, 'Let's talk about what we're doing in the present and in your body right now. Where do you feel that in your body?' We heal from trauma by getting in touch with our body."

Some people feel they can never again experience hope because of their negative beliefs about themselves. "The biggest reframe," for Kristine, "is moving someone out of the role of victim, rescuer, or prosecutor. We too often frame people as *victims* and damaged. I read an editorial that said, 'An abused child is forever broken. They can't ever be healed.'"

She ardently disagrees, drawing on her own personal experiences. "I was sexually abused as a child but don't think I'm forever broken. Only in chap-laincy training did I really became aware of how it affected me. In seminary, we had to tell our life story. I had completely washed away a lot of the sexual abuse history, disassociated myself from it. During seminary, I went back to my mother and said, 'Did this happen?' She said, 'Yes.' I *knew* it! A psycholog-ical theory talks about the *unthought unknown*—as soon as you know it, you knew it all along. So, I went back and recaptured it."

Even if not completely consciously, this abuse had fueled her interest in chaplaincy. "It probably led to my going to seminary. I didn't know it. My parents don't understand why both of their kids became counselors and min-isters. But we are called to these fields through our wounds. I had to do it be-cause I needed so much healing. Not many people are called into chaplaincy who didn't have a pretty tough history as a child." She here echoes Jung's dictum about the importance of being "wounded healers."[1] Such personal experiences spur Kristine and others to "invite patients to reframe *broken-ness* into a source of *wholeness*, compassion, and connection with others."

Reframing miracles and false hopes

Yet at times, hope can morph into unrealistic and unhealthy denial. Many patients or families yearn for a full medical recovery, and believe one will occur, and they push for aggressive treatments that doctors see as futile.

Such patients and families harbor "false hopes" that a "miracle" will tran-spire. Desperation, resistance, and denial run deep when confronting death, leading many patients and families to feel they will defy all odds, and to envision divinely sent miracles. Such confidence in miracles and conse-quent demands for invasive futile treatments exasperate physicians and nurses, who, along with chaplains, respond to these sentiments in better or worse ways.

"Miracle language is very common," Sam Lacey, a Louisiana chaplain, noted. "The biggest problem clinically is if patients are requesting inappro-priate or futile treatment based on the idea that God is going to intervene." Families may insist that a miracle will occur, and they cling steadfastly to this notion, despite staff efforts to alter these perspectives. "When they know death is coming," Brenda Pierson, a pediatric chaplain from the Bible Belt, observed, "some families are open to hearing that a miracle might be just that their child is not suffering anymore and is living in an afterlife. But most say, 'My child is *not* dying. You're *wrong*'—as if death were the enemy of life, not part of life. People keep praying for a miraculous healing, almost never for a good death."

The word "miracle" derives from the Latin *mīrārī* ("to be surprised, look at with wonder"),[2] which is also the root of "admire," "mirror," and "remark-able," and is thus not necessarily religious per se. Yet through the millennia, religions have commonly invoked the term. In the Gospels, Jesus performs miracles—as evidence of God's divinity. In a study of clergy, 98% of whom were Christian, 86% believed God performed miracles. Most would agree with patients saying, "God will cure me of cancer" (86%), pursuing treatment because of the sanctity of life (54%), or accepting every medical treatment possible (53%).[3]

Patients may cite Biblical passages to support their views, and providers then struggle with what to say. "One of the hardest cases we ever had," one physician told me, "was an evangelical patient with terrible metastatic cancer who wanted every aggressive treatment, though he was dying. He said, 'God will save me! I want everything done. That's what St. Paul and my Church say.' I said, 'That's *not* what St. Paul says.' We argued about it. Finally, his minister visited and agreed with me, telling the patient, 'That's rubbish.'" Doctors, nurses, and chaplains should generally avoid such direct theolog-ical arguments with patients, but then face challenges of how best to respond.

Such unwavering faith that a miraculous cure will transpire can ignite conflicts among patients and families as well. Juan Rodriguez, the chaplain who developed stage IV cancer and later died, said, "My family are devout Catholics and believe the newborn Jesus is going to bring a miracle and save my life. I feel that that helps them. I do not take away their beliefs that a miracle could happen. Jesus begins his ministry by curing people. Could that happen? Yes. Is it *going* to happen? We cannot say: yes. *Could* it happen? Absolutely! But my family is thereby also *denying what I'm saying and feeling*. I feel like my life has completely stopped and that they are not listening to me, which makes me miserable. I believe in miracles as much as the next person, but miracles come in many forms. A miracle that I would welcome now is just that my body might feel somewhat normal and be able to lay comfortably. It's tough to summon energy, except for trying to find a comfortable place to sit or getting a bowl of soup. It's difficult to read or concentrate, because it's hard to lay on my back, because of my spine. Watching TV is hard; I just can't find a comfortable place. Miracles do happen. I pray that my partner is able to express himself and what he's going through. That would be another miracle— that he feels the freedom to express himself. So, I pray."

Despite the wide range of potential meanings of "miracles," patients' and families' requests for them can still trouble staff. Unsure how to respond, doctors commonly throw up their hands. Lisa Ringel, a Jewish chaplain, relayed how doctors say, "The family is talking about a miracle happening— Call the chaplain!" As a fellow doctor told me, "We think patients are delusional when they say, 'God is going to save me.' One woman had a terrible neck injury and refused surgery and was therefore probably going to end up paralyzed. But she said, 'God is going to save me!' Her family said: 'She is not crazy. This is her faith—her faith is very strong.' So, we said OK. But it makes us uncomfortable! We had the chaplain see them. Often, the chaplain says to these patients, 'God works through doctors, and you should follow the doctors' recommendation.' Sometimes the patient then agrees."

Still, clashes erupt. Physicians and nurses frequently find it hard to challenge the convictions of patients and families who insist that a miracle will occur and/or who then seek evidence. Some physicians find it easier just to go along, continuing to provide aggressive but futile care.

Ideally, a chaplain should not argue with patients, and instead listen, glean what they mean by "miracles," and reframe such wishes—rather than destroying all hope. Chaplains can emphasize how small marvels may be possible, and how providers won't abandon the patient and instead try to eliminate pain and discomfort, and not thwart an unexpected recovery if it occurs.[4] Patients and families may dream of an unexplained, uncanny, or unfathomable event, but other times, the patient or family saying, "God will heal me" may just reflect hopes to survive until an upcoming birthday, holiday, or grandchild's wedding. "Miracles" can therefore represent not divine interventions, but rather small, simple, secular events that may occur despite unlikely odds. Still, staff may misconstrue such patients' or families' comments. Cathy Murray, the chaplain at a Catholic hospital whose boyfriend died in high school, observed, "Parents feel it's their job to have hope until their son or daughter dies. But the healthcare team says, 'This family has *false or unrealistic hope.*' The staff fear that the family, because of this unrealistic optimism, is going to fall apart when the child dies. It can cause conflict with the healthcare team. *Yet the parents were defining 'hope' differently than the medical staff.* Parents have dreams for their child, even if only for a peaceful death. But the healthcare team thinks families define hope only as 'hope for a cure.' That's not, however, necessarily what parents are wishing for. Most parents said, 'I'm not looking to the healthcare team to give me hope, but I don't want them to take my hope away!' " Cathy tries to redefine expectations so that the family and the team can work together.

At times, patients *do* beat the odds, even if such occurrences are not divinely sent. Cathy, for instance, described what she termed "a Christmas miracle... A young 21-year-old woman had liver disease and was admitted to the ICU on Christmas Eve. If she didn't have a liver transplant within 24 hours, she would die. Her family lived several hours away. I introduced myself, and asked how she wanted to spend the time. First, she wanted to pray. She led the prayer. Then, she wanted to play a game: Life. So, her nurse, the patient, and I played Life. Players go through what they are going to do in life: Are they going to go to college, get married, have kids? As we're playing, knowing she might not survive the night, she started talking about her life plans. She and her boyfriend already planned how many kids they were going to have, what the names were going to be. It was a very profound experience.

"Later that night, to our surprise, she got a liver! She lived another year, and accomplished some of the things she wanted to do." Cathy was astonished and saw it as a "miracle"—even if not from a divine force—a reason not to surrender hope.

Yet chaplains as well as physicians can still find these conversations difficult, walking a fine line between supporting patients and not eviscerating dreams. End-of-life issues can be frustrating and painful to discuss. "One of the biggest challenges is talking to people about death and dying," added Marvin Beck, a chaplain at a small community hospital. "The elephant in the room is when the patient is 88 and has cancer and is still getting aggressive chemo. Chaplains are the ones who ask, 'Do you have a will? Have you talked about what you would want in terms of 'do not resuscitate' [DNR]?'"

These situations can, however, profoundly disconcert chaplains. As Marvin Beck added, "A 94-year-old patient was full code—intubated, catheter, the whole nine yards. I said to the doctor, 'Isn't somebody talking to them about comfort care?' The doctor said, 'We talked to them, but they're *praying for a miracle.*' I sat and prayed with them, and said, 'We're getting in the way of what God's plan here may be: We're keeping your loved one alive.'" Marvin's conversation helped this family begin to accept the inevitable.

In responding to "miracle language," providers hence have to be careful. "I do not feel comfortable if patients ask me to bless a plan for futile care because they believe a God-given miracle will occur," Sam Lacey, a Louisiana chaplain, reported. But chaplains can also assist by encouraging patients and families to imagine what a miracle might be. "It would be hard if a patient asked for a miracle and wanted me to ask for it, too. If I agreed, it would be disingenuous. So, I say, 'I wish this could be the case,' trying to convey that it's not for me to say, while not lying."

Outside clergy can also get frustrated and respond in poor ways. "One family wanted everything done for their child because they believed a miracle would save him," a pediatrician told me. "Their priest got angry at them: 'If you really believe a miracle will happen, let's just unplug your child now! Then we'll *see* if that miracle happens!' That was the wrong approach: We need to be respect families' beliefs about miracles—sit down, talk with them, and try to understand."

Chaplains and providers strive to recast families' desires for miracles in various ways. Upset and overwhelmed, facing deeply emotional, not just intellectual, concerns, patients often come to apply and interpret religious doctrine, but can potentially change, guided by chaplains or other staff. "One woman wanted everything done for her father," another physician told me, "because she was 'born again' and believed he wouldn't go to heaven unless he had accepted Christ into his life—even though he was not very religious. This daughter insisted that we do everything for her father. But he was in stupor—unresponsive."

"How did you resolve the situation?" I asked.

"One day, his arm twitched. I said, '*That* is his sign that he agrees.' Luckily, she was able to accept that."

9

"I pray to the God I don't believe in"

Creating prayers

Everyday en route to work, I stroll by a small pond in Central Park, admiring towering maple, birch, pine, gingko, and cypress trees, their leaves and branches sprouting and spreading toward the sky. The clear water sparkles, reflecting white clouds and the bright blue sky seeming to stretch on forever. I inhale the sweet scents of fresh-cut green grass, pink and white blossoming cherry and apple trees, and rich, mossy earth. I close my eyes for a moment and express thanks for the blessings I have in my life—my health, family, and friends.

After speaking to chaplains, I have come to see these expressions as forms of prayer.

Countless patients pray, but many questions about it arise. Prayer is associated with spiritual well-being, faith, and assurance, yet is often misunderstood by providers.[1] Medically ill older adults pray more than others.[2] Eighty-nine percent of patients, but only 58% of providers thought that it was very important for patients, for instance, at the end of life.[3]

Chaplains regularly create a wide variety of prayers, drawing on each patient's particular beliefs and existential and psychological needs. Patients differ in how, when, and why they engage in this activity—the purpose, content, timing, and form, whether silent or spoken—that connects people to something spiritual beyond themselves, however they conceive it.

Routinely, chaplains give extemporaneous prayers, saying, for instance, "May Janet, here in the hospital, feel less pain and be surrounded by her loved ones. May the higher powers, who create and oversee all, help her, and give the doctors all the knowledge and skill they need to aid her."

Even patients who say they are not "religious" nonetheless pray. This term has a wide variety of meanings. According to Cathy Murray, the chaplain at a Catholic hospital, "Even agnostic patients say, 'Yes, please pray with me.' It's a stressful time."

Doctor, Will You Pray for Me?. Robert L. Klitzman, Oxford University Press. © Oxford University Press 2024.
DOI: 10.1093/oso/9780197750841.003.0009

People pray at their own times and in their own ways. "I'm a traditionalist, do the holidays, and very much believe in God, *but am not religious*," a 60-year-old woman who had breast cancer told me. "I'm proud of being Jewish and believe in some spiritualism. Whenever I'm in trouble, I pray. I think He has a path for everybody. But I don't go to temple. My mother always said, 'You don't have to go to synagogue or temple. You can pray in the house.' So, I pray a lot at home. I probably *should* go to temple, but unfortunately don't. I don't know why not. I used to go. I belonged to a temple for 40 years, but just stopped. I'm working, and getting older, and am happy to come home and stay in. I shouldn't.

"I pray for my health, that we should all be well," she explained. Her husband "fell and hit his head, and had major brain surgery. It was terrible. So, I pray to God that he will be well. Given the world we live in today, I pray *constantly* that the world is going to be good. I worry about my grandchildren growing up—that they'll be protected and OK. I pray, before I go to bed, that I wake up in the morning! But I'm *not* a religious person, unfortunately. I *should* be, but I'm not."

The fact that she prays multiple times a day but insists she is "not religious" underscores how blurry these terms can be. Her comment that she "should go to temple" suggests, too, how leaning toward or away from religion is not entirely self-willed, and can result from complex feelings and cause internal conflict. She illustrates, too, how people's descriptions of their beliefs, behaviors, and sense of belonging do not always fit neatly into boxes, and can differ from what an outside observer might assume.

Prayers can take many forms, varying in *to whom* they are directed (to "God" per se or not), *for what* (whether for disease, strength, reassurance, and/or guidance), *what* is said (whether prespecified, established language or spontaneous), *when* (whether regularly and/or at set times or only when a crisis hits), whether it is consciously *planned* or not (i.e., "finding myself doing it"), and *what to call it* (whether "prayer" or not).

Prayers can be articulations of humility and hope—both of which can aid in overcoming crises. Indeed, the core of Alcoholics Anonymous, which is far more successful than psychotherapy or medication in treating addictions, is the Serenity Prayer: "God grant me the serenity to accept the things I cannot change; the courage to change the things I can; and the wisdom to know the difference."[4]

The content and form of prayers spread across a wide continuum—from reciting psalms and specific ancient hymns to simply voicing gratitude. As Olana Ramerez, for instance, a Latina with HIV from injecting drugs, mentioned, she prays in Spanish and does so as if she's "talking to a person."

Many doctors, though by no means all, are in fact open to prayer in some form. Several years ago, I wrote an article for the *New York Times*, briefly mentioning a few of these issues[5] and received a flood of responses. One doctor replied, "Deep down inside I am a very pessimistic agnostic, and yet the closest to religious I ever become is when I pray with my patients, which I do whenever requested. I have seen it work very well in the sense of enhancing a patient's well-being and morale, and once or twice I would attest that it has kept someone off of mechanical ventilation. When I have a patient who is ill, I will take help from any source—seen or unseen—to make him or her better, or at least comfort them in their remaining time."[6] The impact of prayer may result solely from the placebo effect, but that in itself can be beneficial. Not all actions have placebo effects—the patient has to believe that the intervention will help. Certainly, for believers, such actions can thus potentially be positive.

In response to my article, other atheistic and agnostic doctors wrote that despite their own personal views, they commonly tell patients, "I wish you a quick recovery," "I will send you good wishes," or "May your faith heal and give you courage"[6]—essentially de facto prayers. These statements, akin to "prayers," raise questions of how we define this term.

Prayers created by chaplains, such as Sister Francine, voicing hopes that the patient will heal, can make meaningful connections—symbolic, but strong, and potentially salubrious when confronting crises.

Praying for divine intervention

While prayer helps millions of people psychologically, many people want or believe it can do more—by prompting divine intervention. Innumerable patients pray for strength and perseverance, yet some claim that these supplications can directly alter physiology through divine intervention. Others disagree. One nurse I spoke to, with a family history of breast cancer, is open to ESP and believes in prayer, though not in God directly intervening as a result. "I'm a theologian, but don't bank a lot on prayer for divine intervention. Miracles are rare—few and far between—as sporadic for the person who prays as for the person who doesn't.

"Still, prayer helps," she reflected. "Whether or not there's a God, prayer benefits the person who prays. Prayer doesn't heal physically, but can certainly *help heal the soul and spirit, and reduce feelings of isolation.* The power to cure is totally different."

However, other patients, and even some doctors, feel that prayer can do more. "Everyone sent me prayer cards and Mass cards," Roxanne, the Brazilian gastroenterologist with abdominal cancer, stated. "I was in everyone's prayers. It must have worked: I had more energy, which never diminished." She and many other patients believe that prayer can in fact directly improve the physical healing process through God's intervention, directly altering the disease process itself. She also made a religious pilgrimage to Lourdes, which she felt gave her additional strength.

Supporters of such so-called intercessory prayer argue that having someone pray for you, even if you don't know about it, can, in and of itself, directly alter your biological processes, curing disease beyond the placebo effect. Yet while a few studies suggest possible support for these beliefs to small degrees, these investigations have been limited in size and not always replicated.[7,8] Importantly, numerous studies show that such interventions do not in fact work.

While knowing that other people are praying for you can strengthen your sense of social support and thus be beneficial indirectly, some patients nonetheless believe more. Jacob, a Jewish radiologist with melanoma, informed several Jewish friends of his diagnosis in order to get them to pray for him. They did so, which he believes succeeded. "I called up five people whom I consider very holy. They follow Jewish law, without fanfare or publicity. I figure *they've got God on their side.* I know it helped because, knowing they were doing it, I was functioning better . . . Prayer works! That's part of Jewish belief: You can change the way the world is going."

The lack of proof does not dissuade believers in intercessory prayer. "How do you think it works?" I asked a physician and rabbi who believed in it.

"I don't know. It just does!" He paused. "Through God!" He required no additional explanation. Those who believe in such intercession require no scientific evidence or mechanistic explanation, even if they are scientifically trained. They separate phenomena into two distinct realms: what is knowable and what it not.

Yet I have been surprised by who does and does not believe in such "power of prayer." For instance, a medical professor I know, from a prominent WASP family, became depressed for the first time in his life after he had a heart attack. He described a medical colleague who "came to believe in the 'power of prayer' to treat disease. He did not become obsessive about it, but it meant a lot to him. He would just 'sit' with patients . . . He got a theology degree, and now gives talks on the power of prayer. Some doctors won't send him patients anymore. But he is incredibly attached to this idea. And I'm attached to *him*. There's no question: You certainly can call on things that you might not be able to describe, but which make people feel better." In part, the cost is low and the potential advantage high.

"I'm not atheistic, but also not particularly tied to doctrine," he continued. "I'm a practicing Episcopalian and a regular communicant at my church—we have a great church that's half-Black, half-white. I've chaired committees there.

"My wife is the granddaughter of a missionary but is far more of a *doubter* than I am. She comes to church because I want her to, not because she feels like going. I also treat Christian Scientists. A college friend was a Christian Scientist, which impacted me. There's 'craziness' to it: They delay giving their children medicine. But we have some things in common."

As a successful physician and scientist, his openness to the power of prayer surprised me. He was far more receptive to a broader array of religious ideas than are many other physicians, and I would not have predicted his views, further illuminating for me how much we can fail to surmise others' beliefs.

Clearly, though, prayer can serve symbolic, but nonetheless forceful and important, functions, especially in times of crisis, providing important psychological balm.

During the COVID-19 pandemic, particularly in its earliest stages, the symbolic nature of prayers took on special function and significance. "Figuring out what spiritual care means in the context of COVID was really hard," William Gibson, the humanist chaplain, admitted. "I don't know that we did. We had some success. Much of our work is talking with people about their suffering and what they're going through, and what meaning they're making of it or not. We could do some of that with families by phone. Initially, we were also not allowed to use up personal protection equipment and go into patients' rooms. And critically ill patients were more sedated than usual."

In these contexts, prayers gained added import. "Catholic priests spent time standing outside peoples' rooms, praying for them," William reported. "That's not a big part of my practice, or a huge secular Jewish thing. But I did that because it turned out to be meaningful to families—to know that I had gone and said whatever prayers I could from their tradition that I could say with integrity—were kosher enough for me—to tell them that I said the Our Father, and offered a Christian blessing outside their loved one's room. I'd let the family know I'd done that, or even called them from there, standing there in place of the family who couldn't be there. Before we figured out that arrangements like that would work or be meaningful, I felt powerless—even more so than usual."

Prayers can thus take many forms and provide many balms.

10

"The voice of the voiceless"

Aiding vulnerable patients

Chaplaincy departments, while striving to serve all patients who might benefit, generally have limited resources and unfortunately miss many individuals and groups, especially vulnerable ones. "We tend to provide care to the people who need it the *least*," William Gibson opined, "and systemically miss those who need it *most*." Various groups, including patients who are unable to speak, have mental health problems, have different cultural backgrounds or languages, or are LGBTQ+, face obstacles in obtaining optimal healthcare.[41] These groups vary but confront related challenges, misunderstandings, prejudice, stigma, and discrimination from providers, and face barriers in receiving optimal spiritual and other care.

Non-vocal patients

As an intern, I once treated an elderly woman who had had a stroke and lost all ability to talk. The police picked her up at 2 a.m., wandering the streets in her nightgown, confused and unable to give her name or address. She remained in the hospital for weeks and became the ward mascot, smiling, waving to everyone, and helping the nurses tie rubber bands around stacks of test tubes—but unable to utter a word. Eventually, with help from the police, we were able to identify her, but I will never forget her predicament: how the sudden loss of language impeded her life.

For various reasons, numerous hospitalized patients cannot speak, posing challenges for chaplains and other staff. Such patients have spiritual needs that frequently get overlooked. "Non-vocal patients on mechanical ventilation have high self-ratings of spiritual distress," William Gibson explained. "But the staff will just tell chaplains, 'A patient in Room 2 is going through a lot, but can't talk, so skip her.' I tell the nurses, 'We can use speech therapy

Doctor, Will You Pray for Me?. Robert L. Klitzman, Oxford University Press. © Oxford University Press 2024.
DOI: 10.1093/oso/9780197750841.003.0010

techniques and try to communicate with her and get her some care.' We give non-vocal ICU patients pictures to point to, to indicate how they're feeling. The most common feeling they point to is frustration. The second is love. We try to give them a lot of love. Hopefully, they just feel cared for."

Yet in-depth communication with such patients about complex topics presents difficulties. "Intubated patients hooked up in the ICU are hard," Margaret Dixon, the Pennsylvania chaplain, explained. "I feel a little bit at sea with a patient with a tube down his throat, who is struggling to communicate. It's hard for me to go into these rooms. I wonder how I would be if *I* had a tube down my throat, and wires going into me, tracked on a heinous machine. Miserable! I try to explore where my faith would be with that. The other day, a verbal patient said to me, 'It just works for me to feel that God is in control of this, and that I don't have to control everything. I can't control everything. It's going to be what it's going to be.' I'd like to think that's how *I* would be."

These interactions can be arduous for patients, too. At times, humor can help. As Margaret continued, "One patient was intubated and couldn't talk, but was awake. He had a board of alphabet letters and just pointed to them. I asked, 'How are you? How is it going?' He's pointing to T-H-I-S. I said, 'This?' I-S. 'OK. This is?' . . . He wrote: N-O-T. S-E-X-Y. I laughed so hard. He laughed, too—as much as he could."

Patients with mental health problems

Psychiatric problems can pose challenges as well. Psychiatry has long viewed religion with suspicion, yet psychiatric patients face existential and spiritual quandaries that the current psychopharmacological era may miss. Psychiatric hospitals, especially, may lack sufficient numbers of chaplains. In addition, serious medical, rather than psychiatric, diagnoses are assumed to raise more religious, spiritual, and existential issues. "Our psychiatric hospital has 300 beds and only one chaplain," Sam Lacey, a Louisiana chaplain, explained. "There's no way one chaplain could cover 300 patients!"

Patients with suicidal comments pose particular challenges. If a patient mentions such thoughts, the chaplain must report these to the medical staff. Patients may then feel, however, that their trust has been violated. "As soon as a patient discloses suicidal ideation, everything changes," William explained.

"I have to tell the medical team, but continue to provide spiritual care. I hear their pain and have to prepare them for the fact that somebody's going to come to sit and watch them, as if they've committed a crime.

"An ER patient told me that aliens had planted a device in his head," William continued. "He rigged up an appliance at home to put the right amount of voltage into his brain to electrocute it out. I was worried it could kill him. But he said he wasn't crazy, so it was tricky. I tried getting him the help he needs, without him feeling betrayed. But security guards showed up and were very rough. They forcefully took him out of his street clothes and transported him away. All of a sudden, he felt like he committed a crime. He got so spooked that he clammed up and denied everything, and said whatever he needed to say to return home.

"That was one of the very worst moments of my career," William recalled. "I was angry at Security. There are many versions of that—when the patient clearly has a mental health issue, and I'm trying to convince them to seek help, but can't force them."

As part of their delusion, psychotic patients also frequently invoke religious language. Some say they see or hear angels, Jesus or the Devil, communicating directly to them. "Mania with religious ideation is very hard," Cathy Murray noted. "These patients' religious ideation looks like religion but is really mania! We don't want to discount their religious experiences in the middle of full-blown mania, but they do not need to be spiraling out of control. It's not a religious issue, it's mania! I tell trainees, 'You are not helping them by spending hours in a theological discussion about what unforgiveable sin is. You're just building on their mania and keeping them in the same place.' These visits need to be very short. I say, 'I know you're trying to be caring, but you are just helping him spiral, not doing him any good. Stay grounded.' I say to such patients. 'It looks like you're having a lot of thoughts about a very difficult topic. Unforgiveable sin is a struggle for many people. I'll listen to this for a little while, but don't think it's good for you to keep going back. Let's see how long you can stay in a place where you feel forgiveness, not lack of forgiveness.' Listening is also intervention. We need to continually analyze whether what we're doing is working, and not just assume that if we and the patient like it, that it works." She underscores how much chaplaincy, like psychotherapy, involves complex interpersonal dynamics.

She uses centering exercises to bring such patients back to the present moment: "I have a long list of grounding exercises. With a manic patient, I might say, 'Find something red in this room.' The patient will look around and say,

'That cup over there.' 'Good. Tell me about the red.' I try to get the patient back into the present in their bodies and into their senses. 'What color are my eyes?' It brings people back, and not out there in their past or their future. Or I'll say, 'Stamp your feet on the ground. Let's just feel *that*. Doesn't it feel good to feel your feet on the ground? Let yourself feel it.' I've got a list of maybe 26 of these exercises to be in the present in your body."

LGBTQ+ patients

LGBTQ+ patients often face added challenges related to religion, in part given various religious institutions' ongoing homophobia. Most hospice and palliative care staff think that LGBTQ+ patients are more likely to face discrimination: 89.7% think these patients have delayed seeking care because of concerns about discrimination[1], and 43% have observed discrimination against these patients or healthcare surrogates.[2] These stresses can foster mental health problems. LGBTQ+ individuals are two to three times more likely to have depression than the general population, and transgender individuals have even higher rates (48%).[3] LGBTQ+ youth commit suicide at three times the rate of heterosexual youth.[4] In much of society, homophobia is decreasing, but transgender patients, in particular, still face social, psychological, medical, religious, and spiritual hurdles.[5]

LGBTQ+ individuals have frequently felt unwelcome by religious institutions, perceiving religions as "unfriendly," especially Islam (84%), Mormonism (83%), Catholicism (79%), and evangelical churches (73%), and to lesser extents Judaism (47%) and mainstream Protestantism (44%).[6] Among these individuals, 48.6% have experienced microaggressions in religious and spiritual communities, particularly attitudes that homosexuality was incompatible with membership in the community.[7]

Nonetheless, for most LGBTQ+ individuals, spirituality is important, though less than for heterosexuals. In 2014, 55% of LGBTQ adults and 56% of heterosexuals thought about the meaning/purpose of life at least once a week, and 54% of gays, lesbians and bisexuals, and 59% of heterosexuals "felt a deep sense of spiritual peace and well-being."[8] Compared to heterosexuals, LGBTQ+ individuals were less likely to believe in God (77% vs. 89%), to pray daily (38% gay/lesbian, 41% bisexual, and 56% heterosexual), or to be Christian (48% vs. 72%), and were more likely to be atheist (8% vs. 3%), agnostic (9% vs. 4%), or nothing in particular (24% vs. 15%) or to have non-Christian faiths (11% vs. 6%). Among Christians, LGBTQ+ individuals were less likely to be evangelical (17% vs. 25%) or Catholic (17% vs. 21%).[8,9]

Across denominations, conservative churches have vehemently rejected these individuals. Peter Haines, for instance, a gay medical student who reprioritized his life after becoming HIV-infected, told me he sees himself as "personally" religious but not part of an established religious institution, further underscoring how much individuals perceive these institutions in differing ways. "I was brought up Catholic and used to be very religious, but had a lot of problems growing up, and got away from the Church," he said. Now, he joked, he was "religious *only when it's convenient.*"

Yet Peter then described a critical juncture in his life after his infection, when he established a meaningful relationship with Catholicism: "I just needed someone spiritually. I saw a priest, and expected the worst. But he was great, and actually got me to go back to religion. He said, 'In old-school Catholicism, you have fire and brimstone. You'll burn in Hell. But we're not here to judge. We're here to help you get through whatever you need to get through.' He helped me alter my views on Catholicism.

"I'm religious personally, but don't do anything with the community," he continued. "Religion is supposed to be *personal*. It's between you and God or whomever you believe in. So, why do I need to go to the Church to have that personal relationship?" He therefore separated individual clergy from beliefs and broader religious organizations.

"Do you pray?" I asked him.

"Not really. Just those times when I *need* to pray," he laughed, "when I'm having a rough time." Beliefs and religiosity can thus waver over time, and not just in one direction, but rather shift back and forth, depending on events. He would probably not consider himself a None in the strictest sense (highlighting the limits of this category as a single entity) and would probably be unsure how to answer a survey question about whether he had a religious affiliation. He had one, but only some of the time.

Transgender patients can encounter additional challenges. Linda Porter, the Maryland pediatric chaplain and former journalist, "got involved with a transgender clinic because of a specific incident. I was asked to meet with a devoutly Catholic mother whose daughter was transitioning. The mother said it was a 'sin,' and her family 'was going to disown her' if I sided with the daughter and supported the transitioning. I talked with this mother for an hour. Pope Francis has said some very positive things regarding, 'Who am I to judge?,' creating space for other ways of thinking about this. I talked about the God of love—that she could keep loving her child. When this mother first found out she was pregnant, she was filled with love. I told her, 'You didn't know if your child was a boy or a girl. You just loved that baby. It's no different now. You can just keep loving.' But this mother ended up siding with her faith. The parents were divorced, so the daughter went to live with the father. It was awful. I offered to meet with this mother again, but she never wanted to." Unfortunately, chaplains' interventions do not always succeed.

Linda continues to find work with LGBTQ+ patients rewarding but challenging. "One Saturday at 10 p.m., I got paged that a patient wanted a Bible and wanted to pray. If it had just been a Bible, I could have sent someone else to deliver it, but the patient wanted to pray, so I went.

"The patient was transgender but very early in the process. She had a lot of homicidal thoughts about her mother, and other issues. She was raised Catholic but now identified as Wiccan, which I kind of love. We were just chatting about this and that. If anyone was listening, it would just sound like small talk, but there was an unconscious transaction: The patient was implicitly asking, '*Can you hear what I might want to say? Who are you? Can I trust you?*'" Linda here highlights how chaplains' conversations can operate on multiple levels—simultaneously referring to both minimal and larger realms.

"At one point at 10:30 p.m. on a Saturday, she asked me, '*So, if God is perfect, why am I in the wrong body?*' I thought, 'Wow. That's it!' I like that chaplaincy just holds your feet to the fire. You don't get a chance to really think through statements like that very much. I took a moment and said that God created her soul, and that her soul was perfect in the eyes of God, but that in creating a body, billions of little things happen as cells divide. Who knows how things happen, but for some reason, her body didn't match what she felt to be her soul. But today, there are ways to correct that and make them match. I said I would think more about it. That was the best answer I could think of on the spot.

"It felt authentic for me to say that her soul was perfect. In the gender clinic, we have a devout Catholic physician who went to her priest and asked if it was OK to work with the clinic. Thank God, her priest was a Jesuit who said, 'Yes, but I wouldn't talk about it too much.' This doctor has now been deeply engaged in the work for 10 years. When people at her church say to her, 'Changing your gender is wrong! It's a sin. This is the way God created you,' she replies, 'If a baby is born with a heart defect, we don't say, "That's the way God made you: with a defective heart."' I thought, 'That's exactly right.'"

Unfortunately, chaplains may not always realize when patients are LGBTQ+; they frequently visit patients without first consulting the medical chart. Moreover, LGBTQ+ patients rarely call chaplains themselves and may therefore get missed. Religious homophobia erects further barriers. "The last person in the world," William Gibson explained, "that a gay teenager, wrestling with 'coming out,' is going to think will be helpful is a religious person. I got a request for a chaplain for an adolescent patient. I think it came from the patient's parents. I went and introduced myself to the patient in a routine way, and the patient rejected me, so I left. But the next day, I looked at her medical record. I don't know why I wouldn't have done so beforehand—maybe that was my mistake. I gathered that the issue was related to her coming out to her family—maybe to herself. And she played softball, which I love.

"I hadn't done my homework and was sad and angry at myself. I had just played into this whole situation: The Christian family finds out the kid's gay, and doesn't like that, so sends them a pastor. I didn't go to 'pray the gay out of her,' but could have connected around softball, and said something to *signal*, 'Hey, I'm here to visit with you, no matter who you are,' to open a door. I didn't do that, and didn't go back. It was a mistake, a missed opportunity— truly substandard spiritual care. They just didn't get any spiritual care. I still regret that and beat myself up about it."

Such difficult cases have, however, motivated chaplains to enhance their skills for future such situations. Trained to address spiritual, existential, and religious issues and to be supportive in open-minded and nondenominational ways, chaplains can aid many LGBTQ+ patients, who face psychic stresses due to not only disease but also discrimination. Yet chaplains and other providers also need to recognize these complex processes and implicit cues, signaling openness and support.

Patients of other ethnicities and races

Disadvantaged minority groups, too, may receive substandard care, sparking chaplains' efforts to bridge these gaps and power differentials. For instance, Adam Quincy, who reads widely about other religions of the world, described how "white male chaplains can face particular challenges with women of color. Providing chaplaincy to African American women is culturally different, unless the chaplain has good cultural and religious sensitivity, and is sure not to have his or her own agenda. Chaplaincy typically does not meet these patients' needs well. The African American community has a deep distrust of the healthcare system, deeply believing that the system is not set up to meet their needs. The impulse behind Black Lives Matter is that, 'My life really doesn't matter, because the healthcare system was set up by white males for white males, and I'm just not of any value to anyone.'

"My experience is that many African American females, in particular, feel non-validated by society. So, walking into the room with a positive attitude—as if you have your act together and that your life is great, and you are going to build or pump them up—is wrong. Think about how that patient feels! *The right way is to walk in there broken*, trying to identify with your deepest state of feeling alienated from society, when you felt least validated, when nobody chose you to be on the kickball team. It's less about your words than your demeanor, tone, and style. You should walk in very slowly, solemnly, carefully, and attentively, speak softly, and take any edge off your voice, because African American women don't perceive themselves as getting that kind of attention. I'll say, 'It's a rough day today, isn't it?'—trying immediately to show that I identify with their struggle. Or, 'Hospitals should be a lot more comfortable than they are, shouldn't they?' Or, 'Have you ever laid in a hospital bed that felt comfortable?' The best time to visit Black females is when you're having the absolute worst day of your career, because they can see it all over you, and will light up and make friends with you. But just make sure you're *broken*. Tell them that you're empathetic and see their situation. Even throw the staff under the bus for a second and say, 'You know, if they responded to these call buttons like they should . . .' But then, of course, circle back and repair that later. If you don't do that at the start, you'll lose them and have to begin all over. I've made that mistake, thinking they're in a good mood, and walking in there like we're going to talk about pop music, when that's just a smokescreen."

Even a chaplain's clothing can affect interactions. "I've seen chaplains dressed in suits and ties like hospital executives." he continued. "What are they doing? Patients are going to think they're a hospital administrator! You want to go in there as a *suffering healer*, so they can see your pain and relate to that." Wounded healers may thus not only bring unique empathy to patients, but be seen by the latter as doing so.

These poignant insights can help not just other chaplains but also doctors, nurses, hospital administrators, and the rest of us as well.

Unfortunately, chaplains remain disproportionately white and Christian and only speak English, and consequently need to be keenly aware of racial and ethnic differences among patients. "We have tons of resources for Catholic, Protestant, and Orthodox Jewish patients—chaplains and Bibles," William Gibson noted. "Catholics can get Communion. We rarely miss the religious needs of an English-speaking Irish-Catholic lady. For Orthodox Jews, we can get Sabbath supplies and a rabbi. We probably miss Spanish-speaking families more, but have Spanish-speaking chaplains, and lots of staff speak Spanish. A nurse may overhear a family's distress and refer a chaplain, but that doesn't happen for *other* languages—anything other than English or Spanish. And there are a ton of Chinese-speaking families, too."

Chaplains therefore try to encourage doctors and nurses to refer foreign and alone patients who may not explicitly ask for a referral but may be in this country by themselves. "When I lecture to the NICU staff, I coach them to look for patients who are likely to get missed," William explained. "Not just refer patients who are dying, or Catholics asking for a priest, but also Chinese graduate students alone here without their families. We can use a phone interpreter or call the family in China, whether they are Christian, Buddhist, or not religious."

Patients of religious views different from one's own

Doctors and chaplains may also overlook or underserve a patient who has views other than their own, with which they are unfamiliar. Most chaplains are Christian, yet patients may be Muslims, Hindus, or atheists.

Hospital chaplaincy departments range widely in whether and how they address various diverse beliefs. William Gibson recognizes that atheists, too, don't self-refer, and that their needs may be neglected. "Atheist and nonreligious secular patients don't realize that we have a humanist chaplain on staff—that chaplains aren't proselytizing. These groups are unlikely to self-refer, and staff are more likely to miss their needs. As chaplains, we're guilty of it. We can get a list of the patients identified with a religious tradition where we know how to help, so we do those. It's low-hanging fruit, but what about unaffiliated patients wrestling with deep, existential questions about why this is happening to them?"

Though most U.S. patients' views lie within the framework of the larger Western, Judeo-Christian traditions, not all do. Increasingly, patients are affiliated with non-Western faiths—including Islam, Hinduism, and Buddhism—that nurses and doctors, as well as chaplains, may little comprehend. As Amanda Shaw, a devoutly Catholic Tennessee psychiatrist, said, "I'm more comfortable talking to somebody about their faith when they're Christian, rather than something else, where I'm going to end up running into areas where I don't quite know what to ask."

Among the world's faiths, similarities as well as differences exist. "It could be helpful to understand differences between Eastern and Western religions," Adam Quincy, who had studied world religions, explained. "Judaism, Christianity, and Islam are very dichotomous and black and white, and tend to have a lot of fixity to them. People tend to be emotionally charged defending them. Eastern religions, though, tend to be more mystical and imagistic, characterized by pantheism, monism, and reincarnation."

Interfaith lectures tend to highlight underlying commonalities of all religions, but key differences also exist that can affect medical decisions. Barriers can emerge, especially regarding Islam. The number of Muslim patients has been increasing in the United States[10] and in the rest of the world. In 2010, among the world's population as a whole, 31.4% were Christians, 23.2% Muslims, 16.4% unaffiliated, 15.0% Hindus, 7.1% Buddhists, 5.9% followers of folk religions, and 0.8% other.[10] But by 2050, due to relative population growth in various countries, the number of Christians and Muslims will become almost equal (31.4% and 29.7%, respectively).[10] However, the United States and numerous other countries confront particular barriers, notably rising Islamophobia, which can impede Muslims' mental health and pursuit of treatment.[11] In addition, these individuals often view illness differently, seeing suffering as redemptive and death as God's will, and have particular dietary needs; whole families may be involved in making decisions.[12] But these patients also vary considerably, based partly on their particular culture and sect.[13]

Chaplains who understand non-Western faiths can play pivotal roles in these patients' care. For instance, one Muslim woman wanted more aggressive treatment for her dying husband, though the doctors considered such efforts futile. Masud Noor, a Muslim chaplain, from Algeria, now working in California, reported that in the husband's chart, the staff wrote that this wife was "in denial, had poor coping skills, and wouldn't accept his situation." After several weeks of mutual frustration and antagonism, a social worker finally arranged for Masud to visit. The wife, it turned out, believed that without the treatment, her husband wouldn't go to Heaven. The staff had failed to appreciate her perspective. Masud told her that God wouldn't want her dying husband to undergo more suffering, which additional treatment would cause. She then aligned with her doctors' views.

"Most non-Muslim doctors do not understand," Masud explained. "Muslims believe that *all events are due to the will of Allah*. So, doctors saying to a patient's wife, 'Your husband has two months to live' rubs the family the wrong way, because they fervently believe that God, *not* the doctor, makes decisions about life. The physician should say instead: 'Among patients with your husband's condition, 80% live for around two months.'"

Masud grew up in the Middle East, where he attended seminary, and then received a master's degree in social science and came to the United States. After a bad car accident, he was hospitalized several days, and a chaplain visited him. Masud felt so assisted that he decided to become a chaplain himself. Eventually a major medical center that treated many wealthy Middle Eastern patients hired him, though most of the patients he sees are not Muslim.

He wore light blue buttoned-down Oxford shirt and khaki pants and loafers and looked like a casual, friendly graduate student. "The work is very gratifying," he explained. "A few days ago, an Egyptian patient in the ICU shook my hand, and said, 'Speaking to you has been the most comforting thing that has happened to me here in the hospital.'"

Yet, as a Muslim chaplain, he faces challenges. "The Prophet, Mohammed, teaches that it is virtuous to suffer," Masud continued, "This life is a trial and error for the next one. The Prophet also says that for every illness, there is a cure, and that saving life is the most important thing. So, DNR orders and withholding care pose problems. Many patients think that withholding *some* care means withholding *all* care. We try to frame it differently. Arab legal scholars say, for instance, that no one can inflict harm or suffering on a patient. Risky treatments and procedures with side effects and little, if any, chance of success can in fact hurt patients. Patients and their families may accept *that* as a reason to avoid additional futile interventions."

Chaplains can also help medical staff interpret patients' statements about pain. "Part of being a patient is being *patient*," Masud continued. "When a doctor asks, 'How are you doing?' Muslim patients may say, 'OK,' even if they are in pain, because it is virtuous to suffer—they will be rewarded because of dying, death, or suffering. At the end of life... many Muslims might not want a lot of morphine, if they can help it, because they want to be able to declare at death, 'There's no God but the one God, and Mohammed is His Prophet.' Just as we would do certain rituals for Catholics, we want the patient to say that."

Unfortunately, ignorance about Islam fuels mutual fear. "Since 9/11 and Trump," Masud added, "many Muslims fear being misunderstood or facing discrimination. When asked their religion on hospital forms, some Muslims write 'none.'"

Enhanced understanding can lower Islamophobia. As Adam Quincy, who reads widely about world religions, observed, "Some Christians say, 'Islam is based on the Ishmael and Isaac problem, so Muslims are bitter and always will be.' Every religion has fundamentalists. I might have a hard time dealing with fundamentalist Baptists. But overall, Muslims are really easy to work with. They're very peaceful, very intelligent, and really good. When you embrace and reach out to them, they embrace you back."

Given the ignorance on the part of staff and the wider public, as well as misunderstanding and discomfort regarding Islam, Muslim patients can face additional obstacles with pastoral care. "Muslims assume that the chaplaincy service isn't for them," William Gibson observed. "They are surprised to learn we have a Muslim chaplain, Jum'ah prayer services, a box of prayer rugs and supplies."

Muslim chaplains can uniquely aid certain patients. For instance, Rashid Ayad, a Muslim chaplain, described a Middle Eastern family who "had traveled all over the world for a 14-year-old son with a tumor on his neck that was bigger than a softball. The doctor called, telling me to talk to this family, because there's nothing further he could do for the child. The child would die on the operating table, attempting to remove the tumor. He was the parents' only child, and in their culture, it was important to carry the family name on. The child was very educated and articulate. He did everything a wonderful young man likes to do. The father said, 'I've been all over the world and paid all this money. Now I've come to America. I'm going home now, broke. I have no money.' And he left the mother and the child in America all alone with no support system. It was terrible. He just walked away. So, I visited the child every day, just to talk with him. He liked soccer. We watched the games, and talked about girls—the good things in life. I wanted to keep it normal. And after these sessions, we would pray together. He was very religious. One day he said to me, 'Imam [religious leader], help me do one thing: Help my mother regain her faith in God so I can meet her in Paradise.'

"Every time I went into the room, she would walk out of the room and just stand by the door with her hands crossed, mad and angry—angry with God. But she would not go far. I talked louder with him, so she could hear. The next day, she stayed in the room, but didn't pray at the end of our session together. She raised her hands just a little bit, but still didn't pray. The third time, she raised her hands and began to pray. I looked at him and he looked at me. He was so happy that his mother was praying again. Three or four days later, he died.

"About a month later, his mother called me from the Middle East and said, 'Thank you.' I said, 'For what?' She said, 'You stood by me and my child when nobody else would. My husband left me. The doctors and the nurses left us. But you came and stayed. Now I go to the mosque and pray and do all the things I used to. Thank you so much for that.' That's more important to me than anything you can pay me. I see I made a difference. To this day, I'm still honored to remember that child and his mother, what they gave."

Specific and solid knowledge of this religion can thus clearly benefit patients and families. It would have been much more difficult for a non-Muslim chaplain to have assisted such a mother to regain her faith. The fact that Rashid was a fellow Muslim built strong trust.

Chaplains who are well versed in Islam can educate other staff. Rashid Ayad, who sees Islam as "the most misunderstood religion in the world, especially in America," perceives a lot of resistance from other faith traditions: "Other religions still have to understand where the Islamic community is coming from in dealing with death and dying. Even chaplains from other faiths may be prejudiced against Islam."

Yet, though possessing important specific expertise, trained Muslim chaplains remain relatively rare. Rashid therefore tries to "tell doctors what they should know about Islam. For instance, Muslim patients pray five times a day. Doctors need to know that if they're going to barge into a patient's room, the patient may be praying. You may think the patient is ignoring you, but he is just praying at a certain time."

Non-Muslim doctors may also fail to appreciate that Muslim patients routinely want to avoid vaccines or other substances made from pig or pig gelatin. Rashid informs doctors that "halal involves not just good food, but intravenous medicine containing pork byproducts. Some Muslims would reject the medications if they knew these contained pork byproducts. By the Quran, they can have it if it sustains their life, but that fact needs to be explained to them."

Muslim patients and non-Muslim doctors and nurses frequently face additional communication barriers regarding healthcare more generally. As Rashid added, "Staff also need to be aware that a Muslim woman might put a sign on their door saying, 'No Men.' The physician could be male and needs to realize that he needs to ask, before entering the room, whether the patient is dressed—have the nurse go in and see if the patient is dressed or comfortable enough with their covering. Many patients want a female physician and have that right. Hospitals should honor that."

Rashid also tell doctors, "Culturally, grief and decision-making might be different. The family makes the decision, and hierarchy is involved. The grandmother or grandfather may be in Saudi Arabia, but helping to decide for the patient here. Physicians want to know who is making the decision, and rely on the patient to make it, but the patient has to get back to them. Doctors don't understand that the elders back in Pakistan are involved. I try to buffer this, and give doctors a handout to educate themselves."

A chaplain can remind doctors and nurses of communication barriers that can exist, more generally, with patients and families from various foreign cultures. For instance, Rashid emphasizes to staff, "It's important not to have so many doctors go into the room at once. One doctor should communicate with the patient or family; others can listen. Sometimes patients get conflicting information, which confuses them. *Many patients or families say, 'Yes, yes, yes,' but in most cases have not understood a word that was said.* They tell me, 'I didn't understand.' I tell physicians to try to keep the primary physician involved, who knows the patient more personally than the team in the hospital. Patients then feel more comfortable and open to say what they want."

A chaplain can also directly assist patients and families when their culture differs markedly from that of the medical staff. As Rashid elaborated, "I also remind patients to be themselves, and talk back to the doctor—explain what they're feeling: 'Don't just sit and be bombarded with so much information that, in the end, you've got to figure out what the prognosis and diagnosis mean. Speak up if you don't understand. Have the doctor write down the long words.' I help families go online and look these up, to at least have a little basic knowledge of what's going on."

At the same time, cultures as well as faiths vary considerably across countries. Islam, for instance, is not monolithic. Muslims hail from different countries, and Muslim cultures in fact range widely. "I've seen Muslim patients from all over the world," Rashid explained, "including the African American community; and others who have gotten away from, their cultural identity and want to be more Americanized. I try to focus on the individual, what their cultural needs are and whether they are Sunni, Shia, or African American. All of us are equal in prayers, religious services, washing before prayer, and liking halal food, if available . . . When they want a bed pointing east, I say, 'Well, the Quran says you can pray flat, standing, sitting, or with your face turned east *or* west, especially if you're sick.' Most of them get it."

In hospitals without a Muslim chaplain, non-Muslim chaplains or providers can incorporate a local community imam. Judeo-Christian chaplains may feel more comfortable working with Protestant, Catholic, or Jewish patients than with Muslims. As Rashid continued, "Chaplains should make sure the patient's family and their imam are involved, or contact a Muslim chaplain. Interfaith chaplains should have a list of local mosque leaders. Family members have a particular mosque, and its imam or his representative can come and help guide them through end-of-life issues."

Yet hospitals often lack trained chaplains from outside Judeo-Christian traditions. An in-house Muslim chaplain brings obvious advantages, but the presence of such chaplains appears to vary with the hospital's size, patient population, and geographical location. "We had a Muslim imam as a trainee," Connie Clark reported. "He is now gone. But it was nice because we have a lot of patients from the Middle East. They connect themselves with community resources here." Yet in certain geographical areas, recruiting Muslim chaplains can be difficult. Brenda Pierson, in the Bible Belt, said, "I wish I could recruit non-Christian, non–Judeo-Christian chaplains. Unfortunately, in this region of the country, I can't. But we do have a couple of community members—imams and rabbis—and several Buddhist temples."

Needs for more diversity remain.

PART IV
APPROACHING THE END

11

"We sang my son into Heaven"

Re-envisioning "Heaven" and grief

I will never forget seeing my mother one last time in her coffin. The rabbi silently led me to the front of the hushed dark beige, dimly lit funeral parlor chapel before the guests had been admitted. He solemnly opened the pine coffin. I peered in. There my mother lay, a thin simple white shroud wrapped around her, as is Jewish tradition. Only the day before, we had spoken on the phone. I leaned over now and kissed her. Her cold skin chilled my lips. I recoiled. She was now a corpse. From deep inside me, tears welled up. I cried, flooded with grief.

Later that day, I helped bury her, shoveling a heavy metal spadeful of dark brown dirt onto her coffin. I turned the rough wooden handle sideways. The clump of earth slowly slipped off, dropped into the dark hole of her grave, fell and landed with a hard loud thud. Then silence. The image of her in that white shroud, and the sound of that dull thump still haunt me.

I wondered where her life had gone—all her wisdom, and the conversations and activities we had shared together over 60 years—my entire life! I alone now possessed our shared memories. If I forget them, they, too, would perish.

Arguably, the greatest mystery that has perplexed humankind is: *What happens to people's spirit or soul when they die*? Does the spirit that animated their soul, however we define that term, wholly vanish? As Victor Simmons, the VA chaplain, told me, "When I talk to a dementia patient whose mind is deteriorating, I ask myself, 'Where is his soul?' I wonder whether the soul deteriorates as well. Such patients sometimes come back, through music or pictures, for a moment of lucidity. What is that? Where is it from?"

In his 1973 Pulitzer Prize–winning book *Denial of Death*, the psychologist Ernest Becker wrote that Americans largely deny death.[1] Patients and families do so in manifold ways, struggling to make sense of their mortality—from confidence that they will see loved ones again in Heaven, to holding far more diffuse notions that some aspect of the self, soul, or consciousness or

Doctor, Will You Pray for Me?. Robert L. Klitzman, Oxford University Press. © Oxford University Press 2024.
DOI: 10.1093/oso/9780197750841.003.0011

just an "energy" persists in some way. Ideas about life continuing after death are ancient and ubiquitous—from Greek myths about Hades to Christian depictions of Heaven and Hell, Reform Judaism's more symbolic and metaphorical notion that we continue on through "our good deeds and in the hearts of those who cherished us," to modern scientific theories about the continuation of energy in the universe. "The ancients said the soul was in the guts," Victor Simmons observed, "because that's where you hold stress. The New Testament describes it in the heart. Today, it's in the brain."

Patients and families routinely grapple with questions about what happens after we die. In making sense of, and accepting the inevitability of, death, chaplains not only talk but also create and perform rituals and gestures that, even if small, can structure and frame these events.

Anthropologists have described the key roles of rituals in social groups— preserving group stability and offering ways of marking and understanding emotionally difficult life transitions such as death and dying.[2,3] All cultures follow bereavement rituals, which honor relationships with the deceased and aid in "saying goodbye."[2] Such practices often involve "rites of passage," helping surviving individuals reconstitute their lives and find a new identity.[4] These events can employ symbols and performance and can be psychotherapeutic and healing.[5]

Certain anthropologists have argued that contemporary American culture has minimized and de-ritualized such bereavement practices, and that rituals surrounding grief have lost meaning, becoming inauthentic and empty and leading to insufficient resolution of grief.[6]

But in hospitals, chaplains now pick up the slack, adopting key functions. While scholars have tended to view bereavement rituals as culturally prescribed, many chaplains are now, on their own, establishing such events for both leaving a patient for the final time and for grieving later. Cathy Murray, for instance, described a 19-year-old man who knew he was going to die imminently and wanted to donate his organs. The donation would occur after so-called brain death, not cardiac death. Doctors would bring him into the operating room [OR], remove his life support, and within five minutes start "harvesting" his organs in order to preserve their viability. The family wanted to be with him in the OR when he took his last breath. The surgeons refused, fearing the family would become distraught and delay the organ removal. Cathy had "tearful negotiations with everyone. The family finally said, 'We understand, and will just stay there for three minutes and leave, no matter what.'" So, they escorted the young man into the OR. Cathy asked the family if he had a favorite song. They said, "Amazing Grace." As the staff withdrew life support, the family and staff all sang the song. The staff all cried. Once they finished singing, his life functions stopped, and the family left."

Afterwards, the mother called Cathy and said, "Thank you for that gift. We will never forget it. *We got to sing my son into Heaven!*"

"We just gave the family the small space and opportunity," Cathy concluded, "to do what was meaningful for them." Clearly, chaplains can play emotionally vital roles.

In grief, beliefs in a hereafter, as defined by traditional religion, nourish many people. A 42-year-old mother I interviewed as part of a study on genetic testing[3] described how she was devastated when her two sons died from a congenital heart disease. Ultimately, she was able to find solace only by coming to feel that she would be reunited with them in Heaven. "That this happened to us *twice*," she told me, "that we buried *two* children, was very hard—*that God would allow that to happen!* I felt extreme anger and grief. My husband and I will always have to carry it with us. I will continue to have to come to terms with it for the rest of my life. Luckily, our church had a very strong priest who was very supportive and helpful. We're both practicing Catholics, and our faith was a huge support, helping us to eventually find peace with our grief. Through our faith, I worked through to a sense of relief—that they were in Heaven, with God—that someday we'll be together again. *That* helps with the grief."

Notions of Heaven and Hell can serve multiple functions—diminishing fears of death, offering reassurance, and motivating good behavior on Earth. These beliefs can infuse varied aspects of daily lives when people are healthy, but especially when death looms. Jacob, a devout Jewish radiologist in Chicago, felt devastated by his skin cancer diagnosis. He was on jury duty when his dermatologist paged him. "I remember his words: 'The biopsy results came back and they're not good. It's melanoma.' I was standing up in the telephone booth in the courthouse. I almost collapsed!"

His religious tenets about an afterlife succored him: "I was scared and thought a lot about dying. The biggest help was religion. Judaism is keenly focused on the next world . . . You're supposed to be looking only at how things could be better, and work toward that goal in this world or the *next* one. In the afterlife, you cannot do mitzvahs or good deeds, so you have to store up as many as possible in this world. You get rewards for the effort you put in . . . So, I was motivated to make every minute count. Death is not supposed to represent a tragedy. You can't do mitzvahs anymore, but the soul is not sad, because it's returned to where it came from. The next world is very real, not theoretical. That gave me a lot of strength and support.

"I gave more to charity, because that's what you're supposed to do when you're in a bad situation. Repentance, prayer, and charity are the Jewish prescriptions for getting out of a bad situation—to get God on your side. God stockpiles these things. He sets Nature going, but then just leaves it alone. We can alter it by our good or bad deeds."

A critic may disparage these beliefs as simplistic wish fulfillments, unfounded, mythological, or naïve, but because they uniquely help numerous patients face horror, they are hard to wholly malign. The promise and lure of Heaven are difficult to overestimate.

Terror of death leads even highly educated patients who had for years eyed religion warily to now embrace conceptions of an afterlife. These beliefs can aid patients psychologically in ways that medical science and even psychotherapy cannot. "I had a patient who was a very bright, high-powered, hard-nosed lawyer," a psychologist recently told me. "She had been raised Catholic but long ago distanced herself from the Church. Then, she developed cancer and was dying, and went back to the Church and spoke with a priest. At every psychotherapy session, she now told me how the priest was helping her in ways that I did not. It was humbling. She now believed in an afterlife—that she would go on. That belief was something that I could not give her." Psychotherapy still often pathologizes religious and spiritual beliefs, or views these warily rather than accepting them at face value. This strategy has certain rationales but may at times fall short in benefiting patients as much as possible.

When confronting these ultimate questions about death and afterlife, individuals, even if raised in one religion, frequently pick and choose concepts from multiple traditions, reformulating their own particular views. Many patients reject Christian teachings about a literal Heaven as a place where one sees or reconnects with departed loved ones, and instead uphold secular scientific facts about our atoms going on to create plants, insects, and other animals.

Chaplains can face challenges, however, when their own personal views collide with those of patients and families who fully trust in a traditional Christian Heaven, where the deceased reunite with their forbears. Margaret Dixon, for instance, does not believe in such an afterlife and has to decide how to respond when patients discuss or ask about it. "Mary Oliver described in *Bone Poem*,[7] she said, "how the rat eats the owl's bones and then becomes the owl—a wonderful cycle of nature. If I have to talk about resurrection, I could talk about it *that* way. We're not disappearing. We become something else. I don't think energy disappears. Energy animates us and our souls to join with the matter of the world and the universe."

She regularly sees patients with similar ideas. "An older Catholic patient was married to a Native American and very thoughtful about Native American culture and nature and how Native Americans hold the cosmos sacred. He felt very peaceful, ready to die, because he had a vision of where he was going: back to the Earth, perhaps the sky."

Unreligious patients, too, can believe in an afterlife. A social worker with cancer whom I interviewed believes, "After this planet, *we go to some other place*—a little less stressful. Really good things happen there. I consider myself 'a spiritual person.' I was raised Catholic, though my mother was Jewish, so we kind of got both religions. But I now don't identify myself with *any* established faith. I need to know science to take care of myself—so I can put my head on the pillow at night and say, 'I did the best I could.'" She relies on science but sees it as consistent with, not inimical to, a concept of Heaven (going "to some other place").

Many people have views about forms of an afterlife outside the Judeo-Christian traditions with which they were raised. Another patient I interviewed, who had breast cancer and underwent a mastectomy, leaned toward a vague form of reincarnation: "It's some kind of a renewal thing—like the American Indians believe."

Still others appeal to notions from science itself for a sense of continuity after death. Roy Gifford, for instance, a retired salesman with a serious chronic disease, trusts the laws of physics. A college science major, he now draws on this background in trying to grasp the metaphysical questions he now confronts, in part to try to make sense of his disease and its potential lethality. "I believe in *the Third Law of Thermodynamics*," he concluded. "Energy can neither be created nor destroyed; it merely goes on in another form. After death, I assume I'll be heading in another direction, one way or the other." He is now medically stable but still feels the hovering threat of death.

The possibility of cessation of all consciousness, of our very sense of self, is anathema and an affront. As Roy Gifford continued, "It's hard for me to imagine a total discontinuation of consciousness. If I thought that that was all there was, I would not have hesitated to terminate the experience, because I saw no point in continuing, it was so bad. So, I conceive of a continuation of consciousness, but I have no concept of what that will be like. It sounds very metaphysical, [American] Indian, and irrational, and I'm otherwise a very rational person. But to me, the idea of death being nothing is offensive.

"My friends who have died are just continuing on in a different form. I assume there's something out there, but I don't get bogged down in any one religious system. I take a little bit from here and there.

"*Still, it's not religious!* It's based not on any kind of religious belief but on a need to feel that this isn't all there is." He and many others find the brute fact of death difficult to accept, but nonetheless remain skeptical, if not antagonistic, regarding established religions.

Still other patients believe that something exists beyond them, even if they are fairly uncertain about the details. Though wary of organized religion, one physician with HIV, for example, "grew up Methodist" and felt that life or "energy" somehow "goes on" in an afterlife, though he had not formulated these thoughts further. "I believe in something bigger . . . I want there to be an afterlife . . . I don't know what . . . It's not necessarily Heaven or Hell."

Chaplains assist patients and families wrestle, however they do so, with these unfathomable issues.

How do *we* continue after *they* die?: Reframing grief

Chaplains help not only when patients die, but also afterwards, as families and staff grieve. Pastoral care providers have learned to approach such bereft family members gingerly, offering assistance only if the grief-stricken family members want it.

All deaths trigger bereavement, but the death of a child can cause even more intense grief than does that of an adult.[8] When the patient is a child, parents may feel enormous loss of not only their offspring but also their profound hopes and dreams about the child's future. Grief-stricken parents can feel like their world has been shattered, as well as intense guilt about not having somehow done more to save their child.

After a patient's death, Brenda Pierson, the pediatric chaplain, for instance, sends five emails to every family and then phones every three months for a year. "With every contact, I offer the family an opt-out. But usually, *we are the few people who still say their child's name*, talk about the child being dead, listen to the parents' stories, do not judge their tears, and are genuinely concerned about them and their other children's well-being." Over time, as their family and friends move on, these patients commonly feel isolated in their despair. Here, too, chaplains can assist. As Brenda added, parents complain that "'nobody says my child's name.' Other people are afraid it will make the patients sad—but they're already sad."

Following a patient's death, hospital staff, too, may mourn and experience guilt as well as fatigue, difficulty sleeping, and other physical and emotional symptoms; at times they may cry.[9] Especially early in their careers, however, doctors and nurses commonly feel awkward remaining in touch with families. Chaplains may be uncomfortable doing so as well, at least at first. "Initially, I was hesitant to reach out to families I didn't know," Cathy Murray reported. "I didn't want to burden them or add to their anguish: How can I call bereaved parents if I hadn't met the child? They'll wonder, 'Who is this stranger?' But I learned that I didn't have to know the patient in order to be a comforting presence. I just needed *to listen*. The fact that we cared meant a lot to them. I would phone the family, introduce myself, and say, 'I'm calling from the hospital to express our condolences, and just wanted to check in with you.' From that point, I just listen, sometimes for an hour. Acknowledging deaths and staying in touch with a family after a funeral, as they grieve, can be crucial. It is devastating to people when they come to you for the funeral and afterward never hear from you."

To help families, chaplains create and practice a variety of rituals. Before the COVID-19 pandemic, Cathy organized "a bereavement camp on Mother's Day weekend. For the first two years after their child dies, we invite families to attend a camp in a lovely location at no cost, through the generosity of donors. We do a memory-making workshop and group activities and provide alone time. Families tell us how meaningful it is."

Within a family, members can grieve differently, commonly without realizing it, generating conflicts. Spiritual care professionals help such family members better understand each other's perspectives. "Many families struggle," Cathy continued. "One spouse may be a more *intuitive* griever who needs to process and cry and emote—often the woman, but not always. The other spouse may be a more *instrumental* griever, doing the linear, 'I'm headed back to work.' They can clash. The wife says, 'He's not even grieving! He's already back at work!' The husband says, 'All she does is cry. I can't stand it!'" Cathy helps, asking them, for instance, "'Would you feel comfortable sharing with your husband what you need for yourself?' She'll say, 'He doesn't listen' or 'I shouldn't have to tell him. He should just know.' I've learned just to back off, listen intently, and support each family member as best I can, given their particular situation."

Such parents can struggle profoundly, but eventually find new ways forward. "One dad, whose daughter died, was literally a rocket scientist," Cathy explained, "very much the linear, 'instrumental griever,' focused on getting back at work as soon as possible. I was hesitant to suggest this, but sometimes if you invite an instrumental griever to try an intuitive style and vice versa, it can help—especially if the two parents are grieving differently.

"So, I invited him to draw what his grief journey had been like. At the next session, he had a drawing and discussed it: 'We were on the superhighway of life, had good jobs and a plan. Then, our child was diagnosed with a brain tumor. The car went off the road. We were derailed, through the guardrail, into the woods. The woods were so dense, I couldn't drive. I just got stuck. But eventually, I found I could drive again—on back roads, slower. I got to a point where I thought the view is actually pretty stunning from here. I'm driving slower, but can appreciate the trees, and the clouds, and my children.'"

Chaplains can guide such parents in reconstructing meaning. These patients may blame themselves and question their role, "feeling 'I must not have been a good parent,'" Cathy explained, "or if it was their only child, they wonder, 'Am I even still a parent?' I try to help, to understand their view of the world. If their view of the world is shattered, how are they going to rebuild it? People search to try to have a sense of what happens. They may draw on an amalgamation of religious and spiritual beliefs, about angels or talking to deceased family members through a medium. I can't ascribe meaning *for* them—that's not going to work—but just accompany them, and maybe pose some key questions.

"I ask, 'What does your grief feel like right now?' A lot of people use an image: 'It feels like my chest is being crushed by a boulder.' So, I use that image: 'We can try to chip away at that boulder, so that at some point maybe there will be only some manageable pebbles you can carry around with you, but you won't always feel crushed.' The point is to help them live this life as fully as possible.

"Some people's view of the world is *not* shattered, because their beliefs work, or they don't have any beliefs to be shattered, and some of those folks seem to cope just fine. Still, at the end, every parent I've ever worked with says, 'But I would trade it all to have my child back.'"

12

"When should we pull the plug?"

Aiding end-of-life decisions

At 78, my father was diagnosed with acute myelogenous leukemia, caused by skyrocketing overproduction of white blood cells. No effective treatment existed, and he would probably die in about 3 months, according to his doctor. But, his physician said, my father could try chemotherapy as an experiment, which might give him a 50% chance of living an additional 3 to 18 months. My father didn't know what to do, and asked me what I thought.

The possibility of his death frightened me. I had only recently completed my medical training and was enthusiastic about the advances of medical science. I encouraged him to try the chemo, yet it turned out to cause him intense pain and ongoing nausea. Three months after starting it, his blood counts improved, but he died. If I had known that outcome in advance, I would not have emboldened him. I don't know if, given the odds, we made the best decision. The question still nags me.

Fortunately, I have not yet had to confront such dilemmas for myself. I only signed an advance directive 6 years later, after my sister's death on 9/11. These documents indicate whether a person wants so-called heroic measures taken at the end of their lives and, if so, which—feeding tubes or machines that breathe for patients who will never awaken. I read the form in the tranquility of my lawyer's office, a soothing air conditioner humming quietly and calmly in the background, sounds of traffic and the rest of the world far away. I ticked off several boxes, indicating that I would not want futile treatments. At least I had now filled out the form, stating my wishes, to help my loved ones when I can no longer state my desires.

Unfortunately, most Americans never fill out these forms, and most such documents, even if completed, end up getting ignored or prove insufficiently specific.[1,2] Yet, end-of-life decisions can cause difficult tensions among doctors, patients, and families. Many patients' and families' religious and spiritual views shape decisions of whether to pursue certain aggressive treatments, and collide with complex medical realities. When families

Doctor, Will You Pray for Me?. Robert L. Klitzman, Oxford University Press. © Oxford University Press 2024.
DOI: 10.1093/oso/9780197750841.003.0012

demand that doctors provide additional medical interventions, despite the futility and the patient's prior preferences, physicians and hospitals frequently yield, partly fearing lawsuits. Unfortunately, it is often in crowded, chaotic ERs that patients, families, and doctors must struggle wrestle with these tensions.

For millennia, theologians and philosophers have wrestled with how to define and understand the two end points of life: when precisely it begins and when it ends. Today, patients and providers grapple daily with these puzzles in determining whether to pursue or avoid certain treatments. Yet since these questions lack definitive answers, patients and families do what feels right or comfortable, and can shift with time, affected by spiritual and religious beliefs.

In part, applying millennia-old religious texts to twenty-first-century technologies is clumsy at best, creating ambiguities in defining and applying tenets. "As patients take their last gasps," a physician who specializes in nutrition told me, "Orthodox Jewish families ask whether TPN [total parenteral nutrition—concentrated nutrients provided through a tube directly into a main artery to keep patients alive] is Kosher. I'll tell them, 'It's medicine.' They say, 'OK.' I sometimes use Yiddish words I know to help gain their trust."

When confronting death in ourselves and our loved ones, not just medically or even spiritually and religiously, but also psychologically and emotionally, chaplains help, partly by assisting with decision-making. Patients and families can clash with doctors in wanting either too much or too little treatment, pushing for aggressive but futile undertakings or rejecting beneficial medical interventions.

In recent years, the use of hospice and palliative care (so-called comfort care) has spread, enhancing the quality rather than the quantity of a patient's remaining life, emphasizing holistic, spiritual, existential, and religious, not just medical, issues. Hospice care aids people approaching death, partly by avoiding aggressive treatments to extend life at all costs when horrific side effects will likely ensue instead.

Yet both palliative care and hospice care confront barriers; even many doctors misunderstand them. Palliative care "is becoming more understood and integrated," Jack Stone explained. "Ten years ago, people thought, 'The death team is coming in—Team Kevorkian!' Our team has made a lot of bridges and inroads into many units of the hospital that were very resistant. Now there's trust, but it has taken a long time." Still, numerous families hesitate, insisting on aggressive interventions to try to save a loved one's life, even when these will fail.

The Joint Commission on Accreditation of Healthcare Organizations (JCAHO) therefore mandated that spiritual care needs to be available,[3] and recently that staff assess and be sensitive to patients' beliefs.[4] Yet the Commission does not specify *how* such care is to be delivered and by whom, how the information obtained should be incorporated into medical and decisions, and what to do if conflicts arise.

Pastoral care aids patients in coming to terms with death not just intellectually but also emotionally, partly by normalizing the complex feelings involved. "Patients say, 'I don't think I'm going to make it,'" Connie reported, "and they then look at me, wondering how I'm going to respond. I reply, 'I've never talked with anybody in an ICU who hasn't raised that fear.' They say, 'Wow! It's not just me?' Then, we talk about it. They've realized that death is coming, that they're mortal and not going to live forever. It's a potential crisis, whether the threat of death is real or not. That's scary. *Yet even just saying the 'd-word'—death—is very healing and helpful.* I say, 'How are you going to plan to live your life now?' I never know where these conversations are going to go. They're all different. From every one of them, I learn." Even uttering "death" in a sensitive manner can thus further these therapeutic processes.

Countless patients and families reject palliative or hospice approaches, seeing these as "giving up" on life or, as second best, not fully appreciating the potential benefits. Very religious patients often feel that life is precious and God-given, and that only God gives it and should hence be able to take it away. They push to "save life at all costs," emphasizing the "preservation of life," rather than making the patient DNR.[5] For some Orthodox Jewish patients, their rabbi in fact makes their decisions, not themselves.

Chaplains frequently try to shift families' views, but do not always succeed. "I've seen devout Catholic patients in the ICU who are never going to leave the hospital," Jim Adams, a Philadelphia oncologist and "lapsed Catholic," told me, yet "their families want everything done. The patients end up with tubes coming in and out of every orifice and all kinds of extra drugs. We're torturing the patient! But the family wants everything done because they're Catholic. So, we go along with that. In some states, doctors must provide as much end-of-life care as patients and families want, even if it will be ineffective. Sometimes, it takes me 6 months to gain the family's trust and convince them that I'm trying to *help*, not just withhold treatment. Understandably,

many African American patients, given past discrimination, similarly distrust us and want everything done."

Physicians feel disheartened when they view a treatment as futile, but a
patient or family nonetheless pushes to provide it. Often, the medical staff
do not understand why patients and families won't listen. Here, chaplains
can play critical roles, learning and conveying where patients are coming
from, and assisting the medical staff in grasping the patient's backstory. "One
parent just kept saying she wanted everything done for her son, who had irre-
versible brain damage from an accident," Cathy Murray reported. "The team
got worried: She's in denial, and is going to have a very complicated grief
process. The doctors showed her the brain scans and said, 'He's never going
to get better.' But she kept saying, 'Do everything!' I talked with her, and she
told me that two days before this incident, at the dinner table, the news was
on. It was about the Terri Schiavo case, and her son said, 'Mom, I don't get it.
Just because her brain doesn't work right anymore, they want to just throw
her away, and let her die? Don't throw me away because my brain doesn't
work.' So, there was no way this mother was ever going to decide differently
for her son, because he had given her a mandate.

"Once I shared that information with the team," Cathy continued, "they
stopped barraging her with facts and scans, and realized who she was as a
mother—which, to me, is a spiritual part of our being. The team had to just
back off, and support her and the little boy as best they could."

At other times, families may agree to discontinue futile invasive treatments,
but then doubt their decision. Routinely, chaplains help patients and families
with these conundrums. A chaplain may, for example, assure patients, partly
to help them avoid later regretting their decision, that they made the best decision they could, based on the information they had. "Many people second-
guess treatment options," Connie Clark noted. Such patients later "wish they
would have acted differently: 'If I had only known. If only I had done *that.*'
They wish they would have had perfect knowledge. But nobody has that.
So, I say, 'Look. What you did was *the next best step*. You didn't have perfect
knowledge. But in the absence of that, what you did made sense. You did the
best you could.'" In facing such fraught emotional strains, chaplains can thus
provide vital reassurance.

Yet the ever-mounting complexities of these choices make them difficult
to discuss. Chaplains face challenges, for instance, partly because patients
can feel ashamed even to disclose their worries about their fate and possible
demise. "Some patients don't want to express these fears to their family or

even their physicians," Connie Clark explained. "Patients say, 'I don't want to admit to my doctor my fear of dying. He'll think I've given up.' I understand. It's even more of a reason for patients to have an outlet, a neutral place to explore the existential issues that are part of most hospital visits."

Both within and among religions, differences surface. Members of a particular sect do not all necessarily want the same treatment, especially at the end of life. Many patients end up receiving fruitless care because they incorrectly assume their faith dictates it. However, their religion may also in fact advocate alleviation of suffering, which can mean withholding or withdrawing painful, unnecessary interventions.

Other patients and families disagree with doctors and reject medically-beneficial procedures. Jehovah's Witnesses pose these issues starkly. Few religions strain doctors as much. Founded in the 1870s by Charles Taze Russell, near Pittsburgh, Pennsylvania, this religion now has over 8.4 million followers worldwide, including 1.2 million Americans. The sect is probably best known for prohibiting blood transfusions,[6] based on its interpretation of certain Biblical lines. The story of Noah (Genesis 9:4) states, "You must not eat meat with its lifeblood still in it."[7] Leviticus 3:16–17 states "the priest is to burn the food on the altar as an offering made by fire, a pleasing aroma. All the fat is the LORD's. This is a perpetual statute for the generations to come, wherever you live: You must not eat any fat or any blood."[8] Jehovah's Witnesses believe that if they ingest blood, they will be outcast, cut off.

Religious groups differ in their interpretation of these particular Biblical passages. Kosher Jews, for instance, soak meat in brine to draw out blood, but accept blood transfusions to save lives. Jehovah's Witnesses, however, refuse all such transfusions. Difficulties arise, though. Many Jehovah's Witnesses face medical crises and will die without a blood transfusion. At many hospitals, if a Jehovah's Witness patient has a clearly documented refusal, doctors will not give transfusions. The Church has developed a list of acceptable alternative blood products that can sometimes help[9], but these alternatives often fail. Many members of this religion are therefore ambivalent. About half of pregnant Jehovah's Witnesses would in fact like to receive blood, if they would otherwise die.[10] Some Church leaders also say patients can later repent for receiving blood.

Many doctors will transfuse blood if a patient has not clearly documented a preference otherwise, and has not designated a medical proxy, cannot communicate, and will otherwise perish. Moreover, if the patient is pregnant, her refusal to accept blood will endanger the life of her future child, who cannot consent.

But physicians can also face quandaries about how to discuss these challenges with patients and families both before and after. Numerous patients in this religion who want to receive blood if their life depended on it do not want their family or fellow congregants to know this decision. One such woman told a surgical colleague of mine to transfuse her if needed. This doctor did, but the family then asked him if he had. Unsure what to say, he declared, "We have followed your mother's wishes exactly." "A female Jehovah's Witness came in with a massive pulmonary embolism," another colleague recently told me. "We gave her blood thinners, but she then bled into her leg, and her organs were not receiving sufficient blood. To survive, she would need a transfusion, but was barely conscious. One of her daughters, who was also a practicing Jehovah's Witness, said: 'Don't give her blood!' But we contacted the patients' two sons, who said to give her the blood." My colleague was unsure what to do.

This patient had filled out a from saying, "*Do not transfuse me with blood, even if I am dying and would otherwise live,*" but she had not signed it. A nurse had written on the chart "No Blood," but that dictum came from the daughter, not the patient herself.

My colleague wanted to overrule the daughter and transfuse the blood, but didn't know whether he would then tell the patient, after she woke up, what he had done. He decided nonetheless to administer it. "The daughter who opposed the transfusion resigned herself to the decision, but a few hours later was disappointed that her mother wasn't yet fully 'cured' and back to life. It took a day for her mother to respond."

Another colleague was uncertain what to do in the midst of operating on a Jehovah's Witness who had not signed a statement refusing blood, and who now needed a transfusion. The surgeon called the patient's mother from the OR. "Give her the blood!" the mother said. The surgeon was still unsure, but did so. Afterwards, he didn't know whether to inform the patient what he had done. When she woke up, he told her, wary of what she might then say. But she replied, "God is good!"

In life and death situations, patients' and families' views can shift.

13

"Mommy, when I die . . ."

Helping parents and children

When a young child dies, parents' hopes and dreams perish, too, triggering further existential, spiritual, and religious crises. Spiritual care for children raises different considerations than for adults. Cathy Murray described, for instance, a "two-and-a-half-year-old child who had been developing normally and then all of a sudden started losing developmental milestones. The doctors were tearing their hair out because they couldn't figure out what was going on—perhaps some sort of neurodegenerative disease. The child was a beautiful little boy, a little angel. By the time I met him, he couldn't walk, talk, or move. The mother said, 'I don't know if I can do this—*if I can be a mother to a child with no cognitive function.* My husband and I had planned everything out: We have a boy and a girl. I gave up my job to be at home with them. We were going to do playdates, live in the right neighborhood, focus on what we were going to do as a family and what was best for the children.' It was really painful for her. For a parent to be that honest is hard.

"This mother's sister," Cathy continued, "had asked her, 'Do you want me to have a priest come?' This mother replied, 'A priest?' The sister said, 'Yes, for the Sacrament of Reconciliation. You must have done something really bad if God could have done this to your child.' My first instinct was to say, 'Your sister is crazy! God did *not* do this to your child. She shouldn't have said that.' But instead, I held my own emotion back, and just said, 'What was it like when she said that to you?' I was ready for her to cry or get angry. But she said, 'It's a bunch of crap! I know that's not how God works. But I *would* like a priest to come, to do the Sacrament of the Sick for my child, and to talk with him about this.' So, I was grateful for my training, because I could have gone in and said, 'This is *not* how God works.' But that's not what she needed."

Though every death triggers existential questions, a child's demise adds several stresses and complexities. Dying children, teenagers, and young

Doctor, Will You Pray for Me?. Robert L. Klitzman, Oxford University Press. © Oxford University Press 2024.
DOI: 10.1093/oso/9780197750841.003.0013

adults are denied a full lifespan but are seen as innocent of any actions that may have incurred God's wrath. "Some of the hardest cases are young people dying," Jack Stone elaborated. "I now have a patient who's 23, a father of two or three kids, actively dying. I've been helping him as much as I can, but he has unfinished work. It's difficult to see someone whose life is being taken away, cut short, mourning that future, not being with their kids. It's tough to feel that and not get burned out, but rather to acknowledge that the candle of his life burned bright, but was small."

Moreover, children understand religious concepts much differently than do adults. Kids struggle to make sense of the ultimate mysteries of human existence, often in surprising and unanticipated ways. As Linda Porter, the pediatric chaplain and former journalist, explained, "The doctors couldn't tell a 7-year-old what caused her leukemia. So, she thought it came from God, and was angry she was sick. Her parents were divorced. Her father, a very conservative Catholic, told her, 'Maybe God gave you leukemia to see if you were strong enough to be the first woman president!' I thought, 'I can't get caught in that relationship between the father and child.'

"One day, the girl just looked at me and said, 'So, how *do* you die on a cross?' I was unsure what to say. But I will always tell people the truth, as appropriate. So, I said, 'You would bleed. It would be very painful and hard to breathe. At some point, you couldn't breathe anymore, and would die.'

"I tried to tell her, as much as a 7-year-old can understand, why Jesus was killed: Because He was a threat to the Roman Empire. She took it all in. Then I said, 'Would you like to pray?' She said, 'Yes. Can I say the words?' When a chaplain hears that, our little heart goes, 'Of course!' We held hands, and she said, 'Dear Jesus, *thank you for killing yourself so we can be good.*' I realized: This is the Christian message if you distill it down for a 7-year-old. I've been to seminary, and can talk about atonement. But until you talk to people and really listen, you have no idea of what they're thinking." Over their years of practice, chaplains continue to evolve and learn

Concepts of death and Heaven perplex children, who, as the psychologist Jean Piaget showed, think less abstractly and more concretely than do adults.[1] Linda described, too, "a 6-year-old boy whose brother had died 2 years before. They were adopted together, and because of the brother's death, the doctors discovered a genetic disease in the surviving boy, and he received a bone marrow transplant and did well. One day the boy said to his dad, 'Can you die in Heaven?' His father said, 'No, you can't die in Heaven. You live forever.' The boy look disappointed and said, 'I thought my brother could die in

Heaven and come back to me.' We say, 'You die and go to Heaven.' So, could he come back?"

Linda and other chaplains don't "get into heavy conversations with children, unless they take it there. But kids think about death. I don't bring it up with a child if the parent doesn't. And parents just don't go there in front of children. I'm also not good at having the parent stay outside of the room for a few minutes—I haven't yet figured out how to do that. It's not easy. I am afraid I'll feel I'm shooting them away. I have children of my own and think, 'How would *I* react as a mother if a chaplain came in and said, 'Can I speak to your son alone?' I'd say, 'No.' I would not be very nice. So, I assume other parents won't like it; and I just try to flow with it.

"I just talk to kids about what they're interested in," Linda reported. "They don't really bring up the big questions. One 14-year-old boy had bad cancer, and started describing a dream that clearly seemed about death. He was in the ocean and a shark smelled his scent and swam towards him. I thought, 'Holy crap! His mother is in the room, and is not going to like it if I let him keep talking about this.' Fortunately, because of how we were seated, I couldn't see her. I said quietly, 'What do you think that dream was about?' 'It's about me having cancer and I'm going to die.' I thought, 'Wow!' I said, 'OK, tell me more about that. How do you feel about that?' I encouraged him to talk about what the dream meant, holding my breath."

Death remains a taboo topic for many adults as well. "Even in the adult world," Linda continued, "patients and families are all trying to 'protect each other' by not bringing it up. Yet children are smarter than parents think. Kids know what's happening. But their parents aren't talking about it, which means that these kids can't—that doing so will hurt their parents' feelings. When I was 9, I figured out that Santa Claus wasn't real, but I didn't say anything to my parents: I didn't want to hurt their feelings. Kids know they're not supposed to talk about death. *Most of them know that they're dying, but that their parents don't want to discuss it.* So, they try to protect their parents, and their parents try to protect them. So, nobody talks to anybody! Even if I separate them, it's clear I'd better not bring it up. There's a wall." She tries to muddle through, improvising.

Parents also often hesitate to talk to children about siblings' deaths or dying. Linda described, for instance, "a Muslim family in our obstetrical unit. The baby died shortly after birth. Muslims ideally bury the deceased very rapidly. The baby was going to be buried that afternoon. It all happened quickly. A 6-year-old sibling asked, 'When am I going to meet my sister?'

The mother said, 'Oh, not yet. She's still sleeping.' The family was waiting for the father to come back, but the mother's comment made the social workers, nurses, and me very uncomfortable.

"I wondered what the 6-year-old was going to think when she realized what happened—how she was going to understand it. What happens to those short-stopped feelings? How does the mother grieve? They were being discharged the next day, so I don't know." While many chaplains follow up with a family after discharge, doing so can be hard, and not all do so.

Here and elsewhere, a chaplain must decide whether to intervene in parents' relationships with children, and if so how—what to do when parents' actions may not be in the child's best interests. These tensions clearly heighten with death and dying but can surface at other times, too. Parents may, for instance, inappropriately talk about sensitive personal issues when the child can overhear. "Some parents say things they shouldn't in front of their kids," Nancy Cutler, a South Carolina pediatric chaplain, said. "I don't know a good way to shut that down. One mother talked about her bad relationship with her husband and mother. I knew her son, the patient, was listening to every word, even though he was pretending to be asleep. He and his mother did not have a good relationship, probably because she was a lot like *her* mother. I cringed and thought, 'What was she thinking? And why don't I challenge her on any of this?' I wanted to say, 'God, please stop talking in front of your child,' bad-mouthing the other parent. I was born and raised in the South. Southern women are raised to be polite, to a fault." When death hovers, these situations become even more difficult.

Yet chaplains can help children in moving ways. Linda Porter described a hospitalized girl who said, "'I haven't lived. Everybody's going to forget me when I die.' So, we made a video. Everyone who had cared for her said, 'This is what I'm going to remember about you. I'll never forget you.' We FedExed the video to her home, and she got to see it right before she died."

Families may not even want to talk to a chaplain, because they don't want to confront the prospect of a child's death, and instead push to continue aggressive treatment at all costs, even when these interventions are futile. Though parents may want to avoid mentioning their child's possible death, older youngsters with terminal disease may nonetheless wish to discuss this reality, generating conflict. Cathy Murray described, for instance, "an amazing 13-year-old kid with cancer whose mother spent 3 years going around the country to try to find a cure. They ended up in our hospital for the entire last year of his life. She just could not face that her son might die. She could not even talk about it. When the medical team asked me to meet with her, she literally put her fingers in her ears and said, 'La-la-la-la-la. I can't hear you! Don't talk to me. I don't want to talk about this.' She did not want to discuss at all the possibility that the treatment might fail.

"Her son had a very strong faith from his grandmother, more than his mother. He listed his best friend as Jesus. Everything had to be frogs. I asked, 'Why frogs?' He said, 'F.R.O.G.: "Faithfully Rely On God!"'

"I kept visiting his mother, but she never raised anything related to death. I kept it light. Just 'Checking in today. How are things? Can I get you anything?' Finally, a month before her son died, she was able to say to him, 'I'm concerned that the treatment isn't working how we want.' But based on that comment, he was able to say, 'OK. So, Mommy, when I die, I don't want flowers because they're for girls. I want stuffed animals. Then, after the funeral, bring all the stuffed animals here to the hospital, and give them to all the kids.' He had it all planned out but could never talk about it because she wouldn't let him. He could see she couldn't handle it.

"She wasn't Catholic, but one day asked me for rosary beads and holy water. I connected her with the priest, and they became close. The mother said, 'I don't know much about holy water or rosary beads. But I have to know I've tried *everything*.' Other priests might have said, 'You're not Catholic. You don't understand what this is.' But he was wonderful with her.

"Another day, the mother said to me, 'I'm going to go make him a sandwich. Come down to the kitchen with me.' Then, while she was toasting the bread, she started talking. She said that at one point her son had said he had seen angels in the room, which distressed her. She told him, 'Stop it. Don't talk that way.' But I then worked with her. She finally said to him, 'When you talk about angels, it makes me sad, because I think it means you're not going to be here much longer.' He said, 'No, Mom. The angels are here to *help* me. When it's my time to go, Jesus will come for me.' The priest said to him, 'I've never seen any angels. What do they look like?' He said, 'There are six of them in the room. They fit in the room like a puzzle. One is always there; the others come and go. They are beyond beautiful.' Parents can misunderstand what children mean by such terms.

"Over time, I was able to build a relationship with her. Chaplains don't always have the luxury to do that—especially when patients are just in the hospital for a couple of days. The fact that we had a whole year made the difference. I'm not sure what would have happened if I saw them only in the last few days of his life.

"That summer, her son died. She was devastated. I worked with her in bereavement. The following spring, I said to her, 'Why don't we celebrate your son's life on his birthday?' She had honored his wish, and at the funeral had stuffed animals, not flowers, and now decided she would do a toy drive. She had to hire a U-Haul trailer to bring all the stuffed animals, and she distributed them on the unit."

Given parents' desperation and guilt at children's death and children's difficulty articulating their feelings, patients may seek signs from a deceased offspring of forgiveness or ongoing life—whether fully real or not. Cathy described how this mother "planned to get balloons and let them go in her son's memory, after distributing the animals. We met in front of the hospital, and she had three latex balloons—a red one, a blue one, and a Mylar one that said, *God loves you*. She said she couldn't buy a *Happy Birthday* balloon because she wasn't happy. We said a few brief words about her son and let the balloons go. It was beautiful. The next morning, she called me and said, 'That helped me so much. Thank you.'

"But a couple hours later, she phoned in hysterics. I couldn't even understand who it was. I saw it was her number, but I couldn't understand a word she was saying. I thought, '*Oh my God, what have I done?*' Finally, she put her teenage daughter on the phone, who said, 'You're not going to believe this. We were driving down the street where our old house was, where my brother and I grew up, three hours away from the hospital, and there were three balloons caught in the tree there. A red one, a blue one, and a Mylar balloon saying *God loves you*.'"

I asked Cathy, "What do you make of that?"

"It doesn't matter what *I* make of it, but what *she* makes of it. What *she* made of it was that her son was telling her that he forgave her. He had been tired of all the aggressive treatment and wanted to stop a lot earlier than she did, but kept going because she wanted to. She saw those balloons as her son saying, 'I forgive you,' as a sign of comfort."

At times, children's comments can startle and unnerve adults. "Every year, we have a tribute service to honor the children who had died that year, and a bereaved parent speaks," Cathy continued. "One year, the bereaved parent had had a daughter who died at age 4 from a brain tumor. This daughter had a forceful little personality. When you go into surgery, you can't wear anything. But this daughter made the doctors take her in there with ruby slippers on from *The Wizard of Oz*. After she had been gone 2 years, the mother got pregnant and had another daughter. This new little girl never knew her deceased sister, but they talked about this sibling all the time.

"One day when the little girl was 3, they were driving in a part of town where they never went because of too many memories of the older, deceased daughter. There was a garish purple-and-pink Victorian house, and the older, deceased daughter used to say, 'Mom, I'm going to live there when I grow up.' As they're going down that street, the younger girl pointed at the same pink house and said, 'Mommy, that's the house where my sister and I used to play in Heaven before I was born!'"

Mysteries persist.

14

How close or distant to be

Balancing and ending relationships with patients

Late one Friday afternoon during my training as a psychiatrist, a frail, de-pressed elderly woman hobbled into the outpatient clinic, wondering if life was still worth living and contemplating suicide. She was petite, with short hair, wore a pink dress and gold earrings, and had several medical problems. I thought she was probably not a very high risk for actually trying to kill her-self over the weekend, and I decided not to hospitalize her in a locked, sterile ward, but instead let her return to the comfort of her own home. I told her that if she got more depressed, she should come to the emergency room.

But over the weekend, as I brushed my teeth and watched TV, I found my-self thinking and worrying about her, wondering if I should have been more cautious and hospitalized her, and whether I should therefore call to see how she was doing. I didn't have her phone number with me, but could ask di-rectory assistance. Or should I instead just wait until Monday? I wondered whether, if I phoned her, I would be overly revealing my own novicehood and anxiety, and be crossing some professional line or perhaps even end up further worrying her about the potential seriousness of her condition.

But my concern kept nagging me. In the end, I dialed her number, and took a deep breath. In a faltering voice, she told me that she was still depressed, but no more so than on Friday. "I'm really glad you called," she added. "I'm here all alone." She later gave me a small plant for my office, in appreciation.

Drawing boundaries with patients is not always easy. Over time, I have sought to maintain "detached concern"[1]—to remain concerned, but also somewhat detached, to remain objective. But this exquisite balance can be tough to maintain every hour of every day. Trainees, in particular, like me with this elderly patient, sometimes struggle.

Chaplains, too, face difficulties in maintaining appropriate professional distance, and staying neither too close nor too far. Despite their dedica-tion, these providers encounter various challenges, including moral distress, burnout, and rejections from patients and families.

Doctor, Will You Pray for Me?. Robert L. Klitzman, Oxford University Press. © Oxford University Press 2024.
DOI: 10.1093/oso/9780197750841.003.0014

Maintaining professional distance

In varying ways, chaplains may either overidentify or under-identify with a patient. As Kristine Baker, the Texas chaplain who drew on metaphors, observed, "The two big errors chaplains make are thinking that a patient is *just* like them, or is *nothing* like them. I just worked with a trainee who, because of her religious tradition, had a hard time with transgender patients, thinking that she had nothing in common with them. So, I worked with her to see points of identification. Other trainees *over*-identity and end up intervening in ways that are a function of *themselves*. We're not like anybody else, but we also have a little in common with everybody.

"Some trainees need to know how different they are from the patient," Kristine elaborated, "so they don't overidentify, while others need to realize how similar they are with patients who, for instance, are grieving after a miscarriage. Trainees have trouble relating, and say, 'I've never lost a baby.' I reply, 'No, you have never lost a baby, but you *have* lost dreams. You know something about loss.' That's how we can connect with each other."

At other times, spiritual care providers feel others' pain too closely. "Chaplains make the mistake that a lot of people do," Cathy Murray explained. "We get so overidentified with someone that we feel their hurt, loneliness, and pain for them, but leave them there. Hopelessness is always a countertransference response. So, if we feel hopeless, we're projecting our assumption about their future onto them. That's not fair. I tell chaplains to say: 'Yes, it's bad.' There's a lot of suffering in the world, but we can't live there. We don't know what their future's going to be. But some people never get out of that. That doesn't do anybody good."

In drawing on their own personal experiences and views, physicians as well as chaplains need to carefully separate these perspectives and not let them cloud perceptions of what is best for the patient. Connie Clark, for instance, described a physician and father "who chose to remove his child from artificial life support at the end of life, and often uses that story in trying to get other parents to make the same decision. But rather than listening to families, he comes in and tells them, '*I did it*. I know how hard it was. But I think it's time for you to do it, too.' I keep asking him, 'Do you think this story is helpful today?' Yet he keeps doing it.

"I organized a class called 'Grace at the End of Life,'" Connie continued, "about how staff 'do death' here—based on their own death experiences. We talk about even being able to say the word 'dead'—why plain language and allowing a family to hold their *own* spiritual beliefs when their child is ill are important."

Confronting patients' and families' rejections

When asked what their biggest challenges and more rewarding interactions have been, several chaplains discussed getting rejected by patients and/or families, and then having to decide how to respond. Patients and families mostly welcome, and respond favorably to, chaplains, but at times rebuff them.

Patients and their family members may not all agree on whether to accept or refuse a chaplain's visits. Patients may initially decline to see a chaplain but subsequently be persuaded otherwise by family members. As Sister Francine, the nun, reported earlier, when one elderly man said, "We don't need you," his wife convinced him otherwise and he ended up grateful.

Patients or families turn down pastoral care for various reasons: wanting a chaplain of their own faith or gender, feeling angry or wary of religion, minimizing the illness, or misunderstanding what these professionals do. Such responses can sting, especially early in a chaplain's career, but hurt less over time as these individuals learn how best to react.

Countless atheist patients who initially rebuff a chaplain nonetheless ultimately shift and appreciate and benefit from the person—often despite their initial inclination. "When patients tell me they're atheists," Sister Francine, explained, "I just say, 'That's OK. We are happy to talk with everyone.'" Usually, she eventually finds a way to connect with the patient.

Certain patients and families prefer or request a chaplain of their own faith, generally before speaking at length to the chaplain assigned to them. Over time, spiritual care providers alter their practices to present themselves in ways that patients or families might accept. "When I started, we were just supposed to show up—anybody from any religious or non-religious tradition," William Gibson explained, "and just introduce ourselves as a chaplain, and offer support. We didn't need to identify where we were coming from. Let the patient or family choose to accept us or not. Our dress may disclose our religious affiliation. If a Jewish patient says, 'I only want a Jew,' or 'I only want a rabbi'—which is the religion with which I was raised—I tell them I'm Jewish, which usually lowers their guard. Some Christian families really only want a Christian chaplain . . . I then refer them to a Christian colleague."

Yet, particularly at night, a chaplain of every faith is usually unavailable. Chaplains on call must then judge what to say. "I've changed my practice," William continued, "for when a family says in the middle of the night that they want a Baptist or Pentecostal chaplain, and I'm the only one in the hospital, I now introduce myself and say, 'I know you're asking for a Baptist chaplain, and I'm Jewish, but I'm the only one here right now. I want to see if I could still help. If I can't, I'll see if I can track down someone else tonight, but I don't know if anybody will be available. I can try to get someone here in the morning.' I almost reject *myself*, and give them full license to do so. I am not pretending, intruding, or asserting myself. I have found that they then welcome me in. Their guard really only goes up when there's vagueness and ambiguity. I'm clear about the difference from the very start, respecting the family's boundary, and presume that they won't want me. *Since I've made that change, I've never been turned away!* In those situations, families really don't care much about the religious boundaries in the ways they usually do. Not that they don't care about them at all, but they are open—more permeable than usual." Such transparency can serve as a model of openness in other interactions more generally as well.

At other times, a chaplain, rebuffed by a patient on religious grounds, can try to recast the issue. Kristine Baker described a trainee who said, "I can't go see this patient. She wants a born-again Christian." Kristine responded, "Let's talk about 'born again.' Are you going to let one group of people define that for you?'" This trainee automatically assumed what the patient meant. "I said, 'In some ways, we're all born again every day—sleep is a form of death. Instead of assuming you know what she means by 'born again,' get more comfortable with language like that. She's trying to figure out if you're safe: 'Are you going to judge me? Are you in my tribe? Will you respect my values?'"

Other patients and families reject a chaplain because they are atheists and suspicious of religion in general, given that religious institutions have abused, spurned, and dismayed many patients. In the Bible Belt of the South, Brenda Pierson, for example, opined, "My hospital reflects the culture where we live . . . We are moving in a good direction toward being more inclusive and aware that inclusivity is healthy, but we are very much a product of our environment . . . People here utilize and are familiar with evangelical Christian language . . . The Bible is used as authoritative and as club and battering ram." Evangelical language "is used, misused, and abused."

For millennia, churches have caused both good and bad. Victor Simmons described how the Bible, for example, has been employed to justify racism: "During the Civil War, Northern and Southern pastors were preaching opposite messages, both using the Bible as their common text. A lot of our Biblical convictions come from our culture. We mix up culture with conviction." Similarly, "Christian racists go after Jews. I really don't get that. You'd be racist against Jesus!"

Chaplains therefore seek to engage circumspect patients and come to terms with such harm—distancing themselves from it, while still pursuing the potential benefits of religion and spirituality. "Religion is such a double-edged sword," Linda Porter, the former journalist, observed. "They turn God into a bunch of sound bites. But that's not me."

Consequently, when facing rejection on these grounds, chaplains seek to understand and engage the patient's underlying beliefs, to ascertain why— what past bad interactions may have occurred. "Religion is not always a good thing for people," Jack Stone elaborated. "A lot of people have been abused in religion, temples, and churches. Not only physically or sexually, but psychologically and spiritually. So, people might be very scared or put off by a chaplain, or think 'thanks, but no thanks.'"

Still, patients vary in their degrees of skepticism or hostility toward religion. Some patients at first refuse to speak with Sister Francine, for instance, but eventually usually do so, and appear glad. "I visited one family whose child had just died in the OR," she elaborated. "The wife was sitting on the floor, screaming, 'This isn't happening! This didn't happen!' The husband was crying. I sat down beside her but didn't say anything. What could I say? I gave her a tissue. I always carry around tissues." She removed from the pocket of her white cardigan a clear plastic sandwich baggie, containing a few tissues, showing me. "Each morning, I fill it with five tissues. I usually end up using them all.

"After a few minutes," Sister Francine continued, "I told the woman on the floor that I was from the chaplaincy department. She said, 'We don't need you.' I was with a trainee who thought I would then just leave. But instead, I simply sat there on the floor with them and let them grieve. Finally, the mother began to speak about what happened . . . The student has continued to see them—it's been several years. The couple and the student were all Jewish." Even those who seem atheist may benefit from such interactions to overcome existential despair, especially at the end of life.

In responding to a leery patient, chaplains frequently draw, too, on their own personal approaches or religious perspectives. "Because I'm a Buddhist," Jack continued, "I can play the nonthreatening Buddhist card—it's not about precepts to proselytize. We're not allowed to convert people. I don't often get refused, but when I do, My tail's between my legs—it hurts my pride. I understand and respect the patient's decision."

In responding, chaplains try not to take rejection personally, but see it as an important manifestation of a patient's own agency and freedom. "I'm the only person that they can really kick out of their room," Jack Stone continued. "They can't say to the doctors: 'Get out of my room!' or 'No, it's not a good time.' When we chaplains say, 'I got rejected,' 'refused,' or 'kicked out of a room today,' I reply, 'Wow, congratulations!' Because in this small, limited, vulnerable time in their life, wearing only a bathrobe and a number on their wrist and having a roommate, with deprivation everywhere—it's not a healing environment at all!—you gave them autonomy, the opportunity to say 'no.' And you left. Isn't that a wonderful thing?"

In conservative areas such as the South, chaplains occasionally face rejection because of their gender. One male patient told Kristine Baker, the Texas chaplain, for example, that he didn't believe in female ministers. "I'm a white woman and he was an African American man," Kristine explained. "Perhaps white people have imposed their views on him and disrespected him, and he felt that I might do that . . . I said, 'It sounds like you have a lot of strong opinions.' He said, 'I do.' I said, 'I'm always interested in what people believe. Tell me about those strong beliefs.' He said he was 'very conservative.' His tradition opposed ordination of women. I said, 'What was that like, growing up? How did you learn about that?' I just let him talk. He didn't want me to try to convince him that women could be ministers. But he got so engaged with his story that it didn't matter anymore. He felt like I cared about him. And I *did* care about him. I was really curious about his story." Chaplains can thus work to counteract biases by nonetheless attempting to interact with these patients, even about such wariness, hesitancy, or opposition.

Patients can also refuse to speak to a chaplain because they are angry at family members, the cosmos, and/or God but do not want to discuss the situation or probe these feelings. These spiritual care providers are, however, frequently able to help. "A lot of my best visits started with, 'I don't need no goddamn fucking chaplain,' " Kristine Baker continued. "The sister of a man who died recently told me that. I said, 'That is fine. I can leave if you want. I'll be glad to, but I'd like to just be here with you since you've been by yourself and your brother has just died.' She said, 'I hated that fucking idiot!' I replied, 'Wow. You've got a lot of strong feelings. Tell me about that.' She said, 'He abused me. I'm glad he's dead.' She was hinting: 'And now you can leave.' I told her, 'I'm so sorry that happened to you. It sounds like you're relieved.' She said, 'Yes, I'm fucking relieved!' I said, 'I can see why.' She was rough around the edges, tattooed, and used to offending people, kicking them out. But in the end, we made a beautiful connection. She wasn't redeemed, but let me in and began to integrate who she was in front of me, saying, 'I'm glad you're here.'"

Angry at God, other patients remain vehement in refusing chaplains, who simply then leave. As Brenda Pierson reported, "Several families have told me, 'Get out of my room. Get out of my sight. There is no God to me. A God who would let my child die is no God to me!' Sometimes, there's no language at all. Just un-engagement. We respect that and step out. We continue to remain available for the staff. When they can control nothing else, they can control whether I am in the room."

At times, patients and families do not want to see a chaplain because they minimize or deny the disease, responding in short answers to close the conversation. One chaplain, when asked what her hardest or most challenging cases have been, described an Orthodox Jewish woman who had "a son turn completely yellow because of jaundice. I asked her, 'How is everything?' She said, 'We're *fine!*' 'How is your son doing?' 'He'll be *fine!*' she said," with a definite snap to abruptly end the conversation. "I asked my supervisor what to do. She said, 'The mother's not ready yet. When she's ready, she'll let us know, and we will be there for her.' Patients might benefit from talking to us, but not yet want or feel ready to do so, and chaplains need to know how then to proceed."

A patient or family can decline to see chaplains, too, because of misunderstanding these professionals' roles, functions, or identity—the fact that contemporary chaplaincy takes nondenominational approaches, focusing not necessarily on religion per se, but rather on broader issues of meaning, purpose, and hope. Many patients at first rebuff chaplains, seeing the role as more strictly religious per se. At these times, medical staff can help, facilitating such visits. As Cathy Murray said, "Sometimes it's difficult to get in the door because patients or families have some preconceived notion that a chaplain is only going to want to talk about religious 'God' things . . . Once you get in, as long as you honor that person and that person's wishes, it is fine, because we all wrestle with what suffering means, what our life has meant, and whether we have lived to its purpose."

Other patients and families fear that the chaplain will now scrutinize and criticize them and/or their beliefs. As Brenda Pierson reported, "When I was a brand-new chaplain and went into the room and said, 'Hi, I'm your chaplain today,' people automatically felt judged. They'd say, 'Oh, we go to church!' as if I were going to preach to them about Jesus. My guess is that they thought that they weren't being good Christians and that I was there to judge that. I'd say, 'Good.' I never ask people where they go to church. It doesn't matter."

In their responses to such rebuffs, chaplains vary. Initially in their careers, they may find such refusals unsettling, but then gradually develop more confidence and abilities to reply more effectively. Marvin Beck, the New Hampshire chaplain at a small hospital with a supportive CEO, described how "7 or 10 years ago, I would have taken it personally. . . I felt a little more insecure. But, I don't now."

At times, chaplains' gently persistent presence eventually succeeds. Patients seeing a chaplain regularly on wards, and sensing his or her broader role, may change their minds. A well-known Jewish philanthropist had recently been admitted to Sister Francine's hospital. "I introduced myself to her. She said, 'No, thank you. I don't need you.' But every day, I saw her in the hall, and just said, 'How are you doing?' One day, she waved me in and said, 'OK, come in.' Every day since then, we've spoken at length."

These processes can, however, take time. Adam Quincy gave an example of the challenges involved. "A philosophy professor I know was raised Catholic and had a terribly jaundiced experience of Catholicism. Over 10 years, I have won him over by how I've approached it: I respect him and his love for science, his 'you can't prove that God can do this' perspective. When they feel you appreciate it, they're more willing to look at your stuff, and see if they can find *common ground* with you. Here in the South, you won't necessarily get hardcore flaming atheists or Satanists, but functional or operational agnostics who really don't care one way or the other, and just have a bad view of religion and feel it's irrelevant. Usually, they've been hurt by something and never really processed or gotten over it. It's great to take a chance and say, 'Well, it sounds like there's a lot there. What happened?' If you open the door a little bit, they might say: 'I don't know if I really want to talk about it, but the bottom line is that I was raised in the Catholic Church, and a nun used to beat me.' Typically, it's a terrible experience with religion that's caused them to move away from organized religion. Many of these people will say, 'I'm spiritual, and believe in God, but all these guys organizing religion are a bunch of yoyos.' That's why they're apathetic about it."

Yet Adam and other chaplains tend to welcome such challenges. "I don't want to walk in the room and the patient is perfectly religious," Adam explained, "and just recites what he or she knows. I want something more difficult and richer because I then get to learn something about myself, and about people and chaplaincy."

The fact that many patients who initially decline a chaplain nonetheless end up appreciating such a visit suggests that they often had misunderstandings about these professionals. Chaplains' inventiveness and persistence—in spite of such negative reactions—repeatedly impressed me.

A small study of several Australian chaplains found that patients may reject them because of concerns that the conversation will be too "intimate" or because the patient does not speak English,[2] but additional reasons clearly exist, along with strategies for responding.

The men and women with whom I spoke also help make sense of data reported in other research, showing that most hospitalized patients, when queried, said they did not want to see a chaplain, but that those who ended up doing so were later more satisfied with their care than were those who had not received such a pastoral care visit.[3] Patients may not want to talk to a chaplain but are more satisfied with their care if they nevertheless do, because they had *misconceptions* about pastoral care. Misunderstandings of chaplains by physicians have been described[4] but occur as reasons for patients' rejections, too.

Ending visits

Chaplains struggle with not only how to respond to rejections but also how to end visits and interactions that went well—where and how to conclude both individual conversations and longer, ongoing relationships with patients and families. These spiritual care providers come to develop close therapeutic relationships with patients and families regarding emotionally charged issues. The average length of chaplains' visits is 13.6 minutes, with a range of 5 minutes to 3 hours,[5] raising questions about how long should each visit last, and how chaplains should decide. Other types of healthcare providers, including physicians and psychotherapists, too, need to gauge where and how to establish boundaries with patients and when to say "goodbye." Psychotherapy sessions typically have fixed, pre-established lengths (traditionally 50 minutes), and therapists are paid per visit. Though psychotherapy is clinically effective and frequently very cost-effective, insurance companies commonly cover only limited numbers of sessions.[6] Usually, psychotherapists and patients jointly discuss and explore, in advance, patients' eventual termination and plans for life afterwards.[7]

Chaplains face murkier questions and uncertainties, and rely on both verbal and nonverbal cues to gauge how long to remain with each patient and family and how to navigate each relationship. Little concrete consensus exists on lengths of visits. "There's not much definition around what's the correct amount of time to stay," said William Gibson. "In these interactions, there's a lot of *nonverbal intuition, communication, and reading between the lines.* The other day, I visited a family sitting in a vigil with a dying loved one. It wasn't exactly clear *who* had requested me, which is often the case—whether it was the family or the nurse, and whether the family assented. So, I wasn't even sure if this family *wanted* me there. I introduced myself very carefully. They welcomed me in. I spoke with them and offered, at their request, a prayer for their loved one. Then there was some conversation, but also silence. Clearly, I was not the focus of attention. I basically just laid my hand out there for the family and said, 'I don't want to abandon you, or hover, either. I may just take my leave, and let this be time for just you and your family.' They said, 'Yes.' I don't know how useful or meaningful they perceived my visit. They were polite, but might have been hiding their actual, harder feelings about my presence."

Chaplains must determine how to respond to these cues, which may be implicit rather than explicit. These professionals routinely self-reflect to bolster their practice. "I wonder: Was I helpful or am I just kidding myself?" William pondered. "There's a whole balancing act. At times, we can try to clarify that. Other times, it's not appropriate to even try. I just have to hope that I did the best I could, and that it was helpful, and if it wasn't, try to find some peace with that. Everybody is not going to explicitly thank us or even feel grateful."

"It sounds like your interaction with that family certainly didn't hurt," I said.

He remained unsure. "Maybe I didn't do enough, and could have done more," he replied. "If I leave too soon, that worries me. I critique my own practice and am always trying to improve it. After that patient died, I contacted one of the family members, just to see how they were doing. It came from my heart. I wasn't curt, but it wasn't an in-depth call. I didn't ask 'Hey, did you guys like my visit?' That's not right. I think I basically did right by that family. I don't think I'm doing harm, over-intervening in people's spiritual lives or in the ways they're coping. But . . ." He remained unsure.

The amount of time a chaplain spends with particular patients or families ranges widely based on their particular concerns, needs, desires, and receptivity. Visits may average only a few minutes, but occasionally last an hour or more, and chaplains face dilemmas about appropriate lengths of time with certain patients and families. "When to make one's exit is *ambiguous*," William added, "It varies so much. With non-vocal patients in the ICU, the median time is around 20 minutes. Other times, I'm there with families for hours or just for a minute or two—a quick little blessing on whatever's happening. I'm envious of friends in other fields with more clarity—although in a lot of areas, that clarity is probably kind of misleading."

Ending relationships

When patients and families leave the hospital, chaplains confront questions about ending relationships that have sometimes extended over intense months or even years. These professionals often become attached to patients and their families, and boundaries can be difficult to draw and maintain. Millions of seriously ill patients survive their hospital stay but then die at home. Emotionally, for chaplains as well as families, these patients' deaths can be hard. "We get close with some of our patients," William said, "and end up having long-term relationships."

On their own, several chaplains have developed ways of continuing these connections symbolically after discharge by creating memorial objects. Jack Stone, for example, makes posters for not only unresponsive patients (to whom providers and families might thereby feel more connected) but also for other patients to feel an ongoing, supportive bond with him. He explained, "I write all the words and themes that came up in our visits—forgiveness, love, self-care, self-love, trust, faith, or hope—to acknowledge the work we did together. At our final meeting, I give patients or families the poster and say, 'Goodbye. I appreciate the time together we've had. This might be our last visit together, but I want you to know that I made a handprint of myself here—a little tiny token—you can touch my hand. You can hold my hand whenever you need me.'"

He and other chaplains seek to instill among trainees creative methods for addressing these challenges. "I teach younger chaplains to try this," Jack explained, "to learn these processes, *to think outside the box*. It's not always about prayers. And we're not going to fix anyone overnight. If someone's lived with obsessive-compulsive disorder or anxiety their whole life, and are now at the end of life, we're not going to wave a magic wand and take that away. They're frightened, scared, unattuned to talking about their feelings, or lacking the bandwidth to internally reflect or articulate their feelings. But we can *walk with them on the journey*, and experiment and have a sense of play."

Chaplains face dilemmas about whether to continue to call, see, or stay in touch with a patient or family following a hospitalization. Initially, some do so—visiting patients who are now elsewhere. "In the beginning, I would continue to visit my patients who went to hospice," Jack said, "because I had a special connection with them, or they begged me to come. Now, I very rarely do that. Earlier, I *over*-functioned as a chaplain. I can't go to the hospice for all of my patients. There has to be a boundary."

For chaplains, ending ongoing relationships can be personally hard. "I've learned that I don't have to be present for the moment of death," Jack continued. "Initially as a chaplain, I'd keep coming back to the room and checking in. I didn't want to miss the patient dying. When I did miss it, I felt I had missed the precious point. Four or five of my patients have literally taken their last breath in my arms. That is a wonderful blessing. But I never know when that's going to happen. I can't make that happen, and shouldn't have that as a goal. Now, every visit might be my last."

Nonetheless, chaplains can also still poignantly mourn these losses afterwards. William Gibson, for instance, described a patient who died after a double-lung transplant. "I saw him all the way through the surgery. We stayed close and texted—he would give me parent advice. There was a lot of mutuality to the relationship. I'm still grieving. A lot of our best work is with seriously ill people who die. My friends just had our fantasy baseball draft, and I picked the player that I knew this patient would have wanted—it was a little tribute to him. I look for ways to honor patients."

Feelings of closeness can be mutual, as when seen families sometimes request that chaplains speak at patients' memorial services.

Chaplains facing moral distress

Chaplains face challenges in not only getting rejected and ending relationships but also in experiencing moral tensions, for instance, when dealing with child abusers. When forced to act contrary to their values, these providers feel moral distress. Such moral strain has been examined among

nurses, when they are unable to "preserve all interests and values at stake"[8]—
for instance, when told by a physician to administer treatments that they feel
will harm the patient. Nurses are then compelled to place institutional hierarchy and needs over their sense of how best to help the patient.

Chaplains experience particular moral tensions when working with
maltreated children. These professionals see parents abuse children, more so
during the COVID-19 pandemic, since schools were closed and children and
their parents had to stay home, at times in cramped housing. "Children get
sick and may die," Cathy Murray said. "But to work with children who were
intentionally harmed by patients who were supposed to protect them was
very hard for me and for staff. Sometimes we see 'shaken baby syndrome': an
adult shook the baby so fiercely that the baby was injured and usually has
permanent brain damage and ends up dying. We'll know that the man at the
bedside with his girlfriend or wife shook the baby. She says, 'Don't let the police take him away!' The staff and I are thinking, 'Get him out of here! He hurt
his innocent child!' It is tough working with the staff so that they can continue to be compassionate to these adults, until he has been arrested. The reality is that the police aren't going to come into the room to take him away, so
I can reassure the mother about that. I say, 'While we have this time together,
let's focus on this little one.'"

Such abuse disturbs hospital staff, who can be torn about how to respond.
"During the COVID-19 isolation, we have seen an uptick in child abuse,"
Brenda Pierson reported, "Some staff want physical harm to come to the
abuser. But other staff say, 'That poor abuser must be suffering. What abuse
must he have suffered in his early life?'

"My job," Brenda continued, "is to listen and reflect on what the people on
both sides are saying. I don't have an answer, and don't pretend to whip out
Scripture or a spiritual platitude that presumes to have an answer about why
such evil exists. I allow space for whatever is being expressed."

Chaplains regularly aid medical staff with such moral distress. Brenda, for
example, says to staff, " 'Yeah, it's the third one this week, huh?' Or, 'This is the
fifth case in a row you've worked on that's turned out this way.' I'm privileged
to provide spiritual care for staff. The image I have is of people vomiting out
vileness. I'm simply holding the bucket that gets the vileness. I then carry it
out of the room."

The sheer brutality of adults abusing innocent children clearly triggers
questions of why such evil exists and persists. Patients and families frequently ask Brenda, "Why is there evil?" "But I don't hear it as a genuine

question," she reflected. "They're not really asking for an answer. So, I agree with them: 'This is the worst kind of evil.' Depending on the circumstance, I may redirect and reframe or say, 'It's *absolutely* evil. But when you helped that child, he experienced such grace and love from you! I'm grateful you were here with him today.' Or, 'I saw how you interacted with that parent, even though you thought the parent was abusive. That must have taken a lot out of you! Tell me about that.' Often, they cry because during the event, they held in their emotions, and afterward feel free to express it—how helpless, angry, sad, dismayed, and exhausted they feel."

Burnout

In grappling with these and other emotionally draining challenges, chaplains themselves can get burned out. Burnout occurs when employees experience emotional fatigue, lack of personal accomplishment, depersonalization, cynicism, detachment from the work, loss of idealism, and withdrawal,[9,10,11] and has been found in up to 43.2% of physicians.[12] Individuals who feel that their work constitutes a "calling," experience positive outcomes, but also potentially negative ones, including physical and emotional exhaustion, workaholism, and exploitation by organizations.[13]

COVID-19 heightened these stresses for chaplains, patients, families, doctors, and nurses. As Connie Clark described, the pandemic added a "layer of grief onto what was already difficult" and tapped "into unresolved or fresh grief we had of our own loved ones who had died." Chaplains and other staff struggle to maintain a professional stance and check their emotions, but at times these strains can erupt.

Particular cases can trigger outpourings of such feeling. "Last December, right before Christmas, I hit a wall," Connie said. "We had a post-COVID surge and our ICUs overflowed. I looked down the ICUs and all I saw were closed doors with IV poles outside. It was eerily quiet because all the patients were on ventilators.

"One family in particular put me over the edge. I called the daughter, the next-of-kin of a man in the COVID ICU, and asked her how she was doing. She said, 'I'm here at home with my mom and my aunt who both have COVID, and I presume I have COVID, too. My dad is in the ICU. My husband is dropping off food for us on the front porch. I don't think my mom is going to make it.' It was very sad. The next day I got paged to the MICU.

The man's wife had just died at home, and he was crying: 'We were married 62 years. I didn't even get to say goodbye.' We talked a little, and I helped him process that a bit. A few days later, I returned, and he said, 'I'm done. I just got off the phone with my three children. I can't breathe. Everything hurts. This is no way to die.' He had lost his will to live. A few days later, he died. In one week, his daughter and her siblings had lost both their parents. That is just one story of the 235,000 people at the time who had died from the disease. The enormity of the grief and loss just hit me. I had trouble sleeping and eating. I thought, 'I'm *done*. Fried. I can't do this anymore.' I took a day off, but at home I thought, 'One day is not enough. I want to get away from any more sad stories.'"

Connie adjusted her hours, "did yoga every morning, and commuted to work a little later to miss the rush-hour traffic and to be in the hospital at night, which is usually quieter. But even *that* wasn't enough."

Pre-existing staff shortages exacerbated these COVID-19 stresses. "The challenge was that there was not enough staff," Connie continued. "There was so much need, but we could do only so much. A colleague said, 'I'm not sure that there's enough of *anything* to help at this point in time. There's not enough help on this planet to provide what's needed.' Another colleague said, 'If you don't feel a little fried right now, you're not normal.' Every person in this hospital felt the same."

Supportive spouses, colleagues, and bosses are vital. "I'm fortunate," Connie stated. "I'm married to a doctor, so he understands. I can go home and not have to comfort somebody else about *my* bad day. He lives through it, too, and is my main support. I also share an office with amazing colleagues. We help each other. My boss is very supportive, too, and encourages self-care. Her door is always open. And I meditate daily. The lounge outside the ICU has yoga mats, aromatherapy, coffee, and a massage chair for staff. Last September, when I was trying to hold it all together, I sat in that chair for 20 minutes, and thought, 'This is amazing.' So I bought a massage chair for myself at home. Yesterday, I spent 3 hours in it! My husband said, 'You look 10 or 15 years younger.'"

Chaplains also try to reconceptualize their work to focus on smaller accomplishments. "I have to remind myself that my job is not to save the world," Connie continued, "but to do what I can to the extent that I can. I'm only one person. The world is not going to be served if I end up dead from overworking! I continually have to balance that."

Basic staff self-care was crucial even before COVID-19, but became even more so during the pandemic. "I am fulfilled by my work, but some days I feel depleted," Jack Stone admitted. "We need a life outside of the hospital that is full of love, life, compassion, and passion. For me, that is art—painting and drawing—and nature. I fill my soul back up again with the passions that I love. I get rejuvenated."

Moreover, chaplaincy selects for especially dedicated individuals, drawn to this job as a calling, which, over time, proves sustaining. "This type of work is not for everybody," observed Brian Post, a Michigan chaplain department administrator, "but for those of us who find it deeply meaningful, there tends to be longevity. Chaplains don't have a lot of turnover."

Chaplains thus struggle to maintain an appropriate distance from patients, neither too close nor too far, by gently returning when initially rejected, and navigating desires for continued interactions after hospital discharge. Getting too close can trigger burnout. At other times, these providers wrestle to remain present, despite their moral abhorrence, with child abusers. Chaplains must balance competing goals, emotions, and ideals with patients and, as we will see, with staff as well.

PART V
CONFRONTING TENSIONS
WITH STAFF

15

Seeing patients with fresh eyes

"I want to stop my meds and go home," a frail elderly patient once told me, when I was a medical intern. She spoke in a muffled voice from beneath her light blue plastic mask as it hissed loudly. She wore only a thin blue cotton hospital gown, white gym socks, and an oxygen mask and had soft wispy, white hair. Clouds of white oxygen billowed around her.

For a week, I had been working hard to keep her alive. "But if you leave, you will die!" I exclaimed.

"So I will die," she replied, nonplussed. Astonished, I didn't know what to say.

When providers clash with patients and families regarding needs for more or less aggressive treatment, pastoral care can often mediate, providing fresh eyes and perspectives. A spiritual care professional has time to get to know patients and see them from their own perspectives in ways that doctors miss.

In these conflicts, chaplains' openness and lack of a rigid agenda can be especially beneficial. They can, for example, draw on their connections within an institution to facilitate appropriate treatment. Kristine Baker, for instance, described a young pregnant African American woman who "had come multiple times for pain management, but was not being evaluated and getting the care she needed." The staff saw this patient merely as a drug addict. "It was a sad, profound case of racism and still makes me a little teary. I felt I connected with her, and was able to create a respectful bond. She was legitimately angry at the healthcare team, but it just ended up being a spiral.

"Luckily, I had a very good connection with a fantastic maternal-fetal specialist. We had worked together on the Ethics Committee." Kristine now called him to see the patient. "We found out she had a *kinked bowel*, which can come and go, but get stuck. The patient ended up having a pretty profound infection in her gut because it had leaked. But the medical team had not done certain tests, assuming she was just drug-seeking.

"If you frame someone as 'drug-seeking,'" Kristine explained, "it gets horribly amplified and perpetuated. Nobody sees the patient again as a unique

Doctor, Will You Pray for Me?. Robert L. Klitzman, Oxford University Press. © Oxford University Press 2024.
DOI: 10.1093/oso/9780197750841.003.0015

individual who's different. Because of this one specialist, the patient was able to get the treatment she needed for a diagnosis that could have killed her. She had been drug-seeking because she was never getting the treatment! Even if someone is drug-seeking, we still need to give them comprehensive care."

Chaplains can thus help patients whom providers otherwise dismiss because of addiction or other stigmatized behaviors or characteristics, seeing these individuals with fresh eyes, encouraging staff to overcome cognitive biases and so-called group think.[1] "The chaplain's role is very powerful," Kristine stated. "*We can see people beyond labels.* We can come in and see the patient anew. I often have more time than other staff to read the case thoroughly. Staff can get lost in the medical record. If you can bear down, you can see stuff that can profoundly change your perceptions of the patient."

Chaplains feel a strong moral and religious commitment to aid the needy, underscoring the intrinsic value of seeing each individual patient in and of him- or herself. "Theologically, we have a responsibility to those who are most vulnerable," Kristine declared, "because in some ways, they have the most to teach us. We have an obligation to the '*least of these*,' the ones who could be left out, the widows. Scripture supports this. But it's *more* than text. The basic tenets of those texts are not unique to the Judeo-Christian tradition. We could find those tenets in other faiths, too. They're wisdom literature. Yet actualizing it is different from knowing it."

She therefore instructs trainees to determine and serve, in any particular situation, whoever is most in need. "I teach residents that if you go in a room, and can't decide who you are serving, consider: Who is the most vulnerable, the most in danger of not being heard, the person who will be hurt most by power? That's how to decide whose interests we should serve."

The most talkative person in the room may not be the most grieving or distressed one. "'*The least of these*' is an interesting construct," Kristine continued. "When I walk in a room, and the person in the bed isn't very articulate, someone is often pulling me aside. The mother-in-law is telling me what we need to do. The patient is unable to speak, and I have to listen to a lot of voices. But the wife is very quiet, and seems to have some wisdom I'm not getting, because the mother-in-law is talking for everybody."

Yet, chaplains' attentions and interventions cannot always reverse past misfortunes. Some patients don't get better. Their stories don't end well. "They die in pain, or alone," Kristine continued. "A chaotic story, a story of chaos, as Arthur Frank [the medical sociologist[2]]defined it, is a story that doesn't end up turning out well. The patient doesn't feel they have any meaning."

Countless lives lack happy endings. Kristine described a "young woman without a lot of support who had manic episodes and alienated everybody. We can't pretend in the American Dream, that *everything's getting better every day*. Sometimes, we just need to grieve with somebody, and stay with them in their chaos and not put a premature 'happy face' sticker on it." Yet even then, chaplains and others can recast stories and lives—even if at times to only moderate extents.

However, doctors and nurses may not see or question their prejudices, particularly regarding race, ethnicity, or other areas, hampering approaches to patients. As Sharlene Walters, an African American chaplain from Kentucky, described, "A white guy came into our trauma center after a car accident. He didn't have any identification with him and was covered from head to toe with tattoos. The staff treated him as though he was drugged out and had OD'd. They didn't even really want to touch him because he could have *anything*—because of his tattoos. They automatically ordered a drug test. I thought, 'Why do you assume he has drugs in his system?'

"I said, 'My son has tattoos all over him and a Ph.D. I think I know about people who have tattoos.' Sometimes, tattoos tell a lot about a person. Maybe his name is on his body. We found his name. He happened to be a department chair at the nearby state university. He had never touched drugs in his life. So, people are judging. There's prejudice." Besides ethnicity and gender, "there are biases against handicaps, sexual preferences, the way you look. There's fat shaming. It's sad, since this is a place they're coming to for help."

By providing vital information, reconceptualizing the patient's story, and correcting faulty assumptions, chaplains can assist as critical end-of-life decisions get made. Cathy Murray, for instance, described a patient whom the staff had written off due to his developmental disabilities. "He had been living in a group home, and had an accident and came to the hospital. He was not responsive. The medical team said, 'This is futile. We should let this patient go' [that is, die]. Only one extended family caregiver was involved. I said, 'How can you think of letting him go?' I asked the people at the group home to come to a meeting.

"As they talked, all the facts were presented, but I could see we were getting stuck. So, I then asked them, 'Can you tell us about who he is as a person when he's at your group home?' He was in the group home because he couldn't live independently or work for a living. They said, 'He is the *heart* of our group home. He delivers the mail. He has a pet that he loves and who loves him.' The medical team was aghast. They had no idea he had a life he was enjoying, in which he was interacting. All they saw was the person who had been devasted by the medical problems. They just assumed, 'What would this person be going back to?' He 'was just languishing in a group home anyway.' So, sometimes just asking the right question can elicit a fuller, holistic picture of the person."

Providing such fresh eyes can and should inspire doctors, nurses, social workers, and others to be aware of, and question, their own assumptions and potential biases. Chaplains can illuminate the unique identity, personality, dignity, worth, and individuality of each patient in ways that can enlighten not only staff but also families and patients themselves. "As chaplains, *we are collectors of stories*" Jack Stone said. The COVID pandemic initially prevented him from visiting patients with the virus, but he could nevertheless "meet them through their family. I called the families up and said, 'I don't know your family member, but tell me a story. What are their favorite things? Their favorite color? What's important to them? An episode or a memory that really stands out for you? What's their legacy? What are they leaving behind?'

"I would create a poster. I can't encapsulate everyone's life and what they were, but it contains images and words, their name, favorite color, aspects of this particular person."

When he gave the poster to patients, "Most were already sedated, so I couldn't speak or connect with them. But when patients who were awake and conscious saw the poster, it floored them to see their name, and other people's words describing them—as loving, funny, goofy, wise, a great father. The staff also lit up, seeing this person as more than just a number being transferred to their unit to die. That poster gave them an image, a snapshot of what this person's life was, and what is important in their life. When the family was able to come at the very end, in the last 20 minutes of their loved one's life, as the patient was actively dying, seeing that poster above the bed and then being able to bring it home after their loved one died was a memento for them."

Alas, chaplains do not always succeed in altering doctors' perceptions of particular patients. "A homeless man with end-stage renal disease and no family was dropped off at a service station," Kristine Baker reported. "He said, 'I just want to go back to my garage.' But it was just a gas station in a small town—a place he lived because he was homeless. He had a mental disability and the educational level of a fifth grader. Did he really understand what that was going to look like—could he imagine his future if he went back there?

"I said we needed to make the hospital a guardian for him, but the doctor trumped me: She felt we needed to give him autonomy and freedom. I didn't think this patient had the capacity to make this decision, but she just had much more power in the system than I did. I can state what I believe, but if somebody else has more power, I get outranked. We drop people off on the side of the street all the time. We give them bus fare to go somewhere. That happens much more than people realize. Hospitals are not in the business of housing. We can't keep anybody, especially now. We will spend $100,000 or half-a-million dollars on a patient like that, but then just put him on the street. If we just gave them housing, we could save money." Chaplaincy can thus also provide financial savings to the healthcare system as a whole.

Uncovering vital information

In the harried and fractured medical system, chaplains are often the only hospital staff who have time to speak to patients at length in ways that can reveal vital information. The experience of physical pain, in particular, can result from psychic, not just physical injury, but the psychic wounds first need to be identified and exposed. As we saw earlier, Kristine found that a patient's complaint of physical pain arose from his feelings of guilt over his mother's suicide. Such information can help avoid costly, invasive, and unnecessary medical procedures. Victor Simmons, the VA chaplain, described a patient who "came in for intense gastrointestinal pain, and the doctors did every test found, nothing and sent him home." The patient came back, and the same thing happened again. "He returned a third time and said, 'You're wasting your time and mine. You're not going to find anything, but it hurts!' So, I went and heard his story. I was the first one to sit down and just listen and not try to diagnose. I asked, 'When did this pain start?' He gave me a specific date. 'What else happened then?' He paused. 'My wife died of cancer. We had struggled for a year. Then, my daughter got cancer, and passed away.' He wept. 'The pain started the day my daughter died. The day I came into the hospital, my dog died.' I said, 'Your pain makes sense to me: Your guts are in turmoil over all that pain.' 'Finally, somebody gets me!' So, I told the doctors. The case worker arranged for psychotherapy and they discharged him. He hasn't returned."

Chaplains can be especially helpful when biases may hamper medical staff in obtaining critical information and planning for beneficial psychological interventions. Sharlene Walters, the African American chaplain from Kentucky, discussed another patient whom the medical staff saw merely as drug-seeking; Sharlene was able to arrange successful rehab for her. "The staff had little tolerance for her because they felt she was drug-seeking. I asked the patient, 'Why are you trying to kill yourself?' She looked at me and said, 'You have no idea what I'm going through!' A floodgate of tears came, but it was a breakthrough. I said, 'Tell me about the tears.' She said, 'My tears are my pain. My pain from suffering. My tears of anger, of nobody understanding. I just get mad!' There were a lot of domestic issues. Her husband abandoned her. I asked whether she would go into inpatient recovery. She said, 'Yes.'

"What baffled me was that over 3 or 4 years, she had been a 'frequent flyer' at the hospital, but no social worker, psychiatrist, or other staff had talked to her about drug treatment. I found a treatment center for her. That was 6 years ago, and she's been clean ever since."

Chaplains find vital details that can also aid the medical team's decisions about a patient's arrangements after hospital discharge. Connie Clark described, for instance, a "29-year-old woman who was awake and alert, and looked fine" but was having trouble breathing and was DNR. "I asked her how she was doing. She said, 'I was doing great until yesterday.' I said, 'Really? What happened yesterday?' 'My dad called and said, "You're never gonna leave the hospital!"'

"She was the same age as my daughter. My ex-husband would say very hurtful things to my daughter as well. I was in the middle. So, it was the same situation. It was wrong for this patient's father to say that to her, but I didn't want to slam him, or to step into 'mom mode'—because I could feel that kick in. But navigating that is hard.

"This patient decided not to return home to live with her dad, because he was so negative. I spoke with her mom, who was clearly miserable about it, but understood. I told the social worker, 'I didn't see this in your notes, but you might be aware of this psychosocial dynamic.' She said, 'If that kind of verbal abuse is going on, I wonder what other kind of abuse is going on.' She's going to follow up on it.

"The cases that keep me up at night are those that remind me of something in my own life. These issues were not in my lane, so I referred them to the person whose lane they are in."

Helping patients in conflicts with hospitals

Clearly, chaplains can serve as de facto mediators, having time to gain patients' trust and thus discover key information that can help resolve friction with medical staff. Patients and providers in conflict might then each become more open to the other's perspective. In such situations, Connie Clark, for instance, applies an "ethics of love," not just the principle of beneficence—which is often used as an abstract or intellectual principle—but a deeper sense of caring and commitment. For example, for one brain-dead ICU patient, the whole family still wanted everything done, and became very polarized from the staff. "I interrupted a family meeting," Connie reported, "and said, 'Look, I hear how very much you *love* your mom. I hear and honor that. But I hear, too, that the staff here *also* cares very much for your mom. So, everybody is trying to do the same. We are all coming at this from the same perspective!' Suddenly, when 'love' was introduced, the whole mood in the room shifted. 'OK. We've got some common ground here. We're not on opposite sides of the fence.' That was very helpful. There was no more conflict about it. I could then shift the conversation to, 'What's the most loving course of action for your mom right now, given the realities?'

"This situation has been repeated many times," Connie continued. "Families say, 'OK, as long as the staff knows that we just need more time' or 'OK, the doctors can do the procedure tomorrow.' Much of it's just *communication*. Each group assumes that the other one is hearing them, but they're really not. One of the big gifts chaplains can bring is helping to facilitate those interactions, and helping people communicate on emotional, not just intellectual, levels."

Such approaches can ease medical decision-making and resolve strains among families and physicians. Doctors and families may view a patient's symptoms very differently, fostering tensions. "One family appeared to resist having DNR goals-of-care conversations for a young sedated, intubated patient," Connie Clark continued. "Every time the patient's situation looked very dire, she would open her eyes or squeeze her hand. I hadn't met her mom. I only knew what I'd seen in the chart, and that the patient would be discussed at MICU [medical intensive care unit] rounds that afternoon.

"So, I called the patient's daughter and said, 'I'm from spiritual care, and just wanted to see how you're doing. I know your mom's been in the hospital for a while; it must be really hard.' The daughter was really receptive and said, 'Yes, I don't think she's going to live very much longer.' I thought, 'That's not what I read in the notes.' I said, 'What's going on?' She said, 'My mother has these ups and downs. It's a roller coaster.' I asked, 'What's the hardest part for you?' She said, '*I don't want her to die next week, on my birthday*. She always seems to get sick right before my birthday.' So, the family was very realistic about her mother's condition, and had thought it through. I asked, 'What do you think your mom would want?' 'She made me promise not to put her in a nursing home.' I said, 'How do you think she'd feel about being in a hospital for a while?' 'She wouldn't like that either. I just don't want her to suffer.'"

"I was shocked because she was receptive, and the medical team thought that she was in denial about her mom's condition. Later, the MICU attending called me and asked, 'What did you say to her?' All weekend he had frantically called the residents, who said that the family was 'in denial.' 'I just talked to her,' I said. 'Maybe just tell the daughter that you share her concern for her mom, don't want her mom to suffer, and want the care to be aligned with her mom's wishes, and that her mom momentarily opening her eyes does not indicate improvement.'"

Distrust can fester and escalate, especially when staff are less familiar with the patient's culture. William Gibson, who, though now a humanist, was raised Jewish, described, for example, an Orthodox Jewish family whose loved one died on Shabbat in the early morning. "The burial society ordinarily comes to get the patient's remains directly from the room, but were not going to come on Shabbat. The hospital can't, however, let the body sit in the room for 16 hours. But the family couldn't get in touch with anyone from their community to say that it was OK to let the body go to the morgue in the interim. So, the family literally barricaded themselves in the room. The hospital higher-ups had come and gotten involved. Security guards were there and were going to have to remove the family by force. It was ugly. I didn't know what was going to happen.

"But they said the family wanted to speak with 'that young Jewish guy' they had met earlier. Having been there with them, and having this similarity between us, they trusted me. I explained what I understood from the rabbi, and eventually was the key *negotiator* in a way that got them to agree to have the body removed. Something about the way that I had tried earlier to build a caring relationship with them worked, and it helped the hospital help them. That was kind of crazy, but super-rewarding."

In addition, chaplains can assist in anticipating and ameliorating such tensions that might be brewing. These providers hear patient and family dissatisfactions, and can aid doctors and nurses in avoiding conflicts with patients and families, recognizing issues and "danger signs" that begin to percolate up, foreseeing and forestalling these problems.

Helping patients navigate the hospital

Chaplains can also help empower patients and families, giving them a *vocabulary* for maneuvering within the complex, fractured, and dysfunctional hospital systems. As Kristine Baker said, "A chaplain can give patients and families language to get what they want. Patients say, 'I'm taking pain medication but am constipated.' I say, 'Have you asked about it?' Who can advocate for them? Where's their voice? There's a nurse and a charge nurse, a head nurse, an administrator-on-call, and a VP for nursing. How do I help patients know whom they can contact, if need be, to get their needs met?

"A lot of chaplains act like they're furniture decoration," Kristine continued. "But we have a lot to bring that's very essential to healing. Healing is not just about taking drugs. Recently, I've been working with a patient with juvenile idiopathic arthritis, who is now moving into adulthood, struggling. I've been coaching her about how she sees the medical team. I tell her, *'You are the one who's in charge of the medical team.* They're really just consulting with you. You need to say, 'I'm in charge of my care. I'm going to take everything you say under advisement.' That's part of my work."

Due partly to her experiences with her own daughter's medical problems, Kristine realized how much she can and should fight for patients. "My daughter was born with a minor congenital disorder and had eight different doctors. None of them knew the whole situation. It was depressing and sad. I wanted somebody who knew what they were doing, and finally realized that *I had to be her case manager!* I wrote up everything and sent it to the doctors ahead of time. I expected them to read it. I walked in and said, 'Have you read the summary?' A neurosurgeon said, 'I don't know why she's not walking.' I said, 'Have you read the report?'

"I finally realized: *Healthcare is too chaotic.* Some chaplains say, 'I don't have any authority.' But *we are the voice of the voiceless.* Chaplains mobilize patients' authority and power."

In such ways, these spiritual care providers also serve crucial roles that outside clergy do not. Many patients feel uncomfortable discussing religious quandaries and doubts with their priest, rabbi, or imam, who might judge them, but they are more at ease with hospital chaplains, who might be less doctrinaire. As Margaret Dixon explained, "Some religious people prefer to see a chaplain, rather than a priest or rabbi, to examine questions and avoid being judged. Patients in more formal Orthodox faiths tend to want to explore issues in ways that feel safe. One Catholic man with leukemia wanted to see a chaplain, not a priest: 'I was given bad news: Get your affairs in order. I prayed—so hard that I imagined Jesus reaching into my bone marrow, and healing it.' The lab results then improved. He believed that his prayer had helped but that his faith was weak because he had had doubts." He feared discussing these issues with his priest but felt comfortable with the chaplain.

Many outside clergy would gain from better education on how to address the specific dilemmas patients face, regarding, for example, DNR discussions. Marvin Beck, for instance, thought these issues "should ideally be addressed more from a pulpit, but aren't."

Chaplains can play unique roles regarding not only the content but also the *form* of these interactions, serving as "patient navigators." In recent years, airlines and other high-risk industries have worked to establish a "safety culture" in which "everyone in every group at every level of an organization" (e.g., not just airplane pilots) is involved in noticing and communicating about safety concerns.[3] Similarly, optimal involvement of all hospital staff, including chaplains, could potentially not only avoid problems but also enhance patient outcomes. Many chaplains adopt these roles organically, on their own, in informal if not formal ways, both implicitly and explicitly, working closely and collaboratively with the medical team, whether as significant parts of their job or only when needed.

Difficulties surface, however, regarding not only whether chaplains should take on such roles helping patients, but also *how* exactly they do so. At one ICU, staff formally appointed chaplains to be such "patient navigators," to coordinate family meetings and assist patients with obstacles in the healthcare system.[4] Most doctors and nurses in this ICU thought this role was useful for gathering families for meetings, but physicians were more likely than nurses to think so, or to see this role as helpful. Most nurses (80%) and 42% of doctors thought that the chaplain's background was not appropriate for this role.[5] Problems surfaced because these chaplains lacked medical backgrounds, and the boundaries of their navigator role were poorly defined. These chaplains would, for instance, interrupt critical medical situations to tell the nurse that a family meeting had been scheduled. The scope and parameters of these functions and professional boundaries need to be carefully established. Such chaplains would gain from feedback and education about key elements of medical care. As chaplaincy continues to grow, such roles and models of interaction need to be further developed and refined.

Spiritual care versus psychotherapy

Chaplains clearly resemble, but also differ from, psychotherapists. Both fields abet patients' coping and use several similar methods but have different scope and goals. "There's obviously a lot of crossover between what I do and what therapists and social workers do," Connie Clark said, "if the patient is hopeless, anxious, depressed, or poorly coping. But I don't feel threatened by these similarities. If patients connect better with a psychotherapist than with me, that's great."

Chaplains' and psychotherapists' perspectives vary. As Connie continued, "At least until recently, psychiatry saw grief as a pathology, while palliative care viewed grief as a normal part of the process. Not all grief is pathological or needs to be medicated away; patients might just need to talk to somebody. Hopefully, we assess the family before the patient dies to know whether they're at risk for complicated grief, to arrange for supports.

"I would advise: 'Talk with us first. If we can't help, we'll refer you.' But we also have a little bit more flexibility to spend more time, because we don't have the quotas that social workers and other providers have. Sometimes there is a little bit of tension about what level of care the family might need. But it's important that therapists and chaplains work together."

Still, psychological and spiritual issues can blur. "If the person's at all religious or spiritual, these concerns come into play," Sam Lacey, the Louisiana chaplain, said. "If a psychiatrist said a patient's problems are purely psychological or emotional, I wouldn't necessarily feel I had to dispute that. I would use the words 'existential,' 'spiritual,' and 'religious' to signify depth, but the patient makes that assessment."

Similarly, the word "soul" can be seen as psychological or spiritual—with hazy gradations between these different conceptualizations. Indeed, the Greek term "psyche," the root of the words psychotherapists and psychiatrist, means soul, mind or spirit; and the boundaries and uses of these terms can blur. "Is 'soul' really just the self?" Sam asked. "I'm fine with the word 'self,' but 'soul' conveys a deeper sense of 'identity' or 'being,' which makes sense to some people. I wouldn't force that language on everyone. For me, 'soul' does not mean reincarnation or existence outside of the body, but conveys depth of identity." The term can thus suggest not immortality, but the deepest, fullest sense of a person.

Ordinarily, a psychotherapist works one on one with patients and remains in his or her office, far from stressful life events themselves. Couples therapists and family therapists treat more than one person at a time, but are in the minority among mental health providers. Chaplains, however, view and help respond to stresses *in real time, in the place where they are occurring,* not in cool reflection afterwards, and speak with more patients and families each day, though typically more briefly each time. Additionally, chaplains interact with patients' medical teams more than do the vast majority of psychotherapists. By no means am I denigrating mental health providers— they do immensely valuable work—but these professionals' jobs *differ,* and can complement each other.

Chaplains are careful not to act or present themselves as psychotherapists if they don't have the requisite additional formal training. "I provide emotional and moral support, a kind of grief counseling," William Gibson said, "anticipating or preparing for the possibility of a wife dying or becoming debilitated. But chaplains don't want to bill themselves as psychotherapists or provide psychotherapy, even though we draw on a lot of that training."

In hospitals, social workers, too, could potentially address some of these issues but commonly lack time to do so. These chaplains' and social workers' roles clearly complement each other, but the latter often focus on arranging discharge—getting patients, when leaving the hospital, into rehabs or nursing homes. "We overlap a lot," Margaret Dixon said. "Social workers are psychosocial and do discharge planning. But we can do something that social workers don't. One outpatient cancer patient who saw a social worker once a month for a long time quietly said to her one day, embarrassed, 'I pray.' It was obviously a big part of this patient's way of coping. The social worker told me, 'I felt so embarrassed because I had never bothered to ask her about prayer.' Social workers are frequently interested in family dynamics and what's happening at home in more pragmatic ways, and in decisions about feeding tubes and discharge planning. We take what we hear and invest *the pastoral imagination*. If a patient believes that her deceased mother is holding her hand right now, I say, 'Amen.' If she believes her dead ancestors are alive in the trees and are going to absorb her into the tree, I say, 'I love that. Let's talk about that.' Social workers don't really do that." Psychotherapists tend not to take such statements from patients at face value.

Chaplains can thus improve patient care in several ways that have been unappreciated, having more time to interact and abilities to stand outside the medical system per se. Hence, they can bring nonmedical perspectives, garnering patients' and families' trust and getting to know patients in beneficial ways, and learn and convey to medical teams key information that can assist in diagnosis, treatment, and conflict resolution. Given the increasingly fragmented and rapidly changing healthcare system, with mounting pressures, stresses, and time constraints on doctors, these chaplains' roles are ever more vital.

16

"Which ditch do you want to die in?"

Chaplains versus doctors

One of the biggest challenges spiritual care providers face is not feeling well respected or part of the medical team. Doctors frequently remain wary not only about spirituality and religion in medicine generally but also about chaplains. While some physicians and nurses increasingly respect chaplaincy, many remain ignorant—as I had initially been in my training—and cautious. Only after I embarked on this book did I realize how little I had initially known about chaplains. These professionals aid innumerable nurses and doctors, but still frequently feel marginalized by them.

These issues may seem of little relevance to patients but are important, illuminating why patients should not feel discouraged, dismayed, or put off when doctors ignore these realms. Patients may also personally know doctors and nurses as family members, and can encourage them to be more open, rather than closed, about these topics.

"There is a gulf between chaplains and the other health professionals," Sam, the Louisiana chaplain, explained. On some wards, "chaplains are now kind of part of the team, but not really. We are sort of relegated to the side of the room. We don't have a full voice at the table."

"As chaplains," another pastoral care provider told me, "we joke, 'What ditch do you want to die in?'" Such marginalization proves enormously frustrating. Jack Stone sees the chaplain as "the low person on the totem pole. A chaplain might be in the side or corner of a family meeting or rounds and have a small voice, because doctors sideline the emotional, mental, and psychological aspects of what the patient or the family might be going through, compared to the medical issues. That's a disservice."

Chaplains perceive barriers[1] and lack of connection with doctors, who are often unfamiliar with the role of chaplains and don't see it as helpful.[2] Most chaplains (62%) feel they are too infrequently integrated into medical team discussions.[3] Even palliative care physicians, nurses, and social workers, though broadly understanding what chaplains do, are rarely aware

Doctor, Will You Pray for Me?. Robert L. Klitzman, Oxford University Press. © Oxford University Press 2024.
DOI: 10.1093/oso/9780197750841.003.0016

of chaplains' roles in assisting with treatment decisions and communication among patients, families, and medical teams, as well as caring for the medical team itself.[4] Marginalization may be diminishing a bit but remains a major obstacle.

Unfortunately, chaplaincy departments remain under-resourced. Health insurance generally does not cover their services, reflecting and exacerbating these challenges. In July 2020, during the initial surge of the COVID-19 pandemic, the Centers for Medicare & Medicaid Services (CMS), for the first time, established codes for chaplain services—but only for the VA system, and these codes remain non-billable—documenting, but not reimbursing these activities.[5] Elsewhere, insurers reimburse for hospice care based on a fixed overall daily rate, regardless of what particular care or types of providers are involved.[6] Consequently, for hospitals, chaplains remain an added expense that yields no added reimbursement. Partly as a result, at least 30% of hospitals still lack any pastoral care services, and many services are provided by local volunteer clergy rather than board-certified chaplains trained to work with patients of diverse or no religious beliefs.[7]

A critic might ask why hospitals should provide and pay for a chaplaincy department, and why all patients, including non-religious ones, not just those who use the service, should indirectly help support it through general hospital fees. Chaplains seek to help patients find meaning and connection when confronting severe disease and death, but, the argument goes, can't social workers and psychotherapists perform these tasks?

Unfortunately, while a few hospitals may have sufficient numbers of psychotherapists, the vast majority don't. Chaplains not only focus on different realms than do psychotherapists, but can uniquely benefit countless non-religious and atheist patients and their families. Not all hospitalized patients use certain other services, such as social work, clinical ethics, patient translators (for non-English patients), or the hospital's general counsel, but nevertheless they still help pay for these functions through the institution's overall daily rates.

The financial limitations that beset chaplains mirror and affect staff perceptions. Clinicians and patients are often unaware of chaplains' existence or have misconceptions, seeing spiritual care as unimportant or restricted to narrowly defined religious activities.[8] "Some doctors think chaplains only smile and say, 'Jesus' and a prayer," Linda Porter reflected.

Such misconceptions readily engender disrespect. "Doctors will just barge right in," Jack Stone reported, "even in the middle of a prayer or very deep psychological or spiritual moment, and not even apologize. They say, 'We're here and this is our only time,' and that's it. The atmosphere is destroyed. Imagine if, in the middle of a deep therapy session, a group of people barge in, not even sitting down and ask, 'How are you doing today?' I've learned to put my hand up sometimes and say, 'Please, doctor, let me finish. Give me 2 minutes.' Then, they will understand, but I've had to interject and explain that what I'm doing is just as important as any of the medications. I try to educate staff in a gentle way." More mutual appreciation of each other's respective roles can help.

Medical staff also tend not to read chaplains' notes. As Adam Quincy reported, "Studies on charting found that no one on the clinical team ever looked at a chaplain note, or didn't even know where these were, which is disheartening and sad because chaplains spend 2 hours a day charting their visits. Physicians appreciate chaplain notes, but will they read them? They don't necessarily view the chaplain's work as directly relevant or integrated into medical decision-making."

"We are called in too late and underused," Sam Lacey added. "We have skills, and can help with negotiation and conflict resolution with families and patients." Marginalization, wariness of religion, misunderstandings of what chaplains do, and lack of reimbursement fuel these problems. Focused on objective facts and trying to cure disease, doctors frequently deal poorly with death, seeing it as a failure. Therapeutic optimism prevails, geared toward conquering death, not confronting its ultimate inevitability.

Variations among doctors

Nonetheless, doctors do differ in their personal and professional views of religion and spirituality.[9] Hospice and palliative care doctors, for instance, usually incorporate chaplaincy relatively more than do other specialists.[10,11]

Yet countless physicians remain anti-religion. Sam Lacey, for instance, has seen strict biological determinists among neurologists, who view all mental phenomena as ultimately chemical. "I've heard the hardest kind of determinism from neuroscientists and neurosurgeons—that medicine is just scientific and religion is all a lot of bunk, an extreme that I'm not fully comfortable with. They say that everything is just a chemical reaction in the brain, that we have no choice whatsoever in life, that everything is determined. That's a big part of their identity, but doesn't seem right to me. It feels like we *have* a choice. Yet I yield the floor and just listen to their perspective. Other neuroscientists tell me that we still know very little about the brain. So, I raise skepticism: Can you be so confident that everything is that determined?"

In contrast, certain other physicians have profound faith that deeply motivates them. "I am an instrument of God," an Indiana physician who was raised evangelical told me. He now describes himself as a " 'Progressive evangelical.' At my parents' dinner table, I feel like 'the sloppy liberal.' Still, my religion is what drives me in medicine: My job is to relieve suffering here on Earth."

In general, hospice and palliative care physicians, concentrating on comfort rather than further aggressive care, tend to recognize and support spiritual dimensions in medicine more than their colleagues do. As Connie noted, "It's mandated that hospice teams have spiritual care or a chaplain." Hence, as Brian Post, the Michigan chaplaincy department administrator, observed, "Almost every palliative care physician and a lot of oncologists and pediatricians understand the importance of chaplains and spirituality in patient care." But these specialties remain the exceptions. Physicians in these fields, and occasionally in ICUs, where death hovers close, may value and support chaplains relatively more, but wide variations persist.

The cultures of particular hospitals and wards differ, too. "I think I'm holding a minority position," Adam Quincy commented. "I know colleagues are marginalized—'second-class' clinicians or not considered clinicians at all—and are questioned: 'Why are your notes even in the medical record?' But I have seen physicians appreciate what chaplains do. The directors of my medical ICU support chaplains and have been excited to have me there. Chaplains tend to not view themselves as all that helpful, because they don't get a lot of strokes in these environments."

Depending on the individual doctor, ward, hospital, and geographical region, even some non-believing physicians may nonetheless see the psychological, if not the spiritual, benefits of chaplains. "The chaplain on our ward that patients like most, regardless of whether they are Catholic, Protestant, or Jewish, is a Buddhist monk," said Jim Adams, a Philadelphia oncologist and "lapsed Catholic" who now describes himself as a "nonbeliever." This Buddhist chaplain "does meditation with the patients, which they feel is very helpful. I see him in the hall and say, 'Did you see Mrs. So-and-so? I think it may help her.' "

Other physicians may not understand chaplains' activities but nonetheless appreciate them. As Brenda Pierson commented, "One physician tells me, 'I don't know what you do, but I'm glad you do it.' He doesn't need the details; he just wants the outcome." His remark about his lack of knowledge, even in a relatively religious area of the country, further underscores how chaplains need to educate physicians more about these concrete benefits.

Nurses, too, often appreciate chaplains, and this became especially apparent during the early months of COVID. In certain ways, the pandemic brought chaplains and other medical staff closer, jointly confronting threats. During the surge of the epidemic, William Gibson noted, "The staff had a lot going on, but I was surprised: When I had a family's message to relay to a patient, I told nurses I didn't want to make them spend any more time in the patient's room than they needed to. But almost every time, the nurses wanted to deliver the message. It was meaningful to them to read the few sentences I had printed out. One family sent in holy oil that had been blessed. A nurse, who wasn't Catholic, took it and put it on the patient. It was super-meaningful to the family, and to the nurse."

Doctors misunderstanding what chaplains do

Doctors' perceptions of chaplaincy vary by their specialty and tend to be more favorable in palliative care and oncology. Misconceptions persist: Physicians commonly still see chaplains as merely performing rituals around dying. As Jack Stone continued, "Doctors think chaplains are just there for prayers and last rites, giving out Bibles or doing sacraments of the sick—the ritualistic side of death and dying. They think, 'This patient is dying; call the chaplain!'"

Doctors often fail to recognize that chaplaincy addresses not only religion, narrowly construed, but also wider concerns about meaning and connection to something beyond the confines of one's own life. "We have had a hard time explaining what we do," Jack noted, "because we do religious things, but also *spiritual* work."

Increasing public wariness of religion and interpretations of needs for separation of church and state play roles here, too in limiting reimbursement. "I'd love to see more chaplains," Connie Clark said, "but that depends on government regulations. Medicare mandates that hospice teams provide spiritual care have been very helpful. We should get Medicare and Medicaid to reimburse for chaplain services; it's a no-brainer. But there's this feeling that we are providing religious, not existential or spiritual, services. Our country swings between two extremes: On one hand, the U.S. has an absolute fear of intermingling church and state." Yet on the other hand, religious pro-lifers have been gaining political strength.[12] "It would be nice if we could balance out in the center, and recognize that everybody's got some spirituality, and that chaplains are uniquely positioned to help patients think through these beliefs, which can be helpful in suffering." Moreover, while Medicare and Medicaid cover hospice care, the amounts also vary widely by state.[13,14]

Doctors may also mistakenly see chaplains as the same as local leaders of religious institutions in the community. "A lot of physicians confuse us with outside clergy," Connie explained. "They don't understand the difference. There's need for education."

Physicians' own awkwardness discussing these realms can taint their perceptions of chaplains. "Many physicians are so uncomfortable with religion in general and with anything that's not positivistic that they write us off rather than saying it's because *they're uncomfortable* and don't have skills in this area," Alice Montgomery, a Midwest chaplain, said. "Research shows that physicians who are more religious and appreciate their patients' worldviews can be biased, too, and unaware of how their own beliefs impact their care. So, even if they value religion more, they don't necessarily grasp their own limitations. The same with cultural differences and anything that seems magical, crazy, or doesn't align with the current so-called evidence-based approach. They don't appreciate that chaplains can actually bridge these different worldviews."

However, doctors' lack of time for such discussions can impede care and cause conflicts. "Physicians don't have the time to keep the patient as a person," Alice Montgomery added. "Whether because it's not scientific or detracts from productivity requirements, it is leading to more ethics conflicts." Physicians' discomfort and disinclination to recognize or overcome these barriers can cause problems.

But despite their awkwardness and lack of training on these subjects, physicians can powerfully limit what chaplains do. "The doctor has all the power and is responsible for everything," Adam Quincy commented. "He's still the king with his minions. If patients need emotional support or want to talk about spiritual care, they talk to *him*. That model is ineffective and needs to be transformed, because doctors are put in an unfair situation, and chaplains don't know enough about medicine to have really relevant and intelligent input."

Yet time pressures within an institution, not only doctors' own religious practices, can shape how they collaborate with chaplains. As Brian Post, the

Michigan chaplaincy department administrator, explained, "I've worked with physicians who are very clear about the lack of their religious involvement or belief but are nonetheless great collaborators with chaplains. So, it's not as simple as 'physicians who go to church or synagogue are friendly to chaplains.' Some physicians would like to address their patients' holistic experiences but are just on the treadmill of seeing seven patients an hour or getting in trouble."

Physicians' lack of preparedness to deal with these situations can precipitate awkward encounters. Doctors may sense these pitfalls but not know how to handle them in the moment. "I once was wheeling a young child off for surgery," an anesthesiologist I know told me. "I thought there was a good chance he would die in the OR. The parents might never see the child again. They said, 'Will you pray with us?' I wasn't sure what to do; I'm Jewish and they were Christian. So, I said, 'I'll leave you alone to pray together' and left the room. I have always felt badly about that, unsure if I did the right thing. What do you think?"

I replied, "You could have just said, 'I'd be happy to stand here with you'— in support." His poignant question further helped prompt me to write this book.

Doctors not referring patients to pastoral care

Due to these obstacles, physicians and nurses often fail to refer patients to chaplains, or delay doing so. Many hospitals refer to chaplains all patients who reply "yes" when asked at admission if religion is important to them or if they are having trouble making sense of the illness. Other chaplains mostly or only see patients whom a doctor or nurse explicitly refer. Yet such arrangements may not occur when they should. As Rashid Ayad, the Muslim chaplain, remarked, "Many doctors don't call chaplains until the last minute."

Even physicians who appreciate chaplains may insufficiently refer patients to them. "Most doctors respect what we do but don't necessarily think to call on us or seem to have much use for us," Nancy Cutler observed. "They like when we show up. But still, it's hard to appear at the right place and time if nobody calls us. Ten percent of the patients I see are referred, and 90% are from my going around on my own. I'm the only chaplain in my area of the hospital. But if a crisis is happening and they don't call, I don't know to be there. We have worked out a way for them to notify me immediately of all new diagnoses. But if patients have been in treatment for a while, and no-body calls me, I don't know."

Slowly, some physicians' attitudes may be shifting. "One doctor," Nancy continued, "who claims to believe in God nonetheless used to just come in when I was with a patient and just start talking, without saying, 'Excuse me.' I think he's 'on the spectrum'; that's just who he is. But, in the past 2 or 3 months, even *he* has changed and now says, 'Oh, excuse me. Should I come back?'"

On certain wards, chaplains get more referrals from nurses than from doctors. When they arrive on a ward, chaplains commonly ask the nurses, "Is there anyone I should particularly see?" But nurses may not fully grasp the nature of chaplains' work. As one chaplain said, "They'll say, 'See Ms. X. She seems lonely.' But they don't always quite get what chaplains do or whom we could help most."

Just as I, as a trainee, was unsure whether or when to call a chaplain, count-less doctors remain unclear today. Recently, after they heard I was writing this book, several colleagues have asked me, "What should I do with a patient who is a None and is struggling with spiritual issues?"

"Ask if they are interested in seeing a chaplain," I've suggested. "You might also ask the chaplaincy service if they have a staff person who is partic-ularly interested or has experience with patients who are 'spiritual but not religious.'"

Innumerable patients who would benefit from a referral never get one. "We should be referred all end-of-life situations," Connie Clark said. But out-side of palliative care, "we're not. I can often find out, from talking to the nurses and rounding through the units, which patients need attention."

Questions surface, though, of whether chaplains may at times be expecting too much. Doctors should treat chaplains with respect as much as possible. Yet in the rushed, pressured, and resource-strapped world of hospitals, overworked doctors must triage tasks. Doctors' visits and med-ical interventions cannot always wait. Generally, physicians must perform multiple medical tasks during limited hours, while chaplains have signifi-cantly more flexibility and can potentially return to see a patient later, after the doctor has left. Professionals all need to balance their time with patients, relative to other needs and interventions for that patient and others, which can be difficult.

Hospitals should try, too, to allow patients to self-refer, routinely asking not only at admission but also later if they'd like to see a chaplain.

Variations among hospitals

Broader hospitals' contexts, too, affect how chaplains and patients interact. These institutions vary in how they organize and support pastoral care. Chaplains can aid them in numerous ways—helping patients and families discuss and come to terms with disease and death (potentially improving satisfaction with care[15]) and also, secondarily, to understand and commonly avoid aggressive but futile interventions. These spiritual care providers can thus assist with optimal allocation of scarce resources such as ICU beds, which can then best be used by patients who are most likely to benefit from them.

Chaplains strengthen hospitals in smaller ways, too. Marvin Beck, for instance, and his colleagues collect clothes for patients who lose them in the ER. "When patients come into the ER, doctors have to cut all their clothes off. Sometimes those are the only clothes with the patient and no one can bring others. So, every year we collect sweatsuits and winter coats."

Hospitals differ widely, however, in their support of these professionals. In the United States, the presence of chaplaincy services has been associated with institutional location, size, and church affiliation, with smaller, rural, and investor-owned (rather than not-for-profit) hospitals less likely to have chaplaincy services.[16] Teaching hospitals, those with cancer and occupational health services, and those in the South and Midwest (rather than in the West) are more likely to have chaplains. From 1993 to 2003, church-affiliated hospitals were more likely to discontinue chaplaincy services than to add them, while nonprofit institutions were more likely than investor-owned ones to add these services.[16] Institutions with more chaplains per 100 inpatients were less likely as well to use volunteer chaplains.[17] Pastoral care departments also vary in whether they are more professional (emphasizing board certification) or traditional (with chaplains tending to work alone, rather than as parts of interdisciplinary teams, and not being board-certified) or transitional (between these two models).[18]

However, many questions emerge about how these and/or other differences "play out" on the ground, whether a hospital's affiliation may affect not only the presence or absence of chaplains but also how these professionals see and fill their roles. Religiously affiliated hospitals have also been noted to differ from secular hospitals in other ways, such as in providing contraception and abortion.[19] A hospital's size affects various other aspects of patient care, too: High-volume hospitals, for example, have improved survival rates for several conditions, such as breast cancer, possibly due to better infrastructure.[20,21]

Yet across such larger categories, hospitals share similarities as well as differences. Catholic and secular hospitals, for instance, may resemble each other in several regards, but differ in others. "On one level, interacting with patients isn't different," Cathy Murray said. "Your role as a chaplain is to serve patients and their spiritual well-being. They might be Muslim, Jewish, or non-religious, but really it's the same thing: How do they make sense of what's happening, and find the strength to go on?"

Still, religiously affiliated hospitals may appreciate chaplains more. Catholic hospitals, more than secular ones, may, for instance, tend to integrate chaplains into other leadership decisions. "Catholic hospitals have mission leaders in the administration," Cathy said, "who help to ensure the organization is living its mission, and maintaining a Catholic identity."

Her Catholic hospital also gives staff a "work sabbath" once a year, allowing employees to take "an extra paid day away every year, if they choose to—and we go to a lake. It's a day about work–life balance. I lead it." Other hospitals could potentially benefit from such activities as well. Catholic hospitals may tend, too, to provide more explicitly religious services and rituals, though at times more Catholic than interfaith. "We offer Daily Mass, and do 'Blessing of the Hands.' In Mass, we honor employees, with awards, for their values."

Doctors at religiously affiliated hospitals, too, may, overall, appreciate pastoral care. "I've worked for both faith-based and secular institutions," Adam Quincy said. "Doctors at faith-based institutions tend to be a little more *sensitive* to the mission of the institution. One doctor walked up to me at the nurses' station and said, 'You know what? Without hope, my patients can't heal, and you just instilled hope in that patient. I appreciate that.' That blew me away. I lived off of that compliment for months."

Chaplains at secular hospitals may consequently face greater challenges. Connie Clark has experienced only secular academic hospitals. "If you're at a Catholic or religious-based institution, there's probably a greater appreciation of spiritual care," she said, "because it's in the institution's DNA that it's important. At a more secular place, there's more of an uphill battle." She has "worked in three large, secular hospital systems" and encountered the same problems at each.

At secular institutions, both patients and other providers may sense that issues smacking of religion are somehow off limits, even if these perceptions are incorrect. Institutional affiliation can hence shape patients' and families' expectations of chaplaincy services. "I once prayed with the family of a patient who had just been diagnosed with breast cancer," Connie Clark recalled. "I asked if they would like to have a prayer. Her husband looked at me and asked, 'Is that allowed?' Yes, even in this godless university hospital we're allowed to pray."

In secular hospitals, the presence of religion can surprise patients, too. Connie reported, "A patient today said, 'I'm just so surprised I'm getting Communion here at this hospital. My church is across town. And this is a *secular* hospital!'"

Religious affiliation can also affect hospitals' appearance and therefore culture, tone, and attitudes not only directly and explicitly but also indirectly and implicitly. As Brenda Pierson noted, for instance, paintings and sayings of Jesus decorated the hospital where she trained. Such reminders can reinforce expectations.

Secular institutions also differ in their relative numbers of chaplains, and at times have fewer—even just a single such person, who then faces added strains. Brenda said she felt "very sad" for colleagues who "operate as the sole, individual chaplain in a hospital. Their burden seems to me insurmountable. We do things that we can only talk about with other chaplains. We can't talk about these things with our spouses, families, and/or people in church. What we expect and are taught from our faith versus what we experience is jarring. Usually, only another chaplain understands. Chaplains themselves need support."

Hospital leaders, too, range widely. As Brenda said, "Administrators do not always see that spiritual health and physical health are intertwined and intersect, whether in recovery or death."

Still, among secular institutions, differences exist and aspects of a hospital's particular culture can influence the chaplaincy department's ethos and logistics. Some secular hospitals may contain explicit trappings of religion. Cathy Murray described "an adamantly secular major hospital. But in the lobby, a 10-foot marble statue of Christ still towers. Even people with no religion routinely touch the well-worn, now-shiny white foot for good luck."

Individual hospital leaders vary as well in how much they encourage and financially support chaplaincy. "In our secular hospital, the prior CEO gave me a free hand to do whatever I wanted," Marvin Beck reported. "So, we do prayers over the loudspeaker, blessings for our staff, blessings of nurses' hands, and, in October, blessing of the animals for St. Francis of Assisi. On July Fourth we do a blessing for the military and our country. We distribute

Christmas and Hanukah cards. Our chapel has Bibles, Qurans, the Torah, rosary beads, prayer cards, pamphlets, and spiritual readings. We give Communion. We ask, 'Do you want us to call your pastor or rabbi and see if they'll come in and give you a blessing?'"

Variations related to geography

Geographical regions vary in the roles and importance of religion and the distribution of different faiths. More people are "very religious" in the Southwest and Southeast than in New England and the Rockies (45% and 43%, vs. only 26%, respectively).[22] "Nones" account for 28% in the West and 25% in the Northeast, but only 19% in the South. About half of Evangelicals (49%) live in the South.

Attitudes about science, too, shift across regions, even among physicians. "In the South, some religious medical students and doctors remain doctrinaire and even oppose evolution," said Sam Lacey. "In a lecture, I once in passing mentioned evolution. An attending in the audience took great offense and challenged me: 'I think evolution is just a hypothesis. There are other points of view.' I was shocked. He kept faith and science separate. I just said, 'We can talk more afterwards.'"

In their overall attention to spirituality and religion, doctors and institutions differ widely. "There's quite a big range," Amanda Shaw, a devout Catholic Tennessee psychiatrist, told me. "I trained in the South, and then in the Northeast, where there was less attention on spirituality." In secular Northeast hospitals, religion appears less pervasive and tends to focus heavily on adult palliative care.

Across regions, the importance of religion to both staff and patients varies. Amanda Shaw observed that in the Northeast, "Doctors did have chaplains come occasionally for palliative care on our really sick, dying patients, but it was definitely less. We were doing palliative care for one preemie boy born at 32 weeks gestation. I asked the family if they wanted their baby baptized. They said yes, and I got the chaplain to come. But nobody else brought it up. That would be more typical here in Tennessee, where there would be a lot more discussion, at least amongst nurses and doctors publicly, as well as with a chaplain. Here, your doctor may actually attend your church. It's just much more common. I'm surrounded by people who have more similar spiritual outlooks to me. Up there, your doctor is probably not going to be attending your church. Here, doctors are also more likely to ask patients, 'Would you like me to pray with you?'"

In the South and certain other regions, patients may, in addition, request a physician with faith. "Down here, patients often want a doctor who is religious," Amanda remarked. "They say they're looking for a more spiritual or Christian approach. A lot of the patients I see go to church, and bring up church or going to vacation Bible school. It's just a part of the conversation. Somehow it emerges."

Cutbacks and using volunteer chaplains

In their ratios of chaplains to patients both overall and in particular types of wards, hospitals also differ widely. Alas, a considerable number of institutions are cutting back on paid chaplains, depending instead on local clergy as volunteers; these volunteers are often Evangelical and may be trained as clergy in a particular faith, but not as nondenominational chaplains. "Many hospitals have been laying off or not rehiring after chaplains leave," Adam Quincy explained. "The chaplain is last in line for getting paid. So, if anybody's going to get cut, it's going to be the chaplain. One of our state's largest hospices recently fired *all* its chaplains! The next year, they had to hire them all back because it was such a disaster. They didn't realize what chaplains do. Several administrators got fired over that. Many administrators who oversee chaplains' work are involved in their own religious institutions and think, 'We can get people from my church to do this. All the chaplain does is sit and listen and say a prayer.' They use volunteers, especially evangelicals.

"Would you want your physician to be a volunteer?" Adam asked rhetorically. "Patients want their physician to be well trained and well paid. Why would I expect somebody taking care of my soul to be less than that? Chaplains and volunteers differ in skills. The Protestant Evangelical Christian tradition says we're all supposed to be ministers. It doesn't believe in a professional clergy per se, like the Catholic Church does. So, there is a temptation just to have volunteers, which is a great mistake."

Across institutions, rates of board certification also vary. "Here in the South, a lot of the chaplains are not board certified but are former church pastors, and try to 'save them,'" Adam reported. "It is subtle, not necessarily brazen. But hospitalized patients do not want that. They want someone to empathize with their suffering and maybe understand how that relates to their religious tradition. If a patient says, 'I don't know if the doctors are really telling me how serious my condition is,' the chaplain might say, 'That brings up the issue of where we're going after we pass away in this life. Let me ask you: Where do you think your soul is going to be when you pass away?' That's *not* what the patient was asking, but the chaplain turned it into an evangelistic question. That's a key reason not to use volunteers as chaplains. They tend to be highly evangelical and have their own agenda. They just scare the life out of Ms. Jones. The more professional the chaplain, the less likely that happens. Board-certified chaplains are less likely to do that.

"Many Evangelical volunteers feel they're there to save patients from eternal damnation. They still view themselves as they would in Church ministry and evangelize, or think the patient needs to be saved before death. They see themselves as advocates for God. They don't explicitly say, 'I'm here to win them to God,' but I get that sense. That can be offensive."

Hospitals, as well as doctors, thus range considerably in their support of chaplains, and thereby of patients.

Healthcare providers becoming chaplains

Despite wariness of religion and spirituality in much of medicine, several physicians have themselves become chaplains. They soon recognize underlying tensions, not just synergies, between these two roles—implicit and explicit pressures to maintain "separate lanes." These two functions can complement each other but collide as well. These physician-chaplains hence generally strive to keep these two sets of functions distinct. "I wonder sometimes: When am I a pediatrician and when a chaplain?" one pediatrician who became a chaplain as well told me. "I heard that doing both jobs would be hard, but I didn't think it would be difficult for *me*. When I'm speaking to patients just as a chaplain, though, I sometimes have to be careful. I want to say, 'Did you try this or that treatment?' Once in the ER, as a chaplain, I overheard the resident in the next cubicle unable to draw an infant's blood. I went in and did it myself. The chaplaincy department later reprimanded me, saying I should not have done that: 'Chaplains and doctors need to stay siloed' "—to avoid blurring or confusing roles. But the complexities of real-world clinical interactions can muddy these rigid demarcations. He was surprised these two positions were firmly firewalled apart.

Nonetheless, physician-chaplains feel that these roles can mutually en-hance each other, providing certain benefits. Daniela, another physician who became a chaplain, thought that her faith aided her in many ways. "I was once trying to get blood from a tiny elderly woman with no veins. I kept failing. I knew she was religious, so I said, 'Let's pray together.' Suddenly, all these veins were there. They just popped up. I got blood without a problem."

"What do you think happened?" I asked Daniela. "Do you think more veins appeared because you prayed?"

She shrugged, "Who knows?" She smiled and her eyes twinkled, seeming to suggest that she felt a metaphysical phenomenon may have helped. "Prayer *does* have autonomic and neuroendocrine effects," she explained, adopting a more professional medical demeanor, "and prayer releases endorphins." The morning after Daniela drew blood from the patient, she told the resident who would be covering the patient the rest of the day about it. He was Jewish, but eagerly asked, "What was the prayer?"

Physicians who are also chaplains need to be careful, however, not to blur these boundaries too much. "When I was a resident in the VA," Daniela con-tinued, "I saw a Bible by a patient's bed, so we talked about religion. The pa-tient was gay, Baptist, and had AIDS. One day, he told me that his father was coming to visit him in a few hours. Because of the patient's homosexuality, they had been painfully estranged. The patient hoped they could now re-establish a bond, and he asked me to baptize him. I wasn't sure whether to do it. I was hoping that he would reconcile with his father and that baptizing him might help, but it was my last day on the ward, and I didn't know what baptism meant to him, as a Baptist, versus to me. It was also just easier to say no. So I signed out to the next doctor, who would be covering the patient for the next month, that he wanted to be baptized." Daniela seemed to sense, though, that baptizing a patient was somehow outside her role as a doctor, going too far. Physicians could talk to a patient about the latter's religious or spiritual beliefs, but performing an explicit religious ritual extended too far.

Fellow doctors may recognize and accept physicians who are also chaplains or are known to be devout. "I regularly ask all my medical trainees, 'How's your soul?'" another such physician-chaplain told me. I was amazed he would ask such an explicitly theological question.

"How do they respond?" I inquired.

"Most trainees talk about how the work can be morally crushing—how difficult it is in the ER to go immediately from a patient who just died, despite your efforts, to a patient with only a mild rash. Providers don't have time to consider or process the moral and existential strains"—their grief and distress when patients die.

"Do any trainees find your question too personal?" I asked him.

Short, but ebullient, outgoing and brimming with energy, he laughed. "No. They see me come into the room, and know I'm going to ask!" He smiled.

17

When doctors cry

Assisting staff with stress

Occasionally, when I have tried as hard as I could to help suffering patients and their families, but knew I would fail against the inevitable onslaught of disease, tears have begun to well up in my eyes. I hoped that the patient or family wouldn't see me weeping. I was sad, but embarrassed that I was being emotional rather than wholly objective and rational.

"I wonder if it is OK to cry," a physician with advanced cancer once said to me. She was genuinely unsure; doctors are, after all, supposed to be strong, in control. But when she sat alone in her office, aware she might die in a few months, she wanted to weep.

Though feeling burned out from confronting daily death and dread, in addition to mounting bureaucratic demands,[1] doctors often remain wary of emotional, religious, spiritual, and existential issues in medicine. They avoid and feel awkward about these topics, or even hostile toward them.

Even though they sometimes encounter lack of interest or apathy from doctors and nurses in other instances, chaplains assist these providers. Especially during the COVID pandemic, chaplains sought to help.

This topic may seem far afield for patients and families, but it illuminates what they might expect from their doctor, and what their doctor should ideally know and do. The insights here also offer important life lessons that can aid all of us in our relationships, groups, families, and jobs.

When facing wariness from doctors, chaplains at secular institutions have frequently emphasized how they can benefit staff. Particularly since the COVID pandemic, "we've been focusing on staff support," Connie reported, "because the C-suite folks understand that, and see it as immediately valuable. If we can help alleviate staff stress, we can solidly contribute to the bottom line, though it's an indirect metric." Sadly and perhaps ironically, it took the pandemic for many administrators to fully recognize these benefits.

Even prior to the pandemic, physician burnout was mounting,[2] due to rising stresses related not only to patients' sickness and death but also to

Doctor, Will You Pray for Me?. Robert L. Klitzman, Oxford University Press. © Oxford University Press 2024.
DOI: 10.1093/oso/9780197750841.003.0017

increased bureaucratization, longer work hours, and more time spent on computer screens and less with patients.[3,4] Physicians consequently have higher rates of burnout and substance abuse than the general population.[5,6]

COVID worsened these stresses, since ratios of patients to nurses increased two- to four-fold.[7,8] During the height of the pandemic, almost a third of healthcare workers felt stressed and depressed and contemplated leaving the profession, exacerbating staff shortages, especially of nurses.[9] Burnout rates among hospital staff rose about 62%.[10] Such distress can cause post-traumatic stress disorder symptoms, and interpersonal and work difficulties.[11]

While facing personal moral, existential, spiritual, and religious strains, providers commonly struggle to maintain "detached concern" (to both remain concerned about patients and stay at a professional distance, to avoid being either too close to patients or too cold and distant).[12] Medicine routinely has side effects, hurting as well as helping patients, but physicians succeed professionally because of their abilities to forge ahead undeterred. Doctoring can become a mundane, routinized daily grind, yet becoming either too intimate or too distant can aggravate burnout.

Heightened awareness of these larger existential and spiritual concerns can potentially assist healthcare providers. Some physicians draw on spiritual perspectives for support, even if only in the form of mindfulness exercises, and broader humanistic notions about healing, recognizing and valuing these dimensions of their work. Providers who wall themselves off from these larger spiritual and human meanings in their jobs may impede themselves.

Burnout is linked to existential issues of purpose. "We went into this business for certain meaning-making reasons," Jason Cooper, the Connecticut psychiatrist, said. "But now we're employees, factory workers, and money-makers. The marvelous thing about COVID has been the resurgence of a willingness to put oneself in harm's way, and recognition of how *meaningful* the work has become. Spirituality can help, like any social support system can help with burnout."

During the COVID-19 pandemic, 83.9% of chaplains in one study were asked to provide spiritual care for staff, and 58.9% regularly did so.[13] In another survey, 56% reported providing support for healthcare team members.[14] Chaplains did so in several countries.[15]

At the height of the pandemic, however, quandaries arose about how best to address staff stresses. Hospitals needed medical staff on the frontlines but also perceived needs to give them breaks. "Most of the time, doctors down-play their stresses and just plow through," William Gibson stated. "But now, we encouraged them *not* to downplay it. We told physicians to *slow down*: 'Maybe you need to take care of yourself, and not just plow through this.' With COVID-19, we acknowledged how bad things were, and needs for self-care. But I wondered if we should say what military chaplains say, emphasizing resilience: 'You're part of a system that needs you to get back out there. Slap a Band-Aid on it. Get back in the trenches.' Nurses and doctors themselves also didn't think they could just take a break and do a bunch of self-care. We just kind of blessed them in the midst of the struggle. That was complicated."

How chaplains help staff

Physicians' and nurses' own personal past emotional trauma can heighten their empathy, but at times also hamper their work. A chaplain can help staff understand and frame their own and their patients' distress, and convey appreciation. "I often validate and normalize what the team experiences, helping them understand it," Connie Clark said. "COVID-19 added a layer of grief onto what was already difficult, and tapped into the staff's unresolved grief for their own loved ones who died. So, it felt very heavy. There was a lot of grief. With COVID, I told staff all the time that I appreciated them. If there was a death, I said, 'Just know that I recognize this is really hard, and that people understand that, and appreciate what you're doing.' Staff seem to appreciate that."

Chaplains also help doctors and nurses, including trainees, with *moral conflicts*. As William Gibson said, "Today I met with a spiritual medical resi-dent. Her mother taught her about doing the right things, and living a certain way, and working hard, and that if you do, things will generally work out. But it's not happening for her right now, so she's questioning that. Physicians, es-pecially in training, are unlikely to self-refer and/or get referred to a chaplain or psychologist or admit that they're hurting and feeling they're not tougher, or have a spiritual or religious life, and are not just a secular scientific person."

Especially when personal and professional experiences collide, chaplains can provide crucial sounding boards. "One doctor's 8-year-old son died, and she could not do anything to save him," Brenda Pierson said. "That makes her ultra-vigilant in fighting for life at all costs. Over the years she asks me, 'Am I pushing too hard? Am I hearing the parents' voices, not just my own?'"

Chaplains assist staff, too, in processing particularly troubling and wrenching clinical cases. Connie Clark described, for instance, "a very young mom in the coronary ICU who thought she had the flu, but ended up having endocarditis, and died within 48 hours. It was very traumatic. She had two toddler sons. There's a wail that mothers utter when they realize their child is going to die. It just sears your soul. I'd heard it in pediatric units, but never on an adult ward. When her husband entered the room, I heard it. Every caregiver on the unit stopped dead in their tracks. It was unfamiliar. It shocked and upset them, but they couldn't put their finger on it. When the team debriefed, I explained it as 'the sound of someone whose heart has just broken, who has just lost his or her world. Once you've heard that sound, you will never forget it. No one ever does. It requires a moment of silence and respect.' Some of the residents and younger nurses had no idea how to frame that. It was helpful for them to understand. Just by naming it, normalized it for them." Chaplains can help staff process such experiences witnessing psychic pain.

Chaplains can aid medical staff and trainees more, not just when these staff feel existential struggles or are physically ill. Physicians and trainees confront moral distress, for instance, when they must physically injure patients, even though the benefits outweigh the risks. But often no formal such mechanisms exist for addressing these strains. Sam Lacey described, for example, a third-year medical student's reaction to amputating a patient's leg: "We do a lot of amputations at our county hospital, because of uncontrolled diabetes. The surgical team let the student do the actual cutting. She sawed off this patient's leg off above the knee and put the leg in the bag, and went on to the next patient.

"This was routine for everybody. It didn't seem to affect them. But it shook her up deeply. She wanted the team to stop and acknowledge that this was sad, difficult, and strange, but they didn't want to talk about it. There was no venue for processing this. In patient care, lots of heavy emotional things go on unaddressed. Doctors just carry that on their shoulders, and it contributes to burnout."

Alas, staff may not realize that chaplains can assist them. "Staff are continually surprised to know that we're there for them as much as we are for the patients and families," said Adam Quincy. "We try to advertise that more."

Creating rituals

To help staff cope, chaplains create their own innovative rituals that vary in both form and content—in terms of frequency, audience, size, formality, and goals. Especially when one or more patients die at a particular time, chaplains can organize events for staff to mark the pivotal point of transition from battling to save a patient's life to suddenly accepting death. Such deaths create awkward transitions for not only families but also providers. Pastoral care can build a space to help both groups, guiding and structuring these otherwise disturbing experiences. Even small such rituals, practices, and gestures can help. For instance, after a patient dies, some chaplains have the staff hold a few moments of silence, out of respect—unrelated to religion per se. But many doctors, if told to stay an extra few minutes, instead rush off to further waiting patients. Still, other staff may pause for a moment of silence.

Other chaplains create more patient-specific rituals. Linda Porter, for example, writes "Going Home" prayers that families take with them after their loved one has expired. "When a patient dies, it is impossible to walk out of the room for the last time," she explained. "Everyone stands around. The attending usually comes and says, 'I'm so sorry. Your daughter was wonderful.' The parents say, 'What do we do now?' As the family is getting ready to leave, I say, 'Before you say goodbye for the last time, would you like to pray again?' I'll talk to the parents and write a prayer about their child. I create a Going Home prayer. In the prayer, this moment and boundary between this world and the next one is sacred. I don't care what you call it, but religion can wreck these moments. I'll say, 'We've fought heroically to try and save this child's life, doing everything. We've come to love and care about your child deeply. Now the time has come to say goodbye. There may be a mystery about why this happened, but there is no mystery about how much she was loved or how hard she fought.' You can say a lot that is hope and healing.

"I print the prayer on parchment paper, and they take it with them. I want them to have something to read in 3 months when everything falls apart and slips away. This isn't for every family, but for those that have had real bonds. I say, 'You may be leaving our hospital, but will never leave our hearts. We are grateful.'"

Doctors sometimes join Linda and the family in saying the Going Home prayer. "I'll say, 'I've written a prayer for their daughter. Would this be a good time to pray?' The first time I did that, I thought, 'Is the doctor going to flee or stay? We pray, which then makes it possible for the doctor afterwards to leave; and the parents know they're going to be leaving soon, too. It makes the moment sacred."

In secular hospitals, there is a fine line—anything described as "too religious" makes people understandably uncomfortable. Linda remembered, for example, a boy who died "after a virus climbed up his spine and killed him. Our hospital did everything. His biopsies were sent to other hospitals. They never could identify the virus. When I read my prayer for him, eight or nine staff were in the room. They had tears in their eyes. Our hospital is pretty secular and anything that is too religious makes people uncomfortable, and frankly, it makes *me* uncomfortable. I understand a lot of physicians' skepticism towards religion in the hospital, because it can be pretty icky. But it can be done well.

"Several times, a mother or grandmother writes to me 9 months afterward, telling me they read my prayer at the service. It's important to honor these moments, which are intimate, personal. These patients touch everyone. Physicians have appreciated it.

"A Down's patient who died had her 21st birthday in the hospital," Linda continued. "I have a brother who's developmentally disabled, so these kids just go right up to my heart. I wrote a beautiful prayer for her, which her family talked about—not because of the power of my writing, but because it was such a personal prayer that just lifted up the beautiful traits of this child, who was so loving, kind, and such a sweetheart. This girl made everyone around her glad. That's a rare gift. They read the prayer at her funeral." Hospitals and chaplains employ patient and family "satisfaction scales" to try to measure these professionals' effects quantitatively, but these short-answer questionnaires might not capture the depth and emotional importance of such moments, connections, and meanings.

Chaplains also organize and lead staff memorial services for patients, devising novel rituals. These events vary in size from just a single staff member to many, depending on perceptions of staff needs. "We have a program patterned after the Code Lavender Program at the Cleveland Clinic," Brian Post, the Michigan chaplaincy department administrator, said. He "can tell that somebody is having a bad day—maybe a family member, in the midst of their grief and difficulty, just cussed you out, accused you of being an incompetent nurse, and stormed out. Or a patient spit in your face or called you a racial epithet. These things happen to healthcare professionals much more than people realize. A coworker or manager can call for a 'Code Lavender,' and chaplains pull that healthcare professional out of work for a few minutes and give him or her a chance to vent, providing a little extra TLC and some good active listening, and a process for discussing some of the emotions. Code Lavender is for emotional distress in a staff member just like Code Blue is for a patient in cardiac arrest."

Other rituals aid staff, including even ambulance teams, involved with a particular patient. "This week we held a memorial service for a 2-month-old baby who was born at home, addicted to heroin," Brenda Pierson reported. "The people in her house continued to give her heroin. Last week, she died here alone, without family. I held her and sang to her when she died. We included the staff who knew her, and the ambulance team who brought her. In retelling and reliving it, we were taken aback afresh by how it made us all feel. The case was harder than we thought."

Rituals can benefit whole hospital units. Given that staff are busy and rarely, if ever, able to attend simultaneously, these events can be brief and more informal, and at times serve food to further nourish and potentially attract attendees. "We do a program called 'Refreshment for the Soul,'" Brian Post reported, "for any nursing unit that had an exceptionally traumatic patient care experience or rough few weeks. The nurse manager says to me, 'I think we could use a Refreshment for the Soul.' We find a conference room, redecorate it a little, pushing things around, bring in a teapot with a variety of teas, hot chocolate or instant coffee, and home-baked goodies, soften the lighting, put on soft music, and bring in some aromatherapy. For a couple of hours, staff are welcome to come and go, and we're available to talk. It's simple but remarkably effective." While Code Lavender aids only one doctor or nurse, this chaplain's "Refreshment for the Soul" assists many staff.

At times, a chaplain initiates such activities in conjunction with one or more staff members who see the need and have felt unhelped by others whom they have approached. Linda Porter, for example, formed an ongoing support group. "A beautiful 8-year-old child in the PICU was fine in the morning and dead from sepsis that night. A resident went to a priest and got nothing. A PICU nurse told me, 'I just shut down after the ninth death because it was just too much. I was in Vietnam. It was the same for us then.' They just have to keep going. So, I formed a group, which meets a couple of times a year. There are no answers to these questions, but being able to explore the mystery together and talk about it and feelings about traumatic events helps."

These rituals range, too, in structure and in how much they are freeform. With a pediatric palliative care physician, Cathy Murray started a session "called 'What Matters at the End of the Day,' at the end of the rotation for medical residents on neonatal and pediatric ICUs and pediatric oncology. All we had to say is, '*What case is keeping you up at night?*' Then, for the next hour, we just listened. Some doctors were ready to leave the profession; I think we helped them stay. They said, 'I've learned that I love oncology and want the long-term relationship with the child and the family. It's devastating if the child dies, but I really value the relationship.' Some said, 'I've learned that the ICU is where it's at, because I can't stand getting to know this child over weeks and months and then having them die.' Usually in the ICU, you never got to know the child. They were already unresponsive. So, staff were setting up their own psychological self-protection." Cathy often selects "a theme for the month. It might be gratitude or hope. I use a poem, a video, an article, something to get the conversation going. It's not a therapy or complaint session, but a chance to pause and talk about coping."

Chaplains can establish and conduct events for not only front-line clinicians but also *administrators*, including, for instance, nurse managers. Cathy Murray provides "debriefings" for hospital leaders as well. "We offer spiritual grounding once a month to leadership for an hour—a chance to come together and take a step back from pressures to re-energize and remind ourselves why we're in healthcare, and form relationships with our colleagues outside of needing to transfer a patient to their unit." With COVID-19, Cathy scheduled these "debriefings" at different times of the day and included community healthcare providers and social service professionals as well.

On their own, individual chaplains often create new, innovative kinds of rituals that uniquely allow for expressions of grief and distress. They vary in length (from minutes to hours to weeks or months), formality, aims, and specificity. "There are Grand Rounds, so I do *Chocolate Rounds!*" Connie reported. "I walk up to caregivers and staff with a little basket of chocolate Hershey's Kisses and say, 'Hi, are you in need of chocolate today?' They say, 'Yes! I'm *absolutely* in need of chocolate today.' I then say, 'I just wanted to thank you for all that you've been doing. I know it's been rough lately.' Sometimes they'll say, 'Yeah, it has been rough!' 'Really?' I ask. 'What's been the hardest part about it for you?' 'Last week we had three codes and five deaths—three of them were unexpected.' Chocolate Rounds have been very successful."

The contents of rituals

These events have different foci, aims, and functions but often include expressing feelings, offering support, and/or helping staff to reflect on the emotional and existential, not just medical, aspects of difficult cases, and positively reframe feelings. "We also provide debriefings," Brian Post, the chaplaincy administrator, said, "for exceptionally traumatic group experiences, such as a labor and delivery team caring for a woman in a relatively normal full-term delivery who suddenly arrests and dies, which rattles everybody involved. We gather everybody involved and give space for processing the emotions, like a root cause analysis at a Mortality and Morbidity conference, but dealing with emotional, rather than strictly medical, sides of the decisions made. When people try to 'second-guess' the clinical decisions, we redirect them toward, 'There'll be a context for that, but what was it *like* for you? What were you *feeling* when you were making that decision?' Opportunities to talk about those traumatic events collectively with a group of people who went through them are beneficial and reduce long-term sequelae."

These events can singularly help staff sort through confusing and conflicting emotions. "The spiritual grounding and debriefing sessions we offer help people unpack what is happening," Cathy said. "'Is it because you feel moral distress or because you've added to that patient's suffering, or the institution made an error, or you feel short-staffed?' We can work with staff in different ways, trying to strengthen resilience."

In particular, these sessions can help staff *reframe* their experiences and regrets, especially after a patient has died, establishing a helpful sense of community in the face of apparent sheer loss. Rituals can explore and address the moral distress staff feel due to conflicting feelings, and help these professionals remember and reconnect with why they had entered these fields in the first place. As Nancy Cutler explained, "If staff are feeling, 'We did a poor job here. We didn't support the parents well,' or, God forbid, 'We made a mistake,' we need to address that and say, 'What can we put in place to ensure that this never happens again?'" But, Nancy argued, staff also need to say, "'We cared for this child for the past three months, and she touched all our hearts and we are really grieving for this one individual child.' . . . It comes down to: Could people say how they made a difference in this child's care, even if the child died? They might say: 'I made her look beautiful when her parents came to see her for the last time. I brushed her hair, washed her face, and put real clothes on her, not just a johnny.' Or 'I could tell she was in pain. She was grimacing and crying. I advocated that we had to address that.' Or 'We were able to do something special.' We've had graduations in the ICU. For one child, a major Hollywood studio flew in an advance video copy of a new film so he could watch it before he died. If the staff feels 'we did something that really made that child's life better,' that is important for them."

At other times, such sessions might encourage or help staff explore how a patient's death evokes losses in their own lives. "In these sessions," Nancy Cutler continued, "I try to allow staff the space to grieve for the child, but also get a sense of whether they are grieving *their own* mortality. Was this death reminding them of someone in their family?" or did it make them feel that "they did a poor job as a healthcare team?"

Especially during the pandemic, chaplains drew on multiple such techniques, not only positive reframing but relaxation methods as well. "With COVID, nurses say to me, 'It's all bad. Everything is terrible. The world is falling apart,'" Kristine Baker said. "I say, 'Yes, I'm sorry about that. You're doing such a good job. It sounds like it's so hard.' But I try to give staff space to talk about that, and to remember what's going *well*, bring them around at least to *neutral*. I lead 'listening circles' to give staff space to talk about what's bad, but I don't want it to end there. Our bodies need to get back. So, I say, 'Was there any time during the last week that you even felt neutral? I don't need for you to feel good or grateful; that's too big an ask. But can you find a time over that last week where you felt even just in the middle?' Lots can. Even as small as 'looking out the window and seeing birds.' I'll say, 'Tell me about that. What kind of bird?' 'A bluebird.' 'What was it like?' I want to take them back to that experience."

Making commemorative objects

Rituals can involve not just discussion but also construction of objects of remembrance. Chaplains can create patient-specific documents or mementos. "It sometimes helps to do something with your *hands*," Connie Clark said. "I do a 'Time of Remembrance' for staff, bringing a grapevine wreath in the shape of a heart onto ICUs and other units—it's especially nice on the heart units—along with little precut 3-inch narrow ribbons. We do a brief memorial service. I read the names of patients who have died and invite staff to share a memory of that person and tie a ribbon onto the wreath in remembrance.

"As they're tying the ribbon onto the wreath, I'll ask them what they re-member about this individual. Sometimes they won't recollect the name, but remember the bed space. I'll say, 'I can see that this really bothered you. What touched your heart, or bothered you the most?'

"They'll remember that they talked to the patient and established a con-nection before the patient became intubated or died. Or 'It reminded me of when my own dad died.' Sometimes they won't say anything with other staff around, but I follow up with them later."

Yet with these and other rituals, chaplains may need to be flexible, given that staff are frequently overwhelmed with other tasks. "If the ICU is busy, I won't do a group session," Connie continued, "but take the wreath door to door and say, 'I've got a memory wreath. Would you like to remember anybody?'"

Especially during the height of the COVID pandemic, such a ritual aided staff with loss of their own loved ones as well as of patients. "Before the pan-demic," Connie recalled, "it was almost 100% about patients. Afterwards, staff remembered a lot of their own family members who died years ago but were brought to mind by the pandemic. One unit actually filled up their wreath; I had to start a second one because we got so many ribbons on it—which is sad, but also a testament to how used it is."

These rituals can assist staff as well when a coworker perishes. Connie has "done a couple of *special* wreaths. A beloved physician died—a sudden, un-expected cardiac death. The unit was devastated. So he had his own wreath. Everybody contributed to it and people bought not just ribbons but things that reminded them of him, like a special ID badge holder. It now hangs in the breakroom of the unit. We leave the wreaths up, sometimes in the breakrooms or on the breakroom door. Units are proud of their wreaths and know what they represent."

Chaplains draw, too, on relaxation, behavioral, and psychotherapeutic approaches, reconnecting staff with past, more positive feelings they have had. Connie Clark tells medical teams, "You are dealing with so much. Your body, your nervous system, and spiritual system are taking a hit. Would it be OK if we did an exercise where we try to bring your nervous system a little bit out of that?' I always ask permission because some people don't even want to go to neutral. They just want to grieve. They may need to stay in the bottom. That's OK. Maybe we need more time to talk. Ninety-nine percent of the time they say, 'I don't think I can feel any better, but I'm willing to try.' I say, 'Tell me about that,' because people can get a little addicted to their own misery.

I ask, 'Do you think that you will love somebody less if you let go of that misery? Is it a betrayal of them if you're not miserable?' Because that makes grief hard: 'Do you think this person would want you to be miserable in order to honor them?'"

She also engages staff in exercises to center their bodies, as she does with distressed patients, saying, "'Where in your body are you feeling this?' 'In my gut, my chest, my heart.' I say, 'Go back to that place in your body. Let's just sit and stay there a while and feel that. What's it like for you to tell me about this? What do you feel in your body?'

"We have a GPS in our body," Connie continued, "that 80–90% of the time will take us someplace we don't want to go. Because most people have eight kinds of feelings, and six or seven are negative. Eighty percent of the time, our GPS is going to take us to threat, distress, sadness, or grief, so we can't trust it. We have to *change our GPS*, be aware that our GPS is going to take us to distress. That's not good for our bodies."

Chaplains shift approaches over time, depending on staff interest and perceived needs. Cathy Murray, for instance, "tried doing a shorter session for the front-line staff called 'The Spirit of Caring,' which was going OK until COVID hit. If a distressing event occurred on a unit—a long-term patient died or an unexpected death occurred, or a team member has died—we can offer a session to the staff, almost like a *debriefing*, to be able to talk about what's it been like, what's been happening physically, emotionally, spiritually, and what strategies and resources are available. We are now doing that more regularly with the oncology staff, because, unfortunately, they have a lot of patient deaths."

Other chaplains offer longer, ongoing programs as well. "We also had day-long, even 2-day-long sessions for the residents on death and dying," Brenda Pierson said. "I've done role plays with standardized patients about grief, spiritual care, and communication, and sudden death of children who have been with us a long time."

Chaplains usually name and label these rituals (e.g., Debriefings, What Matters at the End of the Day, Refreshment for the Soul, and Chocolate Rounds), suggesting recognition of these activities as specific, special, and distinguished from other endeavors, marking them as "special." This diversity of names suggests, too, how much chaplains are developing these independently.

Though other researchers have attempted to count the number of times pastoral care providers engage in certain activities, including "performing

a ritual," the chaplains here demonstrate the wide breadth, depth, and variability of their activities, highlighting how these events range in both form and
content—in frequency, length, structure, size, audience, and aims.

Chaplains perform rituals to help not only patients and families, but medical staff, too, especially doctors and nurses. Such events can provide ways
of marking and coming to terms with critical life transitions, like death and
dying.[16,17]

All cultures possess rituals surrounding bereavement,[16] frequently
involving rites of passage, facilitating transitions between different phases
of life (such as going from wife to widow)[18] and helping individuals
psychotherapeutically to reintegrate their sense of themselves.[17,19] Though
anthropologists have generally seen bereavement rituals as established by
cultures, chaplains are now often developing these events on their own. While
scholars have opined, too, that American bereavement rituals surrounding
grief have lost meaning, leading to insufficient expressions of grief,[20] spiritual care providers commonly now take on these functions. One such ritual,
Code Lavender, has previously been described,[21] but the chaplains here reveal how additional ones can be used and inspire others.

Challenges in helping staff

Yet obstacles can impede the creation and implementation of such rituals.
Hospital staff, especially physicians, may have limited time for these activities; staff can be too busy or wary. Cathy Murray tries "to find ways to be
visible and present without people asking themselves, 'Why are [chaplains]
here? What did we do wrong? I have to care for the patients, so I don't have
time to talk to you.' It can be 'soft,' like bringing treats, or scheduled, showing
up at your huddles—breaking down barriers of feeling I'm either going to
bother them or be in the way."

Many administrators and others also resist, minimize, or dismiss needs for
these undertakings. Hospitals may purport to support staff but do not always
sufficiently do so, especially concerning spiritual issues. "The hospital would
probably say it supports the medical residents and fellows pretty well," Linda
Porter remarked, "but when you talk to them, they want more."

Nancy Cutler, for example, tried to establish a group for nurses; however,
the ICU nursing director said that these employees should just soldier on: "I
tried doing groups on the ICU with nurses. The nursing director said, 'They

don't need that. We just tell them, "Suck it up. This is how it is." ' I said, 'Would you mind if I just tried? I'd like you to attend as well.' "

Such sessions can lead staff to vent strong pent-up emotions. "We did a session, and new nurses broke down sobbing," Nancy continued, "saying, 'This is the first death I've ever experienced in my life. No one I know has ever died. Other nurses tell me: "Just suck it up." ' They were just in real distress. Luckily, the nurse manager heard that, and told me to schedule more sessions for the nurses. She could see that it was important to them."

Within the longstanding hierarchy of hospital wards, the specific chaplain's status and length of time on a ward can affect receptivity to these endeavors. Linda Porter has "been there long enough now that I'm respected and know the PICU and the oncology attendings, so they're comfortable with me and know I'm 'OK.' I'm not going to make anybody uncomfortable by being too preachy or religious, even though I'm an Episcopal priest."

Chaplains thus devise, on their own initiative, new rituals that vary in form and content, but can help, and serve as models for other institutions, chaplains and providers.

PART VI

GOD 2.0: MOVING
INTO THE FUTURE

18

"Doctor, will you pray for me?"

Improving doctors

A few years ago, I visited Epidaurus in Greece, the home of the largest intact theater from the Ancient World. It is considered to have perfect acoustics: All 15,000 audience members can still hear mere whispers or pin drops from the stage. But outside the theater, with its grand semicircular rows of white marble seats, stood a small, rarely visited museum, filled with stone inscriptions, statues, and tools, all related to medicine, surgery, and healing.

The Greeks believed that Epidaurus was the birthplace of Apollo's son, Asklepios—the god of medicine and healing. Modern medicine still uses the "rod of Asklepios"—a snake entwined around a pole—as a symbol. The theater, it turns out, was in fact part of a hospital complex, the most famous in the Ancient World. For centuries, patients trekked to this sanctuary. Inside stood a hospital, a temple, and the theater. Here, the Greeks sought catharsis, partly through performances of comedy and tragedy, to heal the mind, body, spirit, and soul. This inclusiveness and "holistic" perspective seems right. As Victor Simmons, the VA chaplain, said, "Recovery is holistic when mind, body, and spirit are all working together."

When I became a doctor, I uttered the Hippocratic Oath: "I swear by Apollo the physician, and Asclepius, and Hygieia and Panacea, and all the gods and goddesses as my witnesses, that I will keep this oath . . ." I wondered why we were invoking these gods, in whom no one now believes. The text seemed quaint and anachronistic, unnecessary, even silly. But I have come to see how spiritual, religious, and existential concerns, though most doctors today feel awkward and unprepared to address them, are in fact deeply entwined in medicine. Still, not until after 9/11 and becoming a patient myself did I fully appreciate their importance.

Doctors can frequently address these issues with patients better by not only referring patients to chaplains but also being prepared to discuss these areas themselves, even fleetingly, with patients and families. Several specific sets of improvements are needed.

Doctor, Will You Pray for Me?. Robert L. Klitzman, Oxford University Press. © Oxford University Press 2024.
DOI: 10.1093/oso/9780197750841.003.0018

Doctors should integrate chaplains more on rounds, and recognize chaplains' value. Several years ago, critics successfully pushed physicians to adopt more of a multidisciplinary team approach and include nurses more fully as part of medical rounds and decisions. Similarly, healthcare systems should also now try to incorporate chaplains more.

Physicians should more fully recognize, too, how these conversations can aid patients, especially when death looms, but in other situations, too. Since chaplains are ultimately limited in number, doctors as well should possess skills to address, even if briefly, patients' spiritual concerns, particularly when patients raise these, even if just to make a referral to a chaplain. Alas, *patients and families do not all even know that chaplains exist*, or feel empowered to request one, and would thus benefit from this knowledge and from feeling more comfortable raising these topics.

Patients appreciate, in addition, when their doctor perceives them as individuals, not as anonymous and interchangeable. Physicians should of course have technical expertise in their field, but knowing about their patients as human beings can help as well—whether the patient is facing existential, spiritual, or religious crises, and is religious or spiritual or not. These domains are important parts of patients' social histories; and therefore of doctors getting to know their patients as people.

Several chaplains have sought to educate medical trainees, citing research showing the benefits of spirituality and religion to patients, and trying to address possible barriers. "I tell interns and residents that I'm not here to fight them," Marvin Beck, at a small New Hampshire community hospital, reported, "but that studies show that spirituality and/or religion have health benefits. Patients' blood pressure, breathing, and medical outcomes are better. Their rate of curing is better. They're tied into a community and have support." Given currently under-resourced healthcare systems, these discussions can also help families recognize the disadvantages of costly but unbeneficial treatments.

Yet doctors frequently ignore these spiritual, religious, and existential comments, quickly moving on and responding medically or changing the subject, suggesting that the topic is irrelevant, inappropriate, or of less interest. Healthy medical students and young doctors may be atheist or cynical, but should nonetheless focus on how to best understand and assist their patients. These issues may not be large in these doctors' own lives, but they may be crucial to those they treat.

Doctors should be taught how to address these topics with patients better, and when and how to make chaplain referrals. Such educational efforts can succeed. In one Dutch multicenter trial, for instance, chaplains gave doctors and nurses skills in screening and answering spiritual needs, and enhanced team competences.[1] Patients' ratings of their medical team's attention to their spiritual needs improved. Such training can strengthen doctors' and nurses' appreciation of chaplains' importance.

At a minimum, physicians should be taught to be less awkward, indifferent, or hostile when these topics emerge. Efforts at such training of present and future providers have started, but often minimally, and can be bolstered. "A lot of hospitals and medical schools address end-of-life care," one physician with metastatic breast cancer told me, "but not enough or well enough. No staff is really dealing with end-of-life, except in hospice . . . Our hospital has a rabbi, but I've never seen him." As I saw during my own education, and at many medical schools still, no chaplain ever enters the classroom.

Other healthcare providers, besides physicians, could also benefit from bolstered education about these topics. "I ask psychology students and interns, 'How was spirituality addressed in your training?'" Victor Simmons reported. "One of them said, 'We got the sense: "Don't have anything to do with it. Stay away."' That's not good."

Several efforts have been made and assessed to teach "spiritual care" to healthcare providers outside of pastoral care. One study evaluated 50 healthcare providers (doctors, nurses, and others) at the beginning and end of 400 hours of training[2] and found improvement in comfort and skills. But 400 hours is too long, and hence unrealistic for most physicians. Moreover, teaching "spiritual care," if it means providing significant spiritual interventions and treatment as opposed to just enhancing sensitivity and awareness, may be too ambitious. In addition, shorter questionnaires have been developed to help clinicians obtain a patient's spiritual history.[3,4] In another study, chaplains instructed hospital staff in spiritual care and perceived positive effects, which included reducing obstacles and enhancing team members' competencies and appreciation of chaplains.[1,5] Such training by chaplains can thus potentially help.

Other educational approaches can be important as well—for example, a course in the medical humanities. "Spirituality is just one way of trying to help doctors be humanistic," Sam Lacey said. He tries to help trainees and doctors have "a humanistic approach to their patients' lives—to deal with human beings, not just organs." Such courses include books that provide in-depth patient perspectives and connections to something beyond basic human material needs per se.

Such courses can address some of these issues in secular terms, implicitly and explicitly, but may be insufficient in and of themselves, since they can exclude key elements of patient experiences. Targeted skills are also essential. "We put everything in secular language and call it 'medical humanities,'" Sam Lacey continued, "but I always gear classroom conversations towards *existential* issues. At some point, the conversation inevitably gets to religion, so I try to bring up these issues in a pluralistic way. The students in our classes usually represent three or four different religions and include two or three atheists. We read a book by hospice nurses in which patients describe getting close to death, seeing a light, and communicating with loved ones around the hospital room. I asked, 'How do you read this? What would that mean from a Hindu or Roman Catholic perspective?' I never have a goal of what I want them to think, other than to listen and take patients seriously."

Openness to the potential roles of spirituality in helping patients should, however, not only be taught in classrooms *but also modeled by behavior*. "Students learn best through the apprenticeship mode," Sam added, "watching how senior doctors actually interact with people."

Physicians need training in how to ask questions and feel more comfortable with these topics and with views other than their own, and knowing when to call a chaplain. Medical education should, for example, include case vignettes for student discussion of issues that patients with varying beliefs may raise. Many doctors or nurses know little about beliefs they did not grow up with or explicitly study. What they learn is commonly haphazard, rather than systematic. Jim Adams, the Philadelphia oncologist and "lapsed Catholic," said, "I've only gotten to know about Hasidism, for instance, because I happen to have treated a lot of Hasidic patients over the years. . . . I once had a Hasidic patient who needed to take the elevator to get a CAT scan on a Saturday. I had to call the rabbi to ask if that were permissible. The rabbi said, 'OK, as long as the patient and the family don't have to press the elevator button.' My hospital now has Sabbath elevators that automatically stop on every floor so no one has to press a button. But at that time, we didn't, *and I had no idea what to do!* Whenever I do ask patients if they want to talk to someone about spiritual issues," Jim added, "they almost always say yes." He remains surprised.

Chaplains can help doctors partly by providing a *language* for raising existential concerns without getting religious. "Families want to bring their faith into these decisions but, particularly residents and fellows, who are running most of these family meetings, aren't sure how to incorporate that," Connie Clark explained. "At some point, trainees get a lecture that says, 'You should get a spiritual history and ask whether the patients have religious beliefs that matter to them.' Yet a lot of doctors are uncomfortable and don't know what to do with that information as a next step. If doctors are just willing to ask the questions, though, patients and families feel seen and heard—like you know them as people!"

Chaplains also *model* behavior that doctors can adopt. "If I'm in these meetings, I'll say, 'Where do you suppose God is in all of this?'" Connie continued. "I talk to patients and families so that the doctors can hear and understand how to discuss these topics, and not have to shy away or immediately hand the patient off to a chaplain, but can instead ask these questions themselves. I give them *a language* to talk about it, and help them understand that they can bring up existential issues without getting 'religious' about it."

Though doctors often don't have time for prolonged conversations, a single extra question need not take much time and could aid in understanding and helping patients. Yet doctors' other, medical priorities can themselves become rationales or excuses for avoiding these realms altogether.[6]

Patients and families appreciate even such brief statements from physicians. "I talk to medical students about the importance of *listening*," Sister Francine told me. "*To listen to a patient is giving them a gift.* Often, when someone listens to you, you also then realize what you think."

Even small comments from doctors can help. "My son was in an accident and was Code Blue," one nurse told me. "I was outside the hospital room, praying. His doctor walked out and told me, 'You doing that out here is as important as what we're doing in there.' Eventually, my son came back, but I'll never forget that doctor saying that to me. That one comment was the most important thing anyone has ever said to me.

"Thank God, in the end, my son did OK. I wanted to thank that doctor, and tell him how much I love him for saying that, but I never have. I occasionally see him around, but would feel too awkward saying something." She still hesitates, suggesting how staunchly hierarchies prevail.

Physicians can assist simply by recognizing these topics. Doctors can "talk about spiritual pain," Connie suggested as an example. "Just acknowledge that spiritual distress and pain exist. Ask patients or families to rate it on a scale of zero to ten: 'How would you rate your level of suffering today?' 'I would rate it a seven.' 'Really? Why?' That opens the door. Doctors don't have to be spiritual or religious, but just acknowledge that some other people are." Alice Montgomery, a Midwest chaplain, values simply "having doctors understand that pain is important. It's an easy entrée into these conversations."

In the least, especially for patients who are severely ill and face the prospect of death, physicians should be prepared to offer general, nondenominational support or perspectives. A clinician could ask whether patients would be interested in a referral to help make sense of what they are going through, and potentially get moral support. Doctors can raise these issues in open-ended, secular, and existential ways, through questions such as:

- What sources of strength do you use or draw on? What supports do you have?
- Is a faith tradition part of that? Do you have any beliefs you want me to know about? Many people have religious or spiritual beliefs that are important to them. What is that like for you? Does anything give you meaning or energize you?
- How do you understand your illness?
- Are there things you are looking forward to or want to do?
- Do you have spiritual or religious beliefs that help you understand or make medical decisions?
- Are there any arrangements you think you should make? Do you have a will? Does your family know whether you want to be buried, and if so, where?
- If you would like, we could talk about these issues, or I could arrange for you to talk to one of the spiritual care providers here, if you would like.

Doctors could then refer the patient, if needed. If patients do not want these conversations, physicians should obviously respect these preferences. But many patients find these conversations helpful, often to their surprise. A physician can address these issues to help patients see their problems in larger contexts.

In commenting about these and other domains, physicians should realize, too, the importance of gestures and body language, not only verbal language per se. "When new doctors walk into the patient's room," Jack Stone observed, "they cross their arms, their hands in their white coats, standing over patients, looking down on them, setting up a very intimidating power dynamic. When I ask patients, 'How's your medical team?' they reply, 'My doctors are wonderful. They seem to care about me: *They sat down!* I never saw a doctor sit down with me like that before. They were rushed, but told me they did have a couple of minutes. I felt they really listened.' It's the skill of bedside manners, the actual human connection. After doctors ask how you are breathing and how many bowel movements you had, they could ask, 'How are you doing today?' It doesn't take a lot to establish and nurture that. So, I teach doctors and nurses *to sit down*. If they don't have a lot of time, *say that upfront*: 'I have about 8 minutes. Are there any questions you have?' Sit down not too closely or too far away, but just right, in that middle zone, that sweet spot where 'pastoral touch' can take place."

Even doctors' simple touch or gestures can convey their concern. "I once followed a wonderful teenage boy for a long time," Linda Porter said. "After his leukemia relapsed, his bone marrow transplant was successful, but he was losing the ability to walk. The doctors could never identify the disease, which was moving up his body and would paralyze him before it killed him. There was a full-court press to figure out what was wrong. A famous doctor at our hospital was on service. One doesn't immediately sense his compassion, because he's such a star. But he spoke very candidly to this boy, who then told me, 'When the doctor finished examining me, *he put his hand on my shoulder. I think he really cares!*

"Doctors don't need hours to spend with a patient, which they don't have time to do anyway," Linda continued, "but they can convey a lot through tenderness, a tear, an embrace—that simple gesture, that power of touch, and ability to just sit there for a moment. Parents say, 'When the doctor told me the bad news, she had tears in her eyes, and I knew she really cared.' Doctors think patients want answers, but what patients really want is to know that they matter to the doctor, that they're not 'the medulloblastoma in Room 37.'"

Importantly, physicians should also not be caught off guard, but instead should be prepared to reply in some way to patients' comments about these realms—when patients say, for example, "Doc, will you pray with us?" "Do you believe in God?" "A miracle is going to happen, right?" "God will save me," "I hope I'll be good enough for when I meet God," or "I'm just going to pray" (rather than fully follow treatment). Doctors should be ready to respond when a patient mentions his or her own beliefs and asks about the provider's. Depending on the specific questions, a physician could simply say, for instance, "If you would like, we have chaplains here who could talk to you." Or, "Some people look to a higher power, but it's also important to follow medical advice." If nothing else, physicians should have such scripts comfortably in their repertoire, especially in end-of-life situations, rather than altogether sidestepping these domains.

Patients may perceive a physician's failure to respond to a comment about these realms as disinterest or insensitivity. "When a doctor doesn't follow up on patients' comments about going to church, or religion being important to them," Amanda Shaw, the religious Tennessee psychiatrist, said, "patients experience that as dismissive."

Doctors should strive, too, to avoid insensitive comments. "For difficult end-of-life conversations, hospitals tend to rely on young doctors who are less skilled and prepared and have difficulty with these conversations," Connie Clark observed. "A brand-new resident said to a family member of a new pediatric ICU patient, *'We've got her paralyzed and sedated.'* The family heard 'paralyzed' and went berserk. Afterwards, I told the doctor, 'You don't need to say "paralyzed."' Doctors are so literal sometimes. They're learning so much, and have so much thrown at them."

Physicians may simply not consider the potential inadvertent effects of their words on patients and families. Adam Quincy, for example, recalled an encounter between a doctor and a patient's widow: "The family was coming down the hall and was not expecting the father to die. The doctor was fabulous and did all he could, but now told the family, 'He didn't make it.' The wife collapsed on the floor, screaming and yelling, hitting her head on the ground. I thought we were going to have another death! It was terrible. The doctor's comment was too abrupt and heavy for her to handle. Bad news needs to be delivered sensitively, to prepare families for what you're going to say." Adam then met with, and aided this family.

At times, nurses, too, unintentionally make insensitive comments. When infants or children die, Brenda Pierson observed, "well-meaning nurses or physicians have their own spiritual beliefs, and give those to the family to ease both their own and the families' distress. Nurses say, 'You're young; you'll have another baby,' 'God must have needed an angel,' 'Aren't you glad they're not suffering?' or 'If you had prayed this way, God would have heard you.' Well-meaning people cause harm. Depending who the staff person is, I will go back and say, 'I heard you said this to the family. Would you tell me a little more about that?' I hear how staff members' faith was really the answer to their *own* story, not this particular family's."

Providers should appreciate, too, the complexities, intricacies, and multiple levels of meaning of many patients' questions and comments. Patients who inquire if their doctor will pray for them may be implicitly asking, "*Do you really care about me?* Are you committed to doing everything you can to help me? Will you go the extra mile?" Patients who ask their doctor, "Do you believe in God?" may be wondering, "*Can I trust you?*" Patients may be asking us to draw on whatever healing powers we might possess, symbolized by the purity and sacredness of our white coats, our unique roles as healers or shamans—not just writing prescriptions and electronic medical records—to chant whatever sacred incantations and shake whatever ancient magical rattles we may hold.

Strikingly, physicians are usually unaware that they possess such powers, but patients regularly project these onto us, imbuing us with them. "When my prognosis didn't look good and I was unsure if my cancer would return," one ill physician told me, "My doctor took my hand in hers and said, 'We're doing everything we can to help you.' The warmth of her hand calmed me. But I realized that if her touch affected me so strongly, then *my* touch must also affect *my own* patients. I never knew that." The fact that he was surprised is surprising but revealing, underscoring how much doctors downplay the nonscientific.

Physicians can often frame poor prognoses, in particular, more effectively. "I hear from patients, 'The doctor says there's nothing else we can do,'" Jason Cooper, the Connecticut psychiatrist, said. "But we can do *a lot* of things," making patients comfortable even if unable to cure the disease.

Doctors can also inquire about these topics to encourage and bolster social supports that might ensue. Certain physicians, though they appear to be in the minority, actively look to patients' religiosity as potential sources of strength and assistance. "I may be a little idiosyncratic," Jason Cooper continued, "but whenever a patient is dealing with chronic medical or psychiatric illness—longstanding depression, anxiety, post-traumatic stress disorder, or personality disorder—I look for additional resiliency supports and spirituality, whether it's belief and adherence to organized religion or not. There's nothing like believing in a greater power. Spirituality can be *another* '*arrow*' *in a doctor's or patient's quiver.* I try to get people to have as many arrows in their quiver as possible."

Especially for patients and families who are isolated, with limited outside interpersonal relationships, religious institutions can provide crucial networks. Jason, for instance, treated a schoolteacher with a chronic anxiety disorder and a personality disorder who was trying to cope with her mother's death. "She had a son with an immigrant who was probably a psychopath. Her mother had a mean streak and cut my patient out of her life, excommunicating my patient, who has tremendous guilt and shame over that. My patient has a small group of friends from college but has become more and more isolated. She was raised very Catholic but is really a lost Catholic. In the last three years, though, she started to go back to the church. She doesn't get much out of Confession, but likes being with her people. She's found support that I certainly couldn't provide."

Nonetheless, religious and spiritual issues are not germane for all patients. "For a lot of people," Jason continued, "it doesn't feel relevant, and we don't talk about it." He and other providers therefore gauge patients' and families' openness and interest. "The biggest challenge is *judging your audience*," Jason said. "Many people are desperate but feel these topics are irrelevant, something we're trying to offer that is beyond what they can do. They reject it out of hand. I'm always trying to get people to find things that add meaning to their lives, encouraging them to define spirituality broadly, to help them define a source of meaning or a 'higher power.' It works for some patients, not others."

Patients vary widely not only in what they believe, but also in whether and how much they want providers to explore these topics. "It falls into the three buckets," Jason added. "For the main group, it isn't a source of conversation and doesn't affect what we do. With the second group, which is small, it's important. The third group says, 'Doc, forget about it.' So, I follow their lead. If they don't want to talk about spirituality as a support, we find others that work for them."

Aspects of the particular patient and treatment shape these categories—such as whether the patient's problem is short or long term. Patients facing chronic challenges are often more interested. "Spirituality," Jason continued, "benefits anybody who has had a traumatic life, few supports, health problems, and mental illness. However, you can lead a horse to water but can't make it drink. My long-term patients are different than those who want a quick fix and to then get on with their lives: 'Give me the medicine and some techniques.' They don't want any of this spiritual crapola. It's just not relevant."

Clearly, though, for many patients, these beliefs are highly beneficial. Clinicians can determine whether, when, and how to have patients draw on these activities. "Religion can be adjuvant," Jason elaborated. "I've treated one mental health professional for decades—an alcoholic with chronic pain.

Her life is a constant struggle. She's chronically suicidal. She doesn't act on it, but is a little bit of a wrist cutter. AA has helped. Five years ago, a Seventh-day Adventist couple knocked on her door. This patient was raised Catholic but had a terrible childhood and was not particularly active religiously. But this couple now comes every Wednesday and they read the Bible together, which she finds very helpful. So, when she starts to feel suicidal, I ask her when she last read the Bible with them, and what she learned. When she feels like cutting, can she also open a Bible instead? Most of the time, it works."

Psychotherapy can encourage patients to overcome mental barriers to accessing such unique social supports. "For decades I've seen an Asian woman with paranoid schizophrenia or chronic paranoid disorder," Jason continued. "She feels everybody is always trying to rape, poison, or burn her. She moves from church to church, because after a while, her paranoia gets to her. When she starts to say, 'I have to leave this church because they're going to do X, Y, or Z to me,' I've been able to keep her going there, because it's one of her longstanding supports. I do traditional Motivational Interviewing: trying to assess the pros and cons of what patients are doing, helping them to see their own decision-making." Still, as he readily admits, these suggestions do not work for all patients, and he can't force any to believe.

Doctors grapple, too, with whether they should ever draw on their own perspectives, whether religious or agnostic, and if so, how—whether and how to incorporate their own views. "Patients ask me, 'Am I going to make it?' 'Am I going to die?'" Jim Adams, the oncologist and "lapsed Catholic," reported. "Sometimes I will bring up God and say, 'We're trying our best to help you, but in the end, that may be in the hands of God or a higher power.' But," Jim added, "I have no training on these issues." He remains hesitant, but accepting, toward these subjects.

Importantly, what matters is not the doctor's own beliefs, whatever they are, but rather his or her care, concern, and recognition that patients' beliefs are important to *them*. Nonetheless, doctors who have themselves personally faced these issues and/or are more sensitive to spiritual concerns may be more effective discussing these realms with patients facing life-threatening diseases. A wise pediatrician I know told me how "a 12-year-old-boy with a terrible disease once said to me, 'I hope that I've been good enough when I meet God.' His mother was shocked. But I said, 'I think you will be, and I'll write you a letter of recommendation that you are.'"

"What are your own beliefs?" I asked this doctor.

"I was raised Catholic, but am now an atheist. Still, I think life is a miracle. The fact that we're all *here* is a miracle." He had pondered these issues at length, and he exuded integrity, honesty, and kindness.

"Other people would see you as a very spiritual person," I commented.

He shook his head. "I've seen too much harm done in the name of religion. The worst wars. But," he said, "I've also seen how religion helps people cope."

Physicians who are not "spiritually inclined" may find it harder to communicate with patients about these domains. Yet even if strict atheists, doctors can become more sensitive to the significance of these realms to innumerable patients. Physicians shouldn't make comments that they don't believe, nor should they have these conversations if they don't want to. Atheistic doctors should not tell religious patients, "I will pray for you" if that is insincere; patients may detect the inauthenticity. Nor ideally should such doctors say, "I won't pray for you"; instead, they could use a phrase such as, "I know that religion and spirituality are important to many patients" or "Some patients would like to discuss spiritual issues with someone while here. We have people here trained to talk with patients about these issues, if you would like."

Clearly, doctors should in no way proselytize, impose, or force their own beliefs one way or the other on patients, or tell patients what to believe, or discuss these topics with uninterested patients. Though Daniela Smith, the physician and chaplain, when unable to draw blood, once said to a patient whom she knew was very religious, "Let's pray together," that is a rare exception. Such a statement is generally inappropriate unless special and unusual circumstances exist—if, for example, they have both long been active members of the same church and the doctor knows that the patient is devout. Unfortunately, some healthcare providers may potentially be evangelical and overly zealous. In England in 2009, one National Health Service nurse was reprimanded for offering to pray for a patient, who was "taken aback" by this statement.[7]

Such instances appear, however, to be exceedingly rare. Though opponents of spirituality in medicine fear the possibility of "doctors ramming their own religious beliefs down patients' throats," the physicians I have met have all strained to avoid doing so. Physicians should not let their own beliefs interfere with providing the best possible treatment for their patients. Any doctors who, based on their beliefs, do not want to respect a patient's treatment preferences should inform the patient, and refer him or her to a colleague.

Several states have considered allowing physicians to refuse to perform certain procedures to which these clinicians have religious objections.[8] Many doctors, for instance, oppose physician-assisted death on religious grounds. But doctors should then disclose this fact to patients. Certainly, such doctors should reveal such beliefs if these are relevant to a patient's care.

Doctors should also know their limits and levels of comfort. "When I was really distressed because of bad news I got," said Juan Rodriguez, a chaplain who developed cancer, "one of my doctors said, 'I wish I had the words of comfort that you need right now.' He was acknowledging my despair, not taking it away—because no one can—but just acknowledging it. What he said was profound: He acknowledged my spiritual pain." This doctor's humble admission of his own medical and existential limitations heightened Juan's trust and respect toward him. In such cases, referrals to chaplains could also help.

Enhancing understandings of non-Western beliefs

Raised Jewish, I have never received any formal education about the basic tenets of Catholicism, Protestantism, Islam, Buddhism, or Hinduism. Only by occasionally attending friends' weddings over the years, and traveling to French cathedrals, Turkish mosques, Indian Hindu and Jain shrines, and Japanese Buddhist temples have I begun to learn key elements of these faiths. The vast majority of Americans know essentially nothing about Hinduism, the religion of 20% of the world.[9] Admittedly, it at first seemed strange to me: Do they really pray to an elephant god? It still seems complicated and I do not fully understand it, but I have come to appreciate the richness and insights of its mythology and the fact that it has produced great thinkers like Mahatma Gandhi and Rabindranath Tagore.

Unfortunately, Western doctors and nurses tend to know very little about non-Western traditions, and xenophobia and Islamophobia have been climbing. With patients of non-Western faiths, many physicians thus face particular challenges.

Generally, medical schools teach nothing about these other traditions. Hence, doctors would benefit from having some sense, even if small, of the central elements of at least a few of these creeds to reduce ignorance, wariness, or awkwardness. Especially given mounting Islamophobia in the United States, appreciation of the needs of Muslim patients, for instance, is increasingly important. Still, medical schools generally lack such training.

Medical education should cover these topics more formally and fully. "There's more of a need," said Sam, the Louisiana chaplain, "especially in cities, for training to include religions other than Christianity and Judaism, which aren't included anywhere in the formal curriculum. . . . We have a Diversity Week in the fall and the spring, celebrating different cultures, but that's all." At the same time, covering other religions is "hard, because you don't want it to contribute to stereotyping, or be dry or just some form of 'cultural competency' where everybody just rolls their eyes."

A lecture in comparative religion to increase religious literacy would be ideal, but even that may be seen as too ambitious. Physicians won't be able to know much about all religions but should certainly at least be exposed to basic relevant aspects of the main ones (e.g., Catholicism, Protestantism, Judaism, Islam, Buddhism, and Hinduism). "It's unfair to expect doctors to act like chaplains," Adam Quincy said. "They don't need to have Ph.D.s in world religion or be fluent in all these religions, but need to know a little about key things they should or shouldn't do—some familiarity with the world's incredible religious diversity. Physicians' training shouldn't include all practices, which would bore them to death, but kept at an interesting, helpful, and valuable level for them. Ability to validate a patient's religious identity can be a very quick and powerful way of establishing rapport. It's helpful to know that Sikhs wear turbans and pray 3 hours a day, or that Shintoists believe in fertility but not mortality. There are a staggering 22,000 different Protestant denominations in the U.S. alone, but knowing a little bit of background would help physicians immensely." Such instruction can benefit not only trainees but also doctors already in practice.

Unfortunately, medical staff frequently misconstrue the views of patients of non-Western faiths. "A Muslim patient recently asked me, 'Do you believe in God?'" a Catholic physician told me. "They don't know. It matters to them, to know whether to fully trust us. Muslim patients are often here as refugees in a strange land. This patient's question caught me off guard. I wasn't sure how to respond. I finally said, 'Yes. I'm Protestant, but believe in God.' The patient said 'Thank God!' and then relaxed and trusted me more."

Patients may use such a question to gauge how to perceive their doctor. Physicians who respond meaningfully, however they feel is appropriate, rather than just ignoring or sidestepping such inquisitiveness, can help establish and/or strengthen trust.

Increasingly, physicians themselves have non-Western beliefs, too, especially as the numbers of foreign medical school graduates in the United States continue to rise. But these doctors of other faiths are at times also unsure how to respond to Judeo-Christian patients. "Christian patients ask me, 'Doc, am I going to die?'" a Muslim physician told me. "I answer, because it's authentic for me, as a Muslim: 'It's all in God's hands.' That is what my faith says: 'It is all the Will of Allah.' But some patients don't like that. They get downcast. I don't understand why."

"Probably," I told him, "they feel you're suggesting that you're not going to do all you can to help them, taking away their hope."

"But I didn't say that!"

"Yes, but that's what they may *hear*. Instead, I think you can be true to your faith, but not have patients losing hope, by saying, for instance, 'We're doing everything we can to help you.'"

"So, be diplomatic?"

"Yes." Strikingly, this approach had not occurred to him.

Judeo-Christian patients may also be wary of providers, including chaplains and doctors, from other traditions. Unfortunately, patients may be prejudiced against a doctor whose religious views differ from their own. "Many patients are ignorant," a Sikh physician who wears a large, dark maroon turban and sports a straggly, untrimmed black beard, recently told me. "They assume I'm Muslim, but I am not. Some patients don't want me to treat them. I tell them," he said, with a tinge of irony, "'Fine! Go find another doctor!' It's easier for me that way." Heightened openness to diverse faiths can benefit patients, too.

Overcoming opposition to raising awareness of spirituality in healthcare

Given the strong emotions that religion evokes, both pro and con, even these conclusions may be misunderstood or spurned. Unfortunately, several critics vehemently oppose needs for doctors to become more aware of these patient concerns. Yet such critics commonly ignore patients' needs and create straw dogs. In an article entitled "The Witches' Brew of Spirituality and Medicine,"[10] one clergyman wrote that the idea that physicians will bridge the "rift" between spirituality and medicine "by assuming the role of religious and spirituality authorities is naïve." The languages of science, and of religion and spirituality, are "radically different," and physicians "cannot legitimately incorporate 'relationships with transcendent beings' into their discourse as if there is another source of data like some laboratory result."

But having conversations about "transcendent beings" is not what's needed. Rather, physicians and the rest of us should recognize, rather than simply ignore, the fact that religion and spirituality help many patients. Doctors should by no means become religious "authorities" but should at least recognize these issues when patients raise them, and refer patients, when appropriate, to chaplains. Not all doctors are cardiologists, neurologists, or dermatologists, but medical school gives all physicians certain rudimentary knowledge in each of these fields so they know when and how to refer patients to these specialists when necessary.

Though critics contend that physicians should not provide "spiritual care,"[11] that term can be defined in extreme but overreaching ways. Doctors do not need to provide spiritual care per se, but rather need simply, if nothing else, to become more aware of the importance of these areas to many patients, and be prepared to answer, rather than ignore, the latter's questions even if only briefly.

Physicians should recognize, too, how definitive answers to patients' quandaries in these realms are generally lacking and/or gray rather than black and white. A Protestant chaplain I know regularly tells medical students about being in a hospital room with a Catholic family who had just had an infant die. "A priest walked in and said, 'You are blessed! Your child is now with Jesus in Heaven!' He waved his arms and walked out. That's bullshit! There are no such easy answers here. Instead, we must struggle with these questions and get to the point where we can feel comfortable with them."

Given that only about 60% of hospitals have chaplains, despite The Joint Commission on Accreditation of Healthcare Organization (JCAHO) requirements,[12] and that only 6% of patients in ICUs have seen chaplains,[13] hospitals, which are still largely run by doctors, should also support chaplains more by providing resources and recognition. Chaplains remain in too short a supply.

19

"More than just smiling and saying Jesus"

Improving chaplains

Alas, not all chaplains are equally well trained or effective. Enhanced education and practice can aid not only doctors but also pastoral care providers. A friend recently told me how, when her elderly mother was hospitalized and dying, a young chaplain entered the room: "My mother spoke about the problems of Job. This young chaplain, who looked like she was around 16 years old, didn't know what to say and quickly left."

Spiritual care training has improved over time with expanded attention to multiple faiths, and more chaplains now gaining skills as counselors, but it can be further strengthened in several ways.

Chaplains still learn much on the job over time, especially about how to address complex situations, and these lessons could potentially be distilled and transmitted to novices. "My confidence is much higher after being in the field for a while," William Gibson said. "Initially, I spent a lot of time trying to psych myself up—literally talking to myself in the hallway before going onto the ward, to rehearse what I was going to say. I don't do that as much anymore. I now spend a lot of time reflecting afterwards."

Over recent decades, pastoral care instruction has also changed its processes involved. William, for instance, reported that previously "a lot of chaplaincy educators saw themselves as taking these mostly Christian kids, who believed that everything works for the good—that we just need to be at peace, and see the blessing in everything—and show them, 'No, it's a lot more complicated,' through a lot of in-your-face confrontation, inducing conflict, stoking their anger, letting them feel their rage and act that out, and making them feel the suffering. It was built on group therapy—acting out primal aggression from their family of origin.

"We've moved away from that," William said, "but still have lots of remnants of it. We need to continue to reform that in our field. . . . Lots of

Doctor, Will You Pray for Me?. Robert L. Klitzman, Oxford University Press. © Oxford University Press 2024.
DOI: 10.1093/oso/9780197750841.003.0019

chaplains come to our field because they have traumas in their lives—'big-T' traumas, but also little ones. People that gravitate to this work—myself included—have had horrible experiences in their lives when things were falling apart. So, we're educating people who have backgrounds of trauma, and sending them into difficult situations when they've never done this before—being with families getting the worst news of their life—which itself could be traumatizing."

Further specialized training in counseling would benefit chaplains who lack it. While a number of chaplains have completed education in psychotherapy, such as through master's degrees in counseling, a lot do not. Especially as mental health becomes more biologically focused, chaplains can fill important voids in hospitals, aiding psychotherapeutically. "Many chaplains are now trying to get more specialized counseling training," Brian Post, the Michigan chaplaincy department administrator, said, "because their training was skewed towards theology and traditional seminary training. Quite a few could benefit from some additional preparation in counseling theory and technique."

Psychotherapy and pastoral care can readily complement each other, each focusing on related but different domains. According to Victor Simmons, "Psychotherapists say, 'The way your brain is processing all this isn't working for you. Maybe it's been hardwired over time, and that needs to be redone, or there's a chemical imbalance.' I deal with the fundamental foundational core of a person's belief, and meaning, purpose, and hope. We work together, each on those separate parts."

Chaplains and medical staff should also learn more about each other. "The biggest problem is that chaplains and doctors speak two different languages," Adam Quincy observed. "It's not that doctors ignore us. But if we say to the doctor, 'Mrs. Jones appears extremely depressed today,' the doctor might think, 'Are you diagnosing depression here? That's *my* job.' We each need to learn the other's language. Chaplains may benefit significantly from learning to speak to medical professionals more effectively. It's like doing missionary work: If you're going to convey your message, you have to learn the language. The onus is on *us* to do that, but we're not doing it. We need to integrate and apply what we see into healthcare terminology. Otherwise, doctors don't consider our input. Chaplains make a mistake in wearing their clergy persona, not their healthcare persona. When that happens, a doctor will think our input isn't relevant: 'I don't care where patients went to church or if they believe in God. This is a place of *science*!' If we were a little more fluent in medical terminology, we could speak to these issues more intelligently, and doctors would rely on us."

Enhancing the chaplaincy profession

Several chaplains saw needs as well for other, broader improvements within their field to heighten racial, ethnic, and religious representation, secularism, and professionalization. "Our profession needs to become more diverse," William Gibson stated. "It may never match exactly the demographics of the population, but we have to do more."

Further needs arise for more humanist and secular chaplains. "The U.S. is behind other countries," William added, "in terms of robust humanist and secular chaplains, who are much more established in Canada, the Netherlands, and England."

Increased professionalization and less reliance on local clergy, who are untrained in chaplaincy per se, can also strengthen the field, especially given tightened hospital budgets, which have triggered the use of volunteers, who may be evangelical.

While chaplains can now become board certified, state licensing might also bolster the profession and "go a long way towards credibility," Connie Clark reasoned. "Board certification is rigorous and involved, but uneven because it depends on who's on the particular certification committee. But licensure could potentially include a written test to demonstrate competency."

The field could bolster not only education but also practice. COVID-19 forced the development of innovations, including tele-chaplaincy using electronic audio and/or visual communication. With COVID, "we've had to be creative," Jack Stone explained, "to find means to touch and connect with one another in different ways. We're Zoom churching and having Zoom therapy, though it's not the same. The connection and depth are still there, just through different means. Zoom is not the *same* intimacy as in person, but can be just as intimate, though in a different way."

Still, caution is needed, particularly with tele-chaplaincy that uses audio but not video. "Patients sound very good over the phone," Rashid Ayad, the Muslim chaplain, said. "But when you see them in person, it's different. Helping patients when we can't see them is a challenge. Sometimes, when we call patients, there are distractions in the background. They really don't have time to talk. They're busy doing something else. In person, it's much clearer."

Assessing chaplains

Especially given lack of reimbursement and cutbacks in chaplaincy departments,[1] researchers have been trying to quantify chaplains' benefits, effectiveness, and value. These efforts have had both successes and limitations.

Chaplains can help hospitals and want to do so. In many geographical regions, these institutions face mounting market competition from each other and thus want to measure and raise their patients' satisfaction. As Marvin Beck explained, "One of our hospital's metrics is patient loyalty, whether people are coming back to us. So, I want to give patients a memorable experience. They may forget everything I've said or done, but they'll say, 'I don't know who that Father was who came in'—they frequently mistake me for a priest—'but he was nice.' It's important for us to create an experience in which they like us and are going to come back here and ask for one of us. It happens a lot."

Increasingly, hospitals are using standardized satisfaction questionnaires to evaluate and measure the impact of pastoral care, but these scales have constraints. Efforts to document how chaplains heighten patient satisfaction have produced mixed results. Specifically, in one survey, only 5.6% of patients in a hospital saw a chaplain, and they were more likely to report higher satisfaction on six questions about religious/spiritual and general psychosocial care. However, a larger study found that 26.5% of patients saw a chaplain, but reported *poorer* health and patient experiences,[2] probably since very sick patients and their families are more likely to *both* see a chaplain and have poorer prognoses and hence lower overall satisfaction. A patient's eventual death during a hospitalization, for instance, may override families' prior positive views about the time in the institution. Many factors besides a chaplain's visit may affect measures of a patient's or family's overall experience of a hospitalization.

While generally supporting these efforts at quantification, chaplains perceive challenges, feeling that their work cannot simply be reduced to numbers. Attempts to measure the field's benefits may miss major components of what these professionals do. As one chaplain told me, "Such assessments can help wary hospital leaders, but have perils. Chaplain research is important, but the sole reason has been simply to justify the need for chaplains. You can't justify or quantify our work, because it's spiritual. Don't let that overtake the 'faith' element."

These numerical ratings carry costs if not done well, and these limits need to be well grasped. This pastoral care provider and others averred that the field should "keep God in chaplaincy. Don't let it become strictly programmatic or justifiable based on research only. Chaplaincy represents a faith in God. Chaplains' work can be quantified and justified, but faith cannot be. How can you quantify the amount of work that God does? You might see a result, but can't quantify it. The overall push for measurable spirituality has merit. But you can't let that be the *sole reason* for chaplains. While healthcare is scientifically based, chaplaincy is faith-based."

"What is it about faith," I asked, "that satisfaction scales do not pick up?"

"The *experience* of it. When I'm in a room with a patient or family, the experience is *at that moment*."

"How, then," I asked, "do you feel you know you made a difference?"

"Having somebody tell me, 'Thank you for stopping by and listening to me,' or having the atmosphere of the room change from heavy to light. When I walk in, there's a heaviness and I can literally feel it gradually lifting, and the patient's demeanor becoming much brighter, hopeful, and cheerier. I don't know *how* it happens. It just does."

These difficulties quantifying their work frustrate many chaplains. "Baseball and firefighting have much more obvious success and failure," William Gibson said. "You hit the ball. You extinguish the fire. There are numeric outputs. Chaplaincy is not like that. I totally support trying to quantify it, as far as that will go. But it's often not clear whether I made any difference. It kind of becomes a matter of faith."

Quantifying other, more specific benefits has been elusive. "They've started counting everything," Sam Lacey elaborated, "which can be frustrating. Can you really measure prayer? You can count how many times each chaplain sees a patient or writes in a chart, but that's very rudimentary. The ultimate hope is to convince administrators that chaplaincy visits yield positive patient outcomes, but that'll probably be hard to show."

As Aristotle argued in the *Nicomachean Ethics*, we should not seek more precision about a subject than the nature of the subject allows.[3] We can describe interactions between chemicals far more precisely than those between people's emotions.

Despite these drawbacks, quantitative scales can potentially provide key objective, systematic, and concrete evidence of the field's impact and effectiveness and are worth pursuing. "You can't measure everything, but can nonetheless measure something valuable," Adam Quincy argued. "I've always been uncomfortable with chaplains who feel, 'You cannot measure anything relevant because this is God stuff.' *That's nonsense.* You won't measure *everything* that goes on in interactions, but you can measure something valuable. It depends on your metric and how well you implement it. I want to know: 'Am I making a difference?' It's more than just about having charisma, or patients liking you. What difference are we really making with the patient?"

Still, even Adam, who supports efforts at quantification, recognizes that certain aspects of chaplaincy are difficult, if not impossible, to measure. "I get a lot of intrinsic rewards as a chaplain," Adam admitted. "Most patients say, 'Thank you very much. It was wonderful talking with you. I'm doing much better.' Patients haven't opened up to anybody else, and tell me something painful in their lives that I've processed and connected to the transcendent. We build trust. I see or hear in their voices a lifting of their spirit, mood, and tone. When I see that happening, I know I'm doing a good job."

Critics have argued that medicine has operationalized religion and spirituality in narrow, instrumental ways, emphasizing how these realms can abet patient coping and social supports—partly to study these quantitatively, focusing on procedures and missing key, deeper elements.[4]

Yet chaplains appear to appreciate the fullness of patients' spiritual, religious, and existential lives, without reducing these to statistics. Increasingly, chaplains document their work in patients' medical records to communicate with staff, but struggle with how to explain the contents of interactions, especially given lack of a standardized vocabulary or common language for doing so.[5,6] Ultimately, these assessments are only *indirect* reflections of chaplains' activities. "It's a challenge for chaplains to show we are contributing to the bottom line and to justify additional staff," Connie Clark said. "We're an expensive line item. We contribute to patient satisfaction and patients not being readmitted, but it's hard to trace that directly. A lot of the metrics aren't direct. It's an association by *correlation*, not *causation*."

Another problem is that studies to date have primarily focused on the attitudes and experiences of Caucasian Christian patients, and far less on other groups.[7] As William Gibson observed, "We need more studies on a broader spectrum of other racial, religious, and non–English-speaking patients."

Yet, while prior efforts to quantify certain particular types of the beneficial aspects of chaplaincy have been mixed,[2,8] the individuals quoted in this book suggest other, valuable kinds of assistance they offer.

A better method is to present narratives of successful interactions and of hope. As Sam Lacey said, "The most meaningful approach would be the development not of evidence-based medical indicators, but rather *stories of hope*, of sick children who got better. Then, philanthropic donors will give to that cause." Faith, like love, can't be quantified. "Love, religion, and other very meaningful things are very hard to measure," Sam contended, "and you wouldn't *want* to measure them. We don't live our lives like that. It's misguided."

Instead, he thinks, chaplains should publish qualitative descriptions of their work more fully: "Write more case reports and articles for medical journals and books—chaplains' perspective on cancer or heart disease, which would vary from doctors' or patients'. A chaplain would have a different slant and material because of different conversations."

Unfortunately, this work takes effort and skills. As he added, "Chaplains don't have time." More mechanisms and incentives for doing such research are therefore essential. "Chaplains are not promoted or rewarded for publishing," Sam pointed out, "and typically do not have Ph.D.s." Yet writing such case reports need not take time, and workshops to support and facilitate these can be developed. I have also tried to offer such narratives of success here.

Other studies are needed, too, to examine, for instance, whether quilting, reading, or other group activities that are not explicitly religious provide the same psychological, social, and spiritual support as do religious groups. Such communities undoubtedly vary in what they provide. Do differences exist? If so, how and for whom?

In addition, spiritual care helps patients and families consider all of their medical options carefully, and often avoid invasive but futile treatments, thus saving the healthcare system scarce resources. These efforts should be systematically measured as well.

Chaplains can improve, too, their relationships with hospitals, doctors, and nurses. These spiritual providers feel marginalized and under-resourced partly because they lack professional confidence. They should strive to engage and build trust with healthcare executives, managers, and medical staff, participate in institutional decision-making, and make themselves as visible as possible instead of just "showing up."[9]

With providers and hospital administrators, chaplains should advocate for themselves more as well, and overcome obstacles to doing so. Many chaplains do not feel comfortable or confident promoting these issues. Granted, many doctors are unwelcoming, thinking, "Stay in your own lane." But within hospitals, which are geared toward expensive biomedical interventions, chaplains themselves may also undervalue their own worth. "Maybe because we feel that everybody else has something technical to offer, while we don't," Sam said. "Chaplains have a lot of ambivalence about ambition," Kristine Baker, the Texan chaplain, agreed. "That cripples us a little bit."

Schooled to focus on humility and other people's needs, chaplains may not readily convey the importance of their work to others, undermining others' appreciation of them. "We're trained to be listeners," Margaret Dixon observed, "so we're our own worst enemies, because we don't put ourselves front and center. By the very nature of what we do, we are not the loudest person in the room."

The suggestions here—of demonstrating chaplains' wider functions in fractured healthcare systems, aiding providers as well as patients, assisting in obtaining vital insights and information from patients, and using stories, not just numbers, to convey these goals—can help.

Changing the term "chaplains"

The field should also consider changing the term "chaplain." The term derives from Christianity, to which it once exclusively referred, and is much less familiar to patients and families from other faiths. Muslim countries thus prefer the term "spiritual counselor." Yet that term may be limited, too, since practitioners may not counsel per se. "Spiritual care providers" or "spiritual staff" are other options.

The term "chaplain" offers certain advantages because it is well established. Adam Quincy, for instance, does not want to alter the term and sees "spiritual counselor" as a "real watering down of the gravitas of the word 'chaplain,' which is almost right up there with 'doctor.' We don't want to do away with that. That would be a big mistake."

I asked, "What if patients from other faiths, such as Muslims, think chaplains are just Christian?"

"If you're respectful and sensitive toward them, they will love you," Adam answered, "because they're really looking for acceptance." But that assumes that patients do not first reject the chaplain, put off by the name.

Other people support the term "chaplain" because of its metaphorical implications. "I like the name 'chaplain,'" said Brenda Pierson. "It comes from a medieval word that means 'a cape,' 'to cover.'[10] We cover people with prayer and lots of things. I don't care what the department's name is; it's *the way chaplains live it out.*"

Yet, ongoing consideration of potential alternatives can have important advantages, given the increasing numbers of Nones, Muslims, and non-Christian patients who may not see chaplains as being for *them.* Chaplaincy should also increase public education and recognition regarding the field, and its work and benefits, disseminating information online, in hospitals, and more broadly elsewhere.

20

Finding meaning and hope in a rapidly changing world

After I began research for this book, I visited ancient Christian catacombs in Rome, built in the first through fourth centuries CE outside the historic city walls. Cemeteries haunt me, as stark reminders of death, and these crypts are Christian, while I am not. Yet now, after thinking about religion more, including others than my own, I decided to explore them.

Down dark narrow stairs, I descended through vast underground stories, stretching several kilometers in all directions, filled with tiers upon tiers of tombs, as well as sacred sanctuaries, churches, the tomb of St. Sebastian, famously pierced by arrows, and other early Christian martyrs, carved marble sarcophagi, and the initial burial sites of the first popes. Early Christians dug these enormous labyrinthine catacombs, thinking that the Second Coming and their own resurrections would occur imminently. They would be ready to rise.

Faded frescoes and chiseled carvings covered the ancient rock walls, depicting Jesus Christ's initials and shepherds carrying sheep, symbolizing Jesus aiding his flock of humans. But the most common current symbol of Christianity—the cross—was absent. As lessons for others, the Romans still routinely used roadside crosses to crucify criminals (as Jesus was condemned under Roman law). Only once the Romans ceased using this means of execution did Christians adopt it as a symbol.

These martyrs were slaughtered because they believed that only one God existed and that "everyone is equal." In contrast, the Romans upheld a rigid, class-oriented oligarchy and worshipped many gods—including the emperor himself. To Romans, the idea that Jesus would help the sick and the poor, widows and cripples, was radical and outrageous. No Roman gods aided patients in that way. The Greek Hippocratic tradition had instead created a separate profession of physicians. Yet through the centuries, the Church, though initially eschewing power, eventually sought and obtained immense

Doctor, Will You Pray for Me?. Robert L. Klitzman, Oxford University Press. © Oxford University Press 2024.
DOI: 10.1093/oso/9780197750841.003.0020

political, financial, and military might, arguably becoming the West's most powerful institution.

Here in the dark catacombs, I saw how much a religion may appear a static, unalterable institution at any one point in time, but in fact metamorphosize dramatically over the years—and no doubt it will continue to do so. The change usually takes decades or centuries, and we thus tend not to observe it. Around two millennia ago, Western civilization shifted from polytheism to monotheism, but no objective evidence suggests that either of these perspectives is in fact inherently truer than the other. Rather, each has advantages and disadvantages that fit the particular culture and religion.

Larger world and political shifts transform these traditions as well. Over 1,200 years ago, Christianity and then Islam spread and eventually conquered vast lands across the collapsing Roman Empire. Today, social media is similarly transforming the world. The last major shift in Western religion also stemmed from new technology—the invention of the printing press. Before the fifteenth century, monks had to write out by hand each individual copy of the Bible—a huge, heavy, expensive tome. Forty years after Johannes Guttenberg first mass-produced Bibles, the Protestant Reformation erupted, arguing that individuals should each interpret Scriptures on their own rather than relying on Roman Catholic priests. This movement depended on cheap, widely available Bibles. The Counter-Reformation followed, fueled, too, by books by St. Ignatius Loyola[1] and others. Just as the invention of the printing press triggered the Reformation and Counter-Reformation in the West, scientific and technological advances in electronics, physics, and biology are now fostering new religious and spiritual communities.

Evolutionary psychologists see religion as an adaptive mechanism that united individuals against enemies.[2] Our ancestors evolved in small bands, and group cohesion proved beneficial against other small groups as well as wild beasts. Feelings of shared purpose and belief created and solidified social glue. Those who joined the group survived better than others. Religion welded humans together, rewarding cooperators and punishing others. We evolved, too, to try to understand and solve problems and make sense of our plights.

Evolutionarily, our hardwired impulses toward spirituality and religion and searches for larger purpose and connection constitute valuable but double-edged sets of tools. Through hundreds of thousands of years, humans acquired and spread certain genes that are, on balance, adaptive but can clash with each other and incur costs. Genes that are advantageous in one niche can burden us in others. Unfortunately, humans also possess, biological tendencies toward greed, corruption, and cruelty that at many points have contaminated all religions, even Buddhism, which otherwise promulgates peace. (Myanmar Buddhists, for instance, continue persecuting and slaughtering Muslim Rohingyas.) As individuals and societies, we must thus strive to oppose these harmful urges. Religion should never be used as a justification for hurting other people.

Yet while religion has clearly at times caused damage, patients reveal how it can *also* provide crucial and unique aid. People confronting serious disease, horrific pain, suffering, and death routinely seek meaning and answers to existential quandaries. Spiritual and religious beliefs, and chaplains' abilities to aid and bolster these, are closely tied to resiliency and coping. While critics assail select negative aspects of religion and spirituality, such as promulgation of violence and fears of a mythic Hell, patients and chaplains reveal vital benefits and needs to try to come to terms with profound existential crises and terrors of annihilation, and seek larger answers and understandings of the broader universe. *Though Dawkins and other critics advocate abandoning all religion, seeing it as wholly baleful, patients and chaplains illuminate instead how it possesses both pros and cons*, and is instinctual and inherently human.

Like all tools and human inventions, individuals can use religion and spirituality for either good or bad. Jesus never preached the bloodshed committed in His name. Though some of Mohammed's followers have been terrorists, he himself emphasized other goals. In the Quran, jihads were intended against infidels, not fellow "People of the Book"—Christians and Jews, whom Muslim terrorists now attack. To condemn all religion because of such brutality would be like unilaterally opposing the U.S. Constitution because certain judges have immorally twisted it to uphold slavery and deny voting rights to women and African Americans. The Constitution is by no means perfect, and has at times been misinterpreted,[3,4] but has overall also granted and protected fundamental rights to countless individuals.

Given these pitfalls, however, patients and chaplains today are redefining and reconstructing spirituality and religion, creating alternatives to established institutions, and putting together their own beliefs, revealing what I term a "will for meaning" and a "will for wholeness"—a desire for a sense of coherence about themselves, their fate, and the cosmos. In so doing, patients are also rebutting many arguments lodged against religion. Bertrand Russell, the 1950 Nobel Laureate in Literature, castigated religion and upheld atheism, and Richard Dawkins, Sam Harris, and Christopher Hitchens more recently have looked to him as their predecessor. Emerson and the late-eighteenth century philosopher voltaire attacked church corruption but still believed in God. The late-nineteenth century German philosopher Friedrich Nietzsche attacked the existence of God. But Russell has arguably offered the most thorough and sustaining analytic critique, dissecting opposing arguments. In *Why I Am Not a Christian*, Russell wrote, "Most people believe in God, because they have been taught from early infancy to do it, and that is the main reason."[5] But patients reveal how, psychologically they and others, when confronting existential quandaries, yearn for answers and explanations that make emotional sense to them, even if lacking clear empirical evidence. Moreover, patients' guilt and questions regarding "Why me?" appear deep-seated, arising from unconscious sources, at times against their will. People also hold free-floating notions of justice, which even apes possess[6]—innate drives toward fairness, suggesting that these inclinations in fact have instinctual bases and result not merely from precepts inculcated as children.

"With very few exceptions," Russell added, "the religion which a man accepts is that of the community in which he lives, which makes it obvious that the influence of environment is what has led him to accept the religion in question."[7] Yet as patients here have indicated, over the past half-century, in part given the rise of the internet and globalization, in the United States and most of Western Europe, men—as well as *women*—increasingly *choose* their spiritual and religious views, and shift over time, rather than simply accepting religious dogma unthinkingly from their community. Instead, individuals draw on their own experiences, perceptions, and observations of the world and of others' beliefs to decide what makes most sense to them.

"I think all the great religions of the world—Buddhism, Hinduism, Christianity, Islam, and Communism—both untrue and harmful," Russell continued. "It is evident as a matter of logic that, since they disagree, not more than one of them can be true."[10] However, patients and chaplains vividly elucidate how religions share many common underlying elements.

Partly in response to the problems Russell and his modern disciples mention, religions and spirituality have themselves also changed, making several of his objections obsolete. The circumstances in which he wrote have altered. He mistakenly saw religion as wholly fixed and socially created, rather than fluid, continually adapting, and having profound evolutionary functions and roots.

Science now better explains several natural phenomena traditionally accounted for by religion—the creation of the sun, the moon, stars, humans, and other species—but does not fulfill all human needs. Though Russell saw science as "approaching the stage when it will be complete, and therefore un-interesting,"[8] the subsequent 100 years have highlighted how much we still don't know. Eventually, we may understand everything. One day, in the distant future, perhaps several hundred or thousand years from now, scientists may be able to explain all human experience and the origins and nature of the cosmos.

But at least for now, predictions by Russell and others of soon being able to explain all natural phenomena have proven elusive. We still lack answers to the largest questions—what, if anything, existed before the Big Bang, what lies in the interiors of the smallest atomic particles or beyond the detectable stars, and how chemicals create consciousness and thought. We don't understand what is inside black holes and whether they might eventually help form another universe. One day, physicists may perhaps be able to explain dark energy and matter, quantum phenomena and entanglement (so-called spooky forces at a distance, whereby two particles separated by many light-years still react simultaneously to each other). But so far, these phenomena remain utter enigmas. The history of science consists of slowly peeling away layers of onions, revealing further layers of onions underneath. We should keep stripping away these additional linings, but recognize that ultimate truths usually prove elusive. In his parable of the cave, Plato argued that we see things not in themselves, but merely their shadows on the wall.[9] Belief that we will one day be able to explain everything appears only that—belief. Moreover, we may not survive long enough as a species to understand all of nature's unknowns. Given theories of relativity that time can go backwards, science may one day find manifestations of such phenomena in our daily lives. Yet unknowns and ambiguities persist, and arguably always will. Hubris clouds many atheists' vehement insistence that physics will soon definitely be able to explain everything.

In the meantime, the fact that vast mysteries exist beyond our ken should humble us and caution us about assumptions that we are always "right." As Socrates and Michel de Montaigne, the sixteenth century French essayist,[10] concluded, we only know that there is much we don't know, reminding us to beware of rigid claims of "truth" on either side.

In his recent bestselling books,[11,12] Sam Harris, a prominent atheist, argues that meditation alone suffices to achieve neurophysiological calm to reduce daily routine levels of stress and should thus *replace* religion and spirituality. Yet patients indicate how spirituality usually represents much more. Meditation, Harris argues, can give us a sense of spirituality, which he sees as a feeling of psychological "transcendence," being "I-less"—seeing the "I" as merely a neurochemical phenomenon that does not really exist in and of itself.[13] Countless people pursue mindfulness, but it fills only some, not all, of the functions of spirituality and religion. It provides no moral code concerning, for instance, a sense of justice, responsibilities and respect for others' rights. Perhaps most importantly, it lacks content for which patients and families yearn, especially when facing death and dying. Patients look to spirituality for far more: connections to something that continues beyond them, after their death, even if only symbolically. For such patients and families, the existence of larger, dark unknown and spooky physical forces in the external world can fuel a spiritual sense of awe *beyond* a "psychological state" of meditation alone. As Roy Gifford, a patient with a chronic disease, told me, "I believe in the Third Law of Thermodynamics, that energy in the universe is neither created nor destroyed, but continues on in some form." Our spiritual sense, though experienced in our minds, concerns phenomena and facts outside and extending far beyond us. Spirituality and "higher powers," however individuals define them for themselves, can foster humility, respect, care, and awe as a sense of justice and respect for others.

Given the world's growing political, religious, and cultural divides, with rising hatred, racism, and weapons of mass destruction, such open-mindedness, understanding and toleration of others' views and flexible, nuanced perspectives are ever more essential. In our increasingly polarized political world, and in contrast to recent bestsellers debating whether God is either provable or bunk, patients and chaplains show needs for far more pluralism.

In the midst of deadly religious wars, Montaigne wrote that "each man calls barbarism over what is not his own practice." He urged far more tolerance of each other's beliefs. Similarly, in his book *Religion in Human Evolution*, the late sociologist Robert Bellah examined a wide range of religious traditions—not only Judaism and Christianity, but also Islam, Hinduism, Buddhism, and South Pacific beliefs—and saw not religion "progressing" over time but, rather, needs for pluralism, avoidance of dichotomies of "us versus them," and restraint from using religion to justify violence "toward each other and the environment."[14]

Unfortunately, pundits both for and against religion tend to fight this perspective. Antagonism toward others' beliefs persists. Individuals of diverse convictions regularly attack each other's views as strange, threatening, dangerous, and wrong, rather than appreciating underlying commonalities.

Alas, we face deep competing human tendencies to divide the world into "us" and "them," and to align with those we see as sharing our values, as fellow members of an "in-group." Yet religious and spiritual impulses have also facilitated cooperation and unity across groups from small villages to city-states, countries, and international alliances. For our species to survive, we therefore need to figure out how to channel these innate impulses in order to redefine our in-groups far more widely and inclusively to include everyone and to achieve larger cohesion, reaching out to, rather than attacking, perceived outsiders.

Chaplains provide new models for religion and spirituality. *"We are the harbingers of a new religious order,"* Connie Clark said, "spiritual healers, not tied to a particular religion.

"Chaplaincy offers exciting new ways of thinking about doing church or temple," she continued. "It's not a place *but a state of being*. It ought to transcend physical structures and our own limited understanding of the divine. All of what we experience about God is true, but none of it is complete. It's like the parable of the blind men and the elephant. Each one of us appreciates a piece of it, but none get the whole. We need to talk to see how other people experience it. Otherwise, we are going to forever think that the elephant is just a trunk or a tail."

"But what do you say," I asked her, "to people who feel, 'No, I'm not a blind man. Everyone else is blind. I see it correctly.'"

"I wouldn't say anything to them," Connie replied. "If it makes them happy, that's OK. But they shouldn't tell *me* what to think. Allow me to have my beliefs, too."

To insist, as Dawkins and other critics of religion do, that a patient shouldn't believe what he or she feels uniquely helps him or her is highly presumptuous. Individuals who feel aided by religion and spirituality—as long as their beliefs do not harm other people—should be allowed to do so, unfettered. Indeed, many atheists, for instance, who attack other people's beliefs are in fact physically healthy and have not had to endure severe disease and possible death, as patients have, fostering belief. Efforts to convert individuals to atheism appear akin to those of other religions, and hence problematic.

Who am I, or who is anyone, to say that a person's beliefs, whether Catholic, Protestant, Jewish, Muslim, Hindu, Jain, Buddhist, atheist, or agnostic, are correct or not? No one has grounds for making such a statement. Certainly, not everything stated in the name of all religions is or can be true. I reject, for instance, intelligent design (or creationism—the creed that God designed all species) and intercessory prayer (the belief that people praying for a patient without that patient knowing will improve that patient's biological response to disease), but that doesn't mean we should dismiss the potential value of *all* spiritual notions.

Countless people yearn for definitive answers—hard lines in the sand. When we leap into the Great Unknown, beyond our current knowledge, it feels safer to think that we won't fall forever into an infinite abyss, but will rather land and be able to cling to a comfortable solid ledge of science or God. No "proof" per se exists either way, yet both sides feel unconvinced they have conclusive explanations.

Reasonable stances appear to lie in between. As the philosopher David Hume, the physicist Kip Thorne, and others have argued, mysteries remain. In the interim, many of us feel awe before Nature and the great puzzles of biology, the human mind, and the cosmos. In the face of these immense unknowns, flexible, nuanced views of religion and spirituality appear to make sense. To me personally, agnosticism, rather than atheism, seems most reasonable, appreciating this sense of mystery and awe. I sense that something exists more than our current physics can grasp. I hope that we will one day be able to explain the cosmos (though we would then, arguably, no longer need scientists). But to date we cannot, and our hubris may breed overconfidence.

Religion and spirituality can also inspire us to recognize how much we are all special creatures that each deserve respect, leading many people to do good and avoid doing bad. This ability to inspire moral behavior is longstanding, even if fragile. To be sure, humans can act morally without believing in God or in the potential rewards of Heaven and punishments of Hell. Philosophers from Socrates, Plato and Kant to John Rawls have attempted to establish non-religiously based forms of justice. However, these have not caught on as widely as many of us would like. Hopefully, they can spread further.

"How can you believe in nothing?" several Middle Eastern refugee patients recently asked a physician I know. "If you don't believe in Heaven and Hell, what motivates you to do good and avoid doing bad?" They asked partly as a way to get to know her, wondering, "*Can we trust you? Where are you coming from? What are your intentions? Why are you here with us? What are your motives?*"

"I have strong ideals," she replied. "I believe we should try to help people and make the world a better place." They were initially a bit puzzled, but ultimately seemed to accept her response, partly based on the integrity and sincerity she emanated.

Religion and spirituality are neither necessary nor sufficient for acting morally, but arguably can frequently help and, on balance, have arguably promulgated more good than bad.

Still, partly given past harms, as well as technological advances, the patients and chaplains here limn how spirituality and religion are fluid and dramatically shifting in both content and form, often fulfilling different functions now than in the past, no longer answering riddles that science now explains far more fully. While theologians and idealogues argue for or against God, patients and chaplains shed light on far vaster diversities of beliefs, complexities, challenges, and needs for broader approaches, reconsidering and re-evaluating beliefs and developing new, more fluid, adaptable notions.

Certain religious and spiritual movements are similarly transforming and changing. "Some young Jews find Conservative synagogues not serious enough—dead," one rabbi told me. "The services don't speak to them. Young people want to *feel* something, and bring God into their lives. They become searchers, looking for answers. I believe in organic growth," he continued. "In the 1950s and '60s, congregations all needed a rabbi—an expert. Now, in the Renewal Movement, many people feel they can form their own groups and don't need a rabbi. People make their own decisions of how to connect with God." Millions of Catholics, too, have joined a movement—The Way—to return to and to revitalize the Church's roots.[15]

America is especially fertile ground for new religions. As the late literary critic Harold Bloom described, America is "obsessed" with religion. Unlike all other Western European countries, we lack a single established Church. Catholicism suffuses Italy, France, and Spain; in the United Kingdom, the king heads the Anglican Church. In the United States, however, which lacks a history of such a single, monolithic religion, freedom of religion has flourished, fueling ever new sects. Bloom argues that a distinctly "American religion" exists, based on each individual's own personal relationship and experience with God.

Increasingly, globalization and the internet are disrupting traditional religions, forging new human bonds and allowing people to connect in new ways—from cellphones to social media. In prior eras, people traveled to churches, temples, and mosques to join like-minded individuals who affirmed each other's values and beliefs. Today, millions of people form such meaningful communities online, sharing key values and uplifting messages of hope. Facebook unites large numbers of like-minded people who share inspirational photos, poems, and news of births and marriages as well as deaths and misfortunes, gaining support. "I'm part of an online group for Jewish religious women with special needs children," Sylvia, an Orthodox Jewish woman whose daughter was born with a brain deformity, told me. "We encourage, vent, and pray for each other. It's very inspiring, empathizing with other people who are going to understand you. They know your life, where you're coming from!

"They all have special needs kids—the whole spectrum, every issue you can imagine. Some kids are medically very fragile. One child has cerebral palsy; something went wrong when she was born. The mother said, 'I should have done something differently. I could have . . .' I said, 'It's nothing you did. Even if it were—even if it were the doctor's fault—then ultimately, it was really God!' In a way, I was really talking to myself: I could have done this or that, but if this was the way my daughter was supposed to be born, it wouldn't have changed anything. That doesn't mean 'have an alcohol binge when you're pregnant.' But you do what you can. Afterwards, you realize: It's nothing I knowingly did. It's just the way she was meant to be."

This online group has become Sylvia's major source of support—fellow Orthodox Jewish women sharing their religious and cultural norms and uniquely assisting each other, illustrating how the internet can build and strengthen powerful religious ties. When Facebook users die, their profiles remain, granting them virtual immortality. I still get reminders of birthdays of Facebook friends who are now deceased. On those websites, friends still post loving comments, such as "Missing you on your birthday!"

About two-thirds of Americans using the internet have done so for spiritual or religious purposes—38% have sent and received email with spiritual content and 28% have sought online information about their faith.[16] Internet use does not vary by denomination or amount of church attendance, though those who are "spiritual but not religious" use the web more. Alas, social media can also have perils, fostering "fake news," QAnon, and stolen identities and undermining some users' body image and self-esteem. But the benefits can outweigh these potential risks.

COVID-19 further transformed how people communicate about these areas. "Especially with COVID, people can't go to church or gather in person," Connie Clark added, "which is going to forever change organized religion, I don't see how churches can go back to what they were. They're going to have to change, and have needed to change for a while."

"Post-COVID-19," Jack Stone observed, "Zoom and telecommuting and tele-religion have replaced many face-to-face religious activities." Some people attend church online or forgo services altogether. Jack feels, "We may never fully return."

As we move into the future, patients and chaplains also illustrate needs to expand our vocabulary. Language fails when we try to describe these domains. People have difficulty articulating and comprehending their own spirituality and grasping intangibles beyond words; they differ in how they interpret, apply and communicate their intuitive senses of spirituality and God. We fall back on a handful of terms that inadequately capture inherent inchoate spiritual feelings.

Individuals invoke and define the word "God" to convey a wide spectrum of beliefs beyond words, using this short word as a placeholder for a vast array of ideas, from a single creator with varying degrees of omnipotence and omniscience to vague unknowns beyond our ken. This simple three-letter word, God, can refer to an immortal Being of whom we can have a sense or who is utterly unknown; who is involved or not in human affairs, to differing degrees; and who would have us perform certain actions or not, which themselves range widely. A richer vocabulary would help us.

These beliefs are thus hard to delineate or systematically or scientifically study. To convey these notions, people commonly say that they "sort of," "kind of," or "don't really" believe certain notions. William James described this predicament well in 1902, writing that certain religious states are "ineffable" and defy explanation: "The attempt to demonstrate by purely intellectual processes the truth of . . . direct religious experiences is absolutely hopeless . . . Philosophy lives in words, but truth and fact well up into our lives in ways that exceed verbal formulation."[17] Similarly, Elaine Scarry described how language fails to convey "pain" effectively,[18] hampering our ability to appreciate each other's suffering. Likewise, religious and existential beliefs cannot be fully expressed. Chaplains here help us understand how widely the meanings of words such as "God," "miracle," and "prayer" now range. Yet these definitional vagaries fuel misunderstandings, xenophobia, and failures to appreciate underlying similarities and differences. Heightened acceptance and tolerance of varied and evolving forms of spirituality and underlying positive aspects of belief can benefit us all.

I often wonder what our species would be like if we evolve further and have more powerful brains. What abilities and powers might we possess, and what might we be able to do and comprehend? Could we better grasp the cosmos? Might we seek the benefits of cooperation more broadly, untarnished by greed, and possess innate or learned abilities to respect and aid rather than harm each other? We might better plan for the future and weigh long-term harms of our activities over short-term benefits (burning fewer fossil fuels, for example, and using mass transit more). In the meantime, given threats to the planet, species, and society, the best approach today seems not to reject all religion and spirituality, but rather to try to steer these impulses toward good and figure out how to direct these deep tendencies in beneficial ways and avoid the negatives. We should try to guide and support spiritual and religious forces in positive directions and eschew harmful ones. We should strive to refresh and reconceive religion and spirituality, keeping the good elements while discouraging or eliminating the bad. At worst, efforts to do so will constitute an important social and cultural experiment. I don't mean to be overly utilitarian and instrumentalist, but at this critical juncture in our species' history and tottering world, we need to learn to use our moral compass as much as possible.

The impulses toward a higher purpose (beyond mere sort-term quotidian gain) that have united human groups through our evolution and history, can again powerfully aid our fragmenting world. A reinvigorated sense of such larger purpose can join us, but it will inevitably differ from that in the past. Appreciation of the miraculous creations of nature and species, including our own, can foster humility before the unknown, reminding us that we share and are part of larger natural forces, however we each perceive these, inspiring us to appreciate natural beauty and consequently respect our planet and each other more.

We should be humbled and inspired by the fact that unfathomable billions of galaxies exist, each with billions of stars—vast scientific mysteries beyond our ken that we may one day understand but thus far cannot. In our dangerous, angst-filled world, such appreciation can potentially motivate us to care better for each other, as well as for endangered environments and species.

The personal journeys presented here can also assist us not only as a society but also as individuals, whether as patients, family members, providers, or others. As a doctor, I was initially wary of religion and chaplains but came to see how deeply and genuinely they care, are committed, and can help us confront the most difficult subject, our own mortality—which we frequently deny. As Jack Stone observed, "People don't die in hospitals . . . deceased patients are quietly slipped into service elevators. Death is slipped under the rug."

I will never forget many of the stories and critical *life lessons* that I heard through this journey. Some may be radically novel, but in the midst of daily bustle and stress, these reminders can powerfully strengthen us. These spiritual professionals illuminate how existential and spiritual questions are key components of everyone's life journey, especially when facing death and/or dying, but take vastly different forms, from an array of traditional faiths to the Third Law of Thermodynamics.

In confronting death, many people fluctuate, believing what they "need to at the time." They may feel, for instance, that their faith comes up short and that God has failed His or Her side of the bargain. Others adopt some of the "1,000 kinds" of being spiritual but not religious, even occasionally falling on their knees and praying "to the God I don't believe in."

Chaplains not only bring fresh meaning and hope, and save the health-care system scarce resources, but also help us to interact, address conflicts, reframe problems, respect and be honest with ourselves and others, and heal our hearts and minds. These providers offer specific ways, for example, of better communicating with others about these difficult topics. Many of us carry secret prayers and questions in our hearts. We grapple with seemingly crazy questions, myths, and superstitions that we don't reveal to others. As one mother asked, "Did God give my daughter Down's syndrome because I prayed for her to die?" We ask, "Why me?" even when we know no answer exists. Many people therefore hesitate to talk about these topics even with friends, family, and others. But chaplains show how we can nonetheless help each other address these challenges more effectively.

These chaplains demonstrate, too, precise ways we can negotiate conflicts creatively to resolve disputes, such as by seeking common ground. Connie Clark, for instance, used an *"ethics of love."* I will never always remember Cathy Murray, who drew on the pain she experienced at her boyfriend's death in high school and went on to bring deep sensitivity to patients and families, mediating between surgeons and a family and arranging for a mother to sing a son "into heaven." For a patient with developmental disabilities who had been living in a group home and was now unresponsive after an accident, Cathy knew to ask what he was like when in the home. His doctors then heard that "he was *the heart*" of that institution, delivering the mail, and had a pet he loved and who loved him.

These chaplains reveal, too, how being honest while also respecting others' feelings and views offers benefits. When one mother asked whether a deceased daughter was "in a box," and got upset when a junior chaplain replied, "No, she's in *a bag,*" Kristine Baker understood: The mother wanted to know that her daughter was respected and "covered up." "Almost every question," Kristine reflected, "is actually a statement, not a question." Similarly, when asked by family members if blood had been given to their Jehovah's Witness mother who had secretly wanted to receive blood, the physician replied,

"We have followed your mother's wishes exactly." Chaplains and numerous other providers attend closely to the subtleties of language to avoid potential problems.

These spiritual counselors illustrate as well ways of reframing conundrums. With a patient who asked what benefit there was to his remaining alive, Adam picked up a piece of bread on the meal tray and talked about the value of this basic foodstuff. Such a message may seem simple, but the concreteness of the example in his hand gave it power.

Conflicts can surface as well because we fail to recognize that we use particular words in differing ways. Terms such as *religion, spiritual, atheist, agnostic, prayer* and *God* can be blurry and fluid. Doctors can, for example, get angry when a family seeks a "miracle." But a chaplain can find that the family means merely that the patient will survive until an upcoming wedding or anniversary.

Chaplains show how creating modern rituals, whether doing "Chocolate Rounds" or something with our hands, for example, making commemorative wreaths, can help.

The spiritual care specialists here elucidate as well the importance of nonverbal communication, silence, and tone and not rushing to conclusions—how much we should "ask and not assume," and how "saying something out loud can be healing in and of itself."

These professionals also serve as the "voice of the voiceless." They remind us how much we need to respect others who have faced disadvantages, and how some patients' stories don't end well. I will forever remember Adam Quincy walking into the rooms of female African American patients, appearing "broken" rather than upbeat, to suggest that he recognizes key aspects of the obstacles they face.

The doctors, chaplains, and patients here reveal as well needs to understand others' experiences more fully—how, unfortunately, people often attack each other with their religion, and how little we know of others' beliefs. At times, Muslim patients are afraid even to reveal their religion to the hospital.

In aiding patients and families in considering and avoiding invasive but futile procedures, chaplains can also help reduce unnecessary healthcare system expenses.

Chaplains' visits may not always dramatically alter medical outcomes but nonetheless can help us heal and are vital to innumerable patients or families. Patients, families, and doctors often have little sense of the existence or work of pastoral care. They should recognize that this extraordinary resource exists for discussing their innermost fears, doubts, and questions, but also the fact that, in hospitals, they may need to specifically request it.

On the 20th anniversary of my sister Karen's death on 9/11, I traveled with my sisters and our families to visit her grave, which is beside my mother's and father's in a Jewish cemetery on Long Island. Stressed by several deadlines and chores, I had been feeling a bit burned out at work and took the day off. I had been dreading this anniversary and the painful memories it evoked. The early September morning was clear. The air was still, not too hot and not too cold, a pleasant day with seemingly nothing remarkable about it. Twenty years earlier, Karen had woken up on a morning just like this, thinking it was going to be simply another normal day. Then, within a few hours, the world changed.

The cemetery was quiet. A small office there gave out free copies of tiny booklets containing mourners' prayers, including the Kaddish, the Jewish prayer for the dead. At her headstone, we held the small pamphlets in our hands and chanted together. The Hebrew letter translations and transliterations (the Hebrew spelled out phonetically) were printed in thick, somewhat blotchy ink and looking handprinted, almost handmade— reminiscent of ancient Jewish books. We chanted together. I stumbled through the Hebrew, not understanding most of it. In the translation, the prayer praises God, and it seemed a bit redundant, asking that His name be "blessed, praised, glorified, exalted, extolled, honored, elevated and lauded." The prayer does not mention or refer to death in any way.

But in facing the void that these deceased family members had left in my life, uttering these words was something to do, a traditional, scripted response—even if outwardly I might seem to be just going through the motions. We picked up small stones from the dirt and placed them on each of my family members' graves—a Jewish sign of respect for the deceased, evidence that someone had visited.

As we stood, we talked about memories of these deceased family members and how much the world had changed since their deaths—wars in Afghanistan and Iraq; the elections of Presidents Obama, Trump, and Biden; the advent of smartphones, social media, Amazon, and Google.

Besides their graves are plots reserved for us. I took a picture of my spot—a rectangle of grass like any other—as a *memento mori*. Then, I lay down on the space to see what it felt like. This might seem morbid, but I was curious to sense what it might be like to lie there for eternity. I don't know when I'll end up buried there or what the cause of my death will be, but I thought how grateful I was for many things in my life—my family, my friends, my health. I realized, too, how much the insights from these chaplains, patients, families, doctors, and nurses have altered, strengthened, and helped prepare me for my own eventual demise, whenever that might occur—far more than I ever would have imagined. I felt grateful to them all as well.

The cemetery was peaceful. The grass had recently been cut and was low, fragrant, and sweet. Around me stood maple, pine, beech, and spruce trees. I'd be surrounded by nature. Slowly, I rose to my feet and brushed the brown dust off my clothes. We drove back to the city in silence.

The next day, I hurried back to work and sped en route past the small Central Park pond near my home. The bright sun glittered as ripples spread gently across the silvery blue mirrored surface, surrounded by grass and tall shady trees. All around me, birds tweeted and chirped, piping high notes, rising and falling, long and short into the air. I stopped, breathed in deeply the sweet scents of pine and fresh earth—and smiled.

APPENDIX A

List of frequently appearing chaplains[*]

Adam Quincy: North Carolina Catholic hospital chaplain
Brenda Pierson: Pediatric chaplain in the Bible Belt
Brian Post: Michigan chaplaincy department administrator
Cathy Murray: Chaplain at a Virginia Catholic hospital
Connie Clark: Wisconsin Catholic chaplain
Jack Stone: Buddhist chaplain
Kristine Baker: Rural Texan chaplain
Linda Porter: Pediatric chaplain at a large academic medical center in Maryland, and a former journalist
Margaret Dixon: Pennsylvania chaplain
Marvin Beck: New Hampshire chaplain at a small community hospital
Nancy Cutler: South Carolina pediatric chaplain
Sam Lacey: Louisiana chaplain
Sharlene Walters: African -American chaplain from Kentucky
Victor Simmons: Midwest Veterans Administration hospital chaplain
William Gibson: Humanist Vermont chaplain

*Note: All pseudonyms

Methods

For this book, I conducted 33 formal telephone interviews of approximately 1 hour each with 23 board-certified chaplains. (I interviewed several of the chaplains more than once since they responded at greater length than did others to the questions posed). I recruited participants by emailing an announcement of my research through the listserv of the Association of Professional Chaplains, the leading organization in the field, and by word of mouth. Chaplains who received the announcement and were interested in participating contacted me by email.

Scores of chaplains from across the country responded, saying they would be pleased to speak with me. I sought to include spiritual care providers from a range of geographical regions and religious backgrounds, and conducted interviews until I had reached "saturation"—the point in interview research at which no new information or themes are observed in the data.[1]

As seen in Table B.1, 13 were men and 10 were women; 78.2% were Caucasian, 13.0% were African American, and 4.3% were Latino and "other"; the mean age was 63 (range 42–72). They were from throughout the United States and represented diverse religions (26.1% Protestant; 17.4% Catholic; 26.1% Christian, not otherwise specified; 13.0% Jewish; 13.0% Muslim; and 4.3% Buddhist); 43.5% had master's degrees and 21.7% had doctorates; and 95.7% were board certified. They had practiced for a mean of 18.8 years (range 3–30).

The chaplains were recruited through the listservs of the Association of Professional Chaplains and through word of mouth. Chaplains who were interested in participating contacted me by email.

I drafted the semi-structured interview questionnaire, drawing on the prior literature on chaplains. Questions explored chaplains' views, experiences, and decisions. I conducted all the interviews. Sample questions, asked of all participants, appear in Box B.1.

I held additional informational conversations as background, with 15 chaplains and 12 physicians regarding these issues, to help inform the 33 formal interviews with chaplains. I chose qualitative methods because these can best elicit the full range and typologies of attitudes, interactions, and practices involved, and can inform subsequent quantitative studies. From a theoretical standpoint, Geertz has advocated studying aspects of individuals' lives, decisions, and social situations not by imposing theoretical structures but by trying to understand these individuals' own experiences and perspectives, drawing on their own words to obtain a "thick description."[2]

This book draws, too, on several other recent in-depth qualitative research studies I've conducted of doctors and patients regarding several medical diagnoses, including cancer,[3] HIV,[4] genetics,[5] and infertility.[6] In brief, as described elsewhere, these studies all explored participants' views, experiences, challenges, and decisions concerning conditions they confronted, including their understandings of, and ways of coping with, these conditions, and whether they faced religious or spiritual issues.

Table B.1 Characteristics of sample (N = 23)

Variable	Number	Percentage
Gender		
Male	13	56.5%
Female	10	43.5%
Race & ethnicity		
Caucasian	18	78.2.%
African American	3	13.0%
Latino	1	4.3%
Other	1	4.3%
Age		
Range		42–75 Years
Mean		63 years
Geographical region		
Northeast	12	52.2%
Midwest	4	17.4%
Southeast	3	13.0%
Southwest	3	13.0%
West	1	4.3%
Religion		
Protestant	6	26.1%
Catholic	4	17.4%
Christian, not otherwise specified	6	26.1%
Jewish	3	13.0%
Muslim	3	13.0%
Buddhist	1	4.3%
Highest degree held		
Master's	10	43.5%
Doctorate	5	21.7%
Bachelor's	1	4.3%
Associate	1	4.3%
Unknown	6	26.1%
Years practiced as chaplain		
Range		3–30 years
Mean		18.8 years
Board certified	22	95.7%

Box B.1 Semi-structured interview questionnaire: Sample questions

---

- How did you come to be a chaplain?
- How long have you been a chaplain?
- What kind of work did you do before?
- What kind of work do you now do as a chaplain?
- What have been your most rewarding experiences/cases as a chaplain?
- What were the most difficult?
- Do specific cases/incidents come to mind?
- How do you think chaplains can most help patients and their families? Physicians? Other staff? The hospital? The healthcare system?
- Do you think other chaplains' experiences have been similar or different? If so, how?
- Do you see differences between chaplains in different institutions or geographical regions? If so, how?
- Have you seen religious and spiritual issues affect medical decisions? If so, where and how?
- Do you see room for improvement in how providers address religious or spiritual issues? If so, how?
- Have you tried addressing these issues? If so, how? Has it worked?
- Have you ever faced or addressed burnout among providers? If so, when? What happened?
- What additional thoughts do you have about these issues?

I have published methodological details and other data from these studies elsewhere (e.g., Klitzman[3,4,5,6]), focusing on other topics. The study of genetic testing included 64 participants who had or were at risk for Huntington's disease (21), breast cancer (32), or alpha-1 antitrypsin deficiency (11), including 48 women and 16 men, of whom 50 were white, 8 African American, 3 Latino, and 3 "other."[5] The study on infertility included 37 participants, including 27 assisted reproductive technology providers and 10 patients.[6] The study on HIV included 38 participants (24 men and 14 women).[4] The study of doctors becoming patients due to cancer and other conditions included 50 participants (40 men and 10 women, 49 Caucasians and 1 Latino).[3]

The Columbia University Department of Psychiatry Research Ethics Committee (or Institutional Review Board) approved all of these studies, and participants gave informed consent.

The methods for the studies adapted key elements from "grounded theory"[7] and were thus informed by techniques of "constant comparison," with data from different contexts compared for similarities and differences, to see if they suggest hypotheses. This technique generates new analytic categories and questions and checks them for reasonableness.

I conducted confidential in-depth semi-structured interviews until saturation for major and minor themes was reached. After each interview, I took field notes. Interviews were audiotaped, transcribed, and content-analyzed. Transcriptions and initial analyses of interviews occurred during the period in which the interviews were being conducted, helping to shape subsequent interviews.

In each study, once the full set of interviews was completed, subsequent analyses were conducted in two phases, by research assistants (RAs) and me. In phase 1 of the subsequent coding, we independently examined a subset of interviews to assess factors that shaped participants' experiences, identifying categories of recurrent themes and issues that were subsequently given codes. These coders assessed similarities and differences between participants, examining themes and categories that emerged, ranges of variation within categories, and variables that might be involved. We systematically coded clocks of test to assign "core" codes or categories (e.g., instances of rituals, prayers, rejections from patients, interactions with physicians). While reading the interviews, a topic name (code) was inserted beside each excerpt of the interview to indicate the themes being discussed. We then worked together to reconcile these independently developed coding schemes into a single scheme, developing a coding manual and examining areas of disagreement until reaching consensus between us. We discussed new themes that did not fit into the original coding framework, and modified the manual when deemed appropriate. In phase 2 of the analysis, the RAs and I then independently performed content analysis of the data to identify the principal subcategories and ranges of variation within each of the core codes. We reconciled sub-themes identified by each coder were into a single set of "secondary" codes and an elaborated set of core codes, such as specific types of rituals (e.g., for staff, for patients), prayers (e.g., pre-established or spontaneous), or reasons for rejections (e.g., due to chaplain's religion or gender). These codes assess subcategories and other situational and social factors.

We then used codes and sub-codes in analyzing of all of the interviews. Two coders and I analyzed all interviews. Where necessary, we used multiple codes. We checked regularly for consistency and accuracy in ratings by comparing earlier- and later-coded excerpts. To ensure that the coding schemes established for the codes and secondary codes are both valid and reliable (i.e., consistent in meaning), they were systematically developed and well documented. To ensure trustworthiness, we triangulated the data with existing literature.

Notes

Chapter 1

1. Pew Research Center. (2019). *In U.S., decline of Christianity continues at rapid pace: An update on America's changing religious landscape.* https://www.pewresearch.org/relig ion/2019/10/17/in-u-s-decline-of-christianity-continues-at-rapid-pace/#:~:text= The%20religious%20landscape%20of%20the,points%20over%20the%20past%20 decade. (accessed January 11, 2024).
2. Klitzman, R. (2008). *When doctors become patients.* Oxford University Press.
3. Klitzman, R. (2012). *Am I my genes? Confronting fate and family secrets in the age of genetic testing.* Oxford University Press.
4. Einstein, A. (1926/1971). Letter to Max Born. *The Born-Einstein letters.* Translated from the German by Irene Born. Walker and Company.
5. Klitzman, R. (2019). *Designing babies: How technology is changing the ways we create children.* Oxford University Press.
6. Freud, S. (1927/2019). *The future of an illusion.* Translated from the German by Gregory C. Richter. Beta Nu Publishing.
7. Frankel, V. (1946/2006). *Man's search for meaning.* Beacon Press.
8. Toneatto, T., & Nguyen, L. (2007). Does mindfulness meditation improve anxiety and mood symptoms? A review of the controlled research. *Canadian Journal of Psychiatry, 52*(4), 260–266. doi:10.1177/070674370705200409.
9. Granqvist, P., Mikulincer, M., & Shaver, P. R. (2010). Religion as attach-ment: Normative processes and individual differences. *Personality and Social Psychology Review, 14*(1), 49–59. https://doi.org/10.1177/1088868309348618.
10. Sedikides, C., & Gebauer, J. E. (2021). Do religious people self-enhance? *Current Opinion in Psychology, 40,* 29–33. doi:10.1016/j.copsyc.2020.08.002.
11. Rim, J. I., Ojeda, J. C., Svob, C., Kayser, J., Drews, E., Kim, Y., Tenke, C. E., Skipper, J., & Weissman, M. M. (2019). Current understanding of religion, spirituality, and their neurobiological correlates. *Harvard Review of Psychiatry, 27*(5), 303–316. doi:10.1097/HRP.0000000000000232.
12. Tang, Y. Y., Holzel, T., & Posnter, M. (2015). The neuroscience of mindfulness medita-tion. *Nature Reviews Neuroscience, 16*(4), 213–225. doi:10.1038/nrn3916.
13. Cozier, Y. C., Yu, J., Wise, L. A., VanderWeele, T. J., Balboni, T. A., Argentieri, M. A., Rosenberg, L., Palmer, J. R., & Shields, A. E. (2018). Religious and spiritual coping and risk of incident hypertension in the Black Women's Health Study. *Annals of Behavioral Medicine, 52*(12), 989–998. doi:10.1093/abm/kay001
14. Trevino, K. M., Pargament, K. I., Kraus, N., Ironson, G., & Hill, P. (2017). Stressful events and religious/spiritual struggle: Moderating effects of the general orienting

system. *Psychology of Religion and Spirituality, 11*(3), 214–224. https://doi.org/ 10.1037/rel0000149.

15. Koenig, H. G. (2007). Religion and depression in older medical inpatients. *American Journal of Geriatric Psychiatry, 15*(4), 282–291. doi:10.1097/ 01.JGP.0000246875.93674.0c.

16. Koenig, H. G., George, L. K., & Peterson, B. L. (1998). Religiosity and remission of depression in medically ill older patients. *American Journal of Psychiatry, 155*(4), 536–542. doi:10.1176/ajp.155.4.536.

17. Centers for Disease Control and Prevention. (2022, March 31). *Adolescent Behaviors and Experiences Survey* (ABES). https://www.cdc.gov/healthyyouth/data/abes.htm (accessed January 11, 2024).

18. Knoll, C., Watkins, A., & Rothfield, M. (2020, July 11). "I couldn't do anything": The virus and an E.R. doctor's suicide. *New York Times.* https://www.nytimes.com/2020/ 07/11/nyregion/lorna-breen-suicide-coronavirus.html (accessed January 11, 2024)).

19. U.S. House of Representatives. H.R.1667—Dr. Lorna Breen Health Care Provider Protection Act. December 8, 2021. https://www.congress.gov/bill/117th-congress/ house-bill/1667 (accessed January 11, 2024).

20. Elson, G. (1966, April 8). Is God dead? *Time, 87*(14), 82–87. https://time.com/vault/ issue/1966-04-08/page/98/ (accessed July 20, 2022).

21. Pew Research Center for Religion and Public Life. (2018, August 8). *Why America's 'nones' don't identify with a religion.* https://www.pewresearch.org/fact tank/2018/08/ 08/why-americas-nones-dont-identify-with-a-religion/ (accessed July 20, 2022).

22. Pew Research Center for Religion and Public Life. (2014). *The 2014 U. S. religious landscape study.* http://www.pewforum.org/religious-landscape-study/ (accessed January 11, 2024).

23. Oxford English Dictionary. (2023). Chaplain. https://www.oed.com/search/diction ary/?scope=Entries&q=chaplain (accessed January 11, 2024).

24. U.S. Department of Veterans Affairs. (2024, January 10). *Patient care services: History of VA chaplaincy.* https://www.patientcare.va.gov/chaplain/ (accessed January 11, 2024).

25. White, K. B., Barnes, M. J. D., Cadge, W., & Fitchett, G. (2021). Mapping the healthcare chaplaincy workforce: A baseline description. *Journal of Health Care Chaplaincy, 27*(4), 238–258. doi:10.1080/08854726.2020.1723192.

26. The Joint Commission (2016, April 11; update 2023, July 19). *Does the Joint Commission specify what needs to be included in a spiritual assessment?* https://www. jointcommission.org/standards/standard-faqs/critical-access hospital/provision-of-care-treatment-and-services pc/000001669/#:~:text = It%20is%20important%20 that%20the,end%2Dof%2Dlife%20ce (accessed January 11, 2024).

27. Board of Chaplaincy Education, Inc. (2022). https://bcci.professionalchaplains.org/ content.asp?pl = 25&sl = 26&contentid = 26 (accessed January 11, 2024).

28. Cadge, W. (2012). *Paging God: Religion in the halls of medicine.* University of Chicago Press.

29. Cadge, W., Freese, J., & Christakis, N. A. (2008). The provision of hospital chaplaincy in the United States: A national overview. *Southern Medical Journal*, *101*(6), 626–630. doi:10.1097/SMJ.0b013e3181706856.

30. Balboni, M. J., Babar, A., Dillinger, J., Phelps. A. C., George, E., Block, S. D., Kachnic, L., Hunt, J., Peteet, J., Prigerson, H., G., VanderWeele, T. J., & Balboni, T. A. (2011). "It depends": Viewpoints of patients, physicians, and nurses on patient practitioner prayer in the setting of advanced cancer. *Journal of Pain and Symptom Management*, *41*(5), 836–847. doi:10.1016/j.jpainsymman.2010.07.008.

31. Geertz, C. (1973). *The interpretation of cultures: Selected essays*. Basic Books.

32. Klitzman, R. (1997). *Being positive: The lives of men and women with HIV*. Ivan R. Dee.

33. Klitzman, R. (2021). "Doctor, will you pray for me?" Responding to patients' religious and spiritual concerns. *Academic Medicine*, *96*(3), 349–354. doi:10.1097/ACM.0000000000003765.

34. Klitzman, R. (2022, April). Typologies and meanings of prayer among patients. *Journal of Religion and Health*, *61*(2), 1300–1317. doi: 10.1007/s10943-021-01220-x.

35. Klitzman, R., Garbuzova, E., Di Sapia Natarelli, G., Sinnappan, S., & Al-Hashimi, J. (2022, November 26). When and why patients and families reject chaplains: Challenges, strategies and solutions. *Journal of Health Care Chaplaincy*, 1–14. doi:10.1080/08854726.2022.2150026.

36. Klitzman, R., Di Sapia Natarelli, G., Garbuzova, E., Sinnappan, S., & Al-Hashimi, J. (2023). Muslim patients in the U.S. confronting challenges regarding end-of-life and palliative care: The experiences and roles of hospital chaplains. *BMC Palliative Care*, *22*(1), 28. doi:10.1186/s12904-023-01144-1.

37. Klitzman, R., Di Sapia Natarelli, G., Sinnappan, S., Garbuzova, E., & Al-Hashimi, J. (2023, January 3). Exiting patients' rooms and ending relationships: Questions and challenges faced by hospital chaplains. *Journal of Pastoral Care & Counseling*. doi:10.1177/15423050221146507.

38. Klitzman, R., Garbuzova, E., Di Sapia Natarelli, G., Sinnappan, S., & Al-Hashimi, J. (2022). Hospital chaplains' communication with patients: Characteristics, functions and potential benefits. *Patient Education and Counseling*, *105*(9), 2905–2912. doi:10.1016/j.pec.2022.05.004.

39. Klitzman, R., Sinnappan, S., Garbuzova, E., Al-Hashimi, J., & Di Sapia Natarelli, G. (2022, December 14). Becoming chaplains: How and why chaplains enter the field, factors involved and implications. *Journal of Health Care Chaplaincy*, 1–14. doi:10.1080/08854726.2022.2154108.

40. Klitzman, R., Al-Hashimi, J., Di Sapia Natarelli, G., Garbuzova, E., & Sinnappan, S. (2022). How hospital chaplains develop and use rituals to address medical staff distress. *SSM—Qualitative Research in Health*, 2. https://doi.org/10.1016/j.ssmqr.2022.100087.

41. Klitzman, R., Di Sapia Natarelli, G., Sinnappan, S., Garbuzova, E., & Al-Hashimi, J. (2023, May 13). "Reading" the room": Healthcare chaplains' challenges, insights and variations in entering rooms and engaging with patients and families. *Journal of Health Care Chaplaincy*, 1–15. doi:10.1080/08854726.2023.2210029.

42. Klitzman, R., Di Sapia Natarelli, G., Garbuzova, E., Al-Hashimi, J., & Sinnappan, S. (2023). Barriers and facilitators faced by hospital chaplains in communicating with lesbian, gay, bisexual, transgender and questioning patients. *Patient Education and Counseling, 113*, 107753. doi:10.1016/j.pec.2023.107753.

43. Klitzman, R. (2023, July 14). "It wasn't luck: God wants me here for a reason": Perceptions of luck among US patients and its relationships to other factors among US patients. *Journal of Religion and Health*. doi:10.1007/s10943-023-01859-8.

44. Klitzman, R., Di Sapia Natarelli, G., Sinnappan, S., Garbuzova, E., & Al-Hashimi, J. (2023, September). The effects of contextual factors on hospital chaplains: A qualitative study. *Journal of Pastoral Care & Counseling, 77*(3-4), 137–147. doi: 10.1177/15423050231214459.

45. Klitzman, R. (2023, December). "Why me?": Qualitative research on why patients ask, what they mean, how they answer and what factors and processes are involved. *SSM—Mental Health, 3*, 100218. https://doi.org/10.1016/j.ssmmh.2023.100218

46. Williams, J. A., Meltzer, D., Arora, V., Chung, G., & Curlin, F. A. (2011). Attention to inpatients' religious and spiritual concerns: Predictors and association with patient satisfaction. *Journal of General Internal Medicine, 26*(11), 265–1271. doi:10.1007/s11606-011-1781-y.

47. Peng-Keller, S., & Neuhold, D. (Eds.). (2020). *Charting spiritual care: The emerging role of chaplaincy records in global health care.* Springer.

Chapter 2

1. Klitzman, R. (2019). *Designing babies: How technology is changing the ways we create children.* Oxford University Press.

2. Lehman, D. R., Wortman, C. B., & Williams, A. F. (1987). Long-term effects of losing spouse or child in motor vehicle crash. *Journal of Personality and Social Psychology, 52*(1), 218–231. doi:10.1037//0022-3514.52.1.218.

3. Job 38:4. Holy Bible, King James Version.

4. Boswell, J. (1791/2008). *The life of Samuel Johnson.* Penguin Classics.

5. Klitzman, R. (2012). *Am I my genes?: Confronting fate and family secrets in the age of genetic testing.* Oxford University Press.

6. Didion, J. (2006). *We tell ourselves stories in order to live: Collected nonfiction.* Everyman's Library.

Chapter 3

1. Ramondetta, L., Brown, A., Richardson, G., Urbauer, D., Thaker, P. H., Koenig, H. G., Gano, J. B., & Sun, C. (2011). Religious and spiritual beliefs of gynecologic oncologists may influence medical decision making. *International Journal of Gynecological Cancer, 21*(3), 573–581. doi:10.1097/IGC.0b013e31820ba507.

2. Frush, B. W., Brauer, S. G., Yoon, J. D., & Curlin, F. A. (2018). Physician decision-making in the setting of advanced illness: An examination of patient disposition and physician religiousness. *Journal of Pain and Symptom Management, 55*(3), 906–912. doi:10.1016/j.jpainsymman.2017.

3. Seale, S. (2010). The role of doctors' religious faith and ethnicity in taking ethically controversial decisions during end-of-life care. *Journal of Medical Ethics, 36*(11), 677–682. doi:10.1136/jme.2010.036194.

4. Kelly, E. P., Myers, B., Henderson, B., Sprik, P., White, K. B., & Pawlik, T. M. (2022). The influence of patient and provider religious and spiritual beliefs on treatment decision making in the cancer care context. *Medical Decision Making, 42*(1), 125–134. doi:10.1177/0272989X211022246.

5. Williams, J. A., Meltzer, D., Arora, V., Chung, G., & Curlin, F. A. (2011). Attention to inpatients' religious and spiritual concerns: Predictors and association with patient satisfaction. *Journal of General Internal Medicine, 26*(11), 265–1271. doi: 10.1007/s11606-011-1781-y.

6. Choi, P. J., Curlin, F. A., & Cox, C .E. (2019). Addressing religion and spirituality in the intensive care unit: A survey of clinicians. *Palliative & Supportive Care, 17*(2), 159–164. doi: 10.1017/S147895151800010X.

7. Best, M., Butow, P., & Olver, I. (2016). Doctors discussing religion and spirituality: A systematic literature review. *Palliative Medicine, 30*(4), 327–337. doi: https://doi.org/10.1177/0269216315600.

8. Balboni, M. J., Sullivan, A., Enzinger, A. C., Epstein-Peterson, Z. D., Tseng, Y. D., Mitchell, C., Niska, J., Zollfrank, A., VanderWeele, T. J., & Balboni, T. A. (2014). Nurse and physician barriers to spiritual care provision at the end of life. *Journal of Pain and Symptom Management, 48*, 400–410. doi:10.1016/j.jpainsymman.2013.09.020.

9. Balboni, T. A., Vanderwerker, L. C., Block, S. D., Paulk, M. E., Lathan, C. S., Peteet, J. R., & Prigerson, H. G. (2007). Religiousness and spiritual support among advanced cancer patients and associations with end-of-life treatment preferences and quality of life. *Journal of Clinical Oncology, 25*(5), 555–560. doi:10.1200/JCO.2006.07.9046.

10. Rasinski K. A., Kalad, Y. G., Yoon, J. D., & Curlin, F. A. (2011). An assessment of US physicians' training in religion, spirituality, and medicine. *Medical Teacher, 33*(11), 944–955. doi: https://doi.org/10.3109/0142159X.2011.588976.

11. Robinson, J. D., & Nussbaum, J. F. (2004). Grounding research and medical education about religion in actual physician-patient interaction: Church attendance, social support, and older adults. *Health Communication, 16*(1), 63–85. doi: 10.1207/S15327027HC1601_5.

12. Ernecoff, N. C., Curlin, F. A., Buddadhumaruk, P., & White, D. B. (2015). Health care professionals' responses to religious or spiritual statements by surrogate decision makers during goals-of-care discussions. *JAMA Internal Medicine, 175*(10), 1662–1669. doi:10.1001/jamainternmed.2015.4124.

13. Fine, E., Reid, M. C., Shengelia, R., & Adelman, R. D. (2010). Directly observed patient–physician discussions in palliative and end-of-life care: A systematic review of the literature. *Journal of Palliative Medicine, 13*(5), 595–603. doi:10.1089/jpm.2009.0388.

14. Ehman, J. (2023, July 1 E-dition). References to spirituality, religion, beliefs, and cultural diversity in the Joint Commission's *Comprehensive accreditation manual for hospitals.* https://www.uphs.upenn.edu/pastoral/resed/jcahorefs.pdf (accessed January 19, 2024).

15. The Joint Commission (Last reviewed 2022, July 19). *Spiritual Beliefs and Preferences - Evaluating a patient's spiritual need: Does the Joint Commission specify what needs to be included in a spiritual assessment?* https://www.jointcommission.org/standards/standard-faqs/critical-access-hospital/provision-of-care-treatment-and-services-pc/000001669/ (accessed January 22, 2024).

16. Koenig, H. G., Hooten, E. G., Lindsay-Calkins, E., & Meador, K. G. (2010). Spirituality in medical school curricula: Findings from a national survey. *The International Journal of Psychiatry in Medicine, 40*(4), 391–398. doi:10.2190/PM.40.4.

17. Association of American Medical Colleges. (2024). https://www.aamc.org/ (accessed January 19, 2024).

18. Becker, E. (1974/1997). *The denial of death.* Free Press.

19. Mitford, J. (1963/1978/1996/2000). *The American way of death revisited.* Vintage Books.

20. Sloan, R. P., Bagiella, E., VandeCreek, L., Hover, M., Casalone, C., Jinpu Hirsch, T., Hasan, Y., Kreger, R., & Poulos P. Should physicians prescribe religious activities? *New England Journal of Medicine, 342*(25), 1913–1916. doi:10.1056/NEJM200006223422513.

21. Robinson, K. A., Cheng, M.-R., Hansen, P. D., & Gray, R. J. (2017). Religious and spiritual beliefs of physicians. *Journal of Religion and Health, 56*(1), 205–225. doi:10.1007/s10943-016-0233-8.

Chapter 4

1. Jung, C. (1951/1966). Fundamental questions of psychotherapy. In C. Jung, *Collected works of C. G. Jung* (Vol. 16, 2nd ed.). Princeton University Press.

2. Handzo, G. F., Flannelly, K. J., Murphy, K. M., Bauman, J. P., Oettinger, M., Goodell, E., Hasan, Y. H., Barrie, D. P., & Jacobs, M. R. (2008). What do chaplains really do? I. Visitation in the New York Chaplaincy Study. *Journal of Health Care Chaplaincy, 14*(1), 20–38. doi:10.1080/08854720802053838.

3. Handzo, G. F., Flannelly, K. J., Kudler, T., Fogg, S. L., Harding, S. R., Hasan, Y. H., Ross, A. M., & Taylor, B. E. (2008). What do chaplains really do? II. Interventions in the New York Chaplaincy Study. *Journal of Health Care Chaplaincy, 14*(1), 39–56. doi:10.1080/08854720802053853.

4. Jeuland, J., Fitchett, G., Schulman-Green, D., & Kapo, J. (2017). Chaplains working in palliative care: Who they are and what they do. *Journal of Palliative Medicine, 20*(5), 502–508. doi:10.1089/jpm.2016.0308.

5. Timmins, F., Caldeira, S., Murphy, M., Pujol, N., Sheaf, G., Weathers, E., Whelan, J., & Flanagan, B. (2018). The role of the healthcare chaplain: A literature review. *Journal of Health Care Chaplaincy, 24*(3), 87–106. doi:10.1080/08854726.2017.1338048.

6. Massey, K., Barnes, M. J., Villines, D., Goldstein, J. D., Hisley Pierson, A. L., Scherer, C., Vander Laan, B., & Summerfelt, W. T. (2015). "What do I do?" Developing a taxonomy of chaplaincy activities and interventions for spiritual care in intensive care unit palliative care. *BMC Palliative Care, 14*, 1–8. https://doi.org/10.1186/s12904-015-0008-0.

7. Idler, E. L. Grant, G. H., Quest, T., Binney, Z., & Perkins. M. M. (2015). Practical matters and ultimate concerns, "doing," and "being": A diary study of the chaplain's role in the care of the seriously ill in an urban acute care hospital. *Journal for the Scientific Study of Religion, 54*(4), 722–738. http://www.jstor.org/stable/26651393.

8. Puchalski, C. (1996/2021). *The FICA spiritual history tool: A guide for spiritual assessment in clinical settings.* GW Institute for Spirituality and Health. chromeextension://efaidnbmnnnibpcajpcglclefindmkaj/https://smhs.gwu.edu/spirituality health/sites/spirituality-health/files/FICA-PDF-Final-Nov2020.pdf> (accessed January 12, 2024).

9. Robson, J. P., & Troutman-Jordan, M. (2014). A concept analysis of cognitive reframing. *Journal of Theory Construction & Testing, 18*(2), 55–59.

10. Yeats, W. B. (1893/1902/2011). Earth, fire and water. In W. B. Yeats, *The Celtic twilight: Faerie and folklore.* Dover Publications.

Chapter 6

1. Pew Research Center for Religion and Public Life. (2014). *The 2014 U. S. religious landscape study.* http://www.pewforum.org/religious-landscape-study/ (accessed January 11, 2024).

2. Lipka, M. (2015, May 12). Millennials increasingly are driving growth of 'nones.' Pew Research Center https://www.pewresearch.org/short-reads/2015/05/12/millennials-increasingly-are-driving-growth-of-nones/ (accessed January 25, 2024).

3. Oxford English Dictionary. (2023). Religion. https://www.oed.com/search/dictionary/?scope=Entries&q=Religion (accessed January 9, 2024).

4. Caesar, J. (circa 40 BCE/1976). *The Civil War (Commentarii de Bello Civili): Book 1.* Translated from the Latin by J. P. Gardner. Penguin Classics.

5. Huizinga, J. (1919/1999). *The waning of the Middle Ages.* Dover Publications, Inc.

6. Morreall, J., & Sonn, T. (2014). *50 great myths about religions.* John Wiley & Sons Ltd.

7. Cox, C. W. (2003, April 13). *Religion without God: Methodological agnosticism and the future of religious studies.* The Hibbert Lecture, Herriot-Watt University. chrome-extension://efaidnbmnnnibpcajpcglclefindmkaj/https://s3-eu-west-1.amazonaws.com/img.thehibberttrust.org.uk/Hibbert-Lecture-2003-Dr-James-L-Cox.pdf?mtime=20161116150000 (accessed January 9, 2024).

8. Van Beek, W. E. A., & Blakely, T. D. (1994). Introduction. In W. E. A. Van Beek, T. D. Blakely, & D. L. Thomson (Eds.), *Religion in Africa.* James Currey.

9. Oxford English Dictionary. (2022). Spirit. https://www.oed.com/dictionary/spirit_n?tab=meaning_and_use#21464538 (accessed January 9, 2024).

10. Kellstedt, L. A., Green, J. C., Guth, J. L., & Smidt, C. E. (1996). Grasping the essentials: The social embodiment of religion and political behavior. In J. C. Green, J.

L. Gurth, C. E. Smidt, & L. E. Kellstedt (Eds.), *Religion and the culture wars*. Rowman and Littlefield.

11. Bell, R. (2013). *What we talk about when we talk about God*. HarperOne.

12. Drescher, E. (2016). *Choosing our religion: The spiritual lives of America's nones*. Oxford University Press.

13. Pew Research Center for Religion and Public Life. (2012, October 9). "Nones" on the rise. https://www.pewresearch.org/religion/2012/10/09/nones-on-the-rise/ (accessed January 9, 2024).

14. Hayward, R. D., Krause, N., Ironson, G., Hill, P. C., & Emmons, R. (2016). Health and wellbeing among the non-religious: Atheists, agnostics, and no preference compared with religious group members. *Journal of Religion & Health, 55*(3), 1024–1037. doi:10.1007/s10943-015-0179-2.

15. Murphy, C. (2015, June 2). Interfaith marriage is common in the US, particularly among the recently wed. Pew Research Center. https://www.pewresearch.org/fact ank/2015/06/02/interfaith-marriage/ (accessed January 9, 2024).

16. Emerson, R. W. (1838/1983). The Divinity School Address. In J. Porte (Ed.), *Emerson: Essays and lectures* (p. 71). Library of America.

17. Emerson, R. W. (1841/1951). Self-reliance. In I. Edman (Ed.), *Emerson's essays* (pp. 34–35). Harper Perennial.

18. Bloom, H. (1992/2006 [2nd ed.]). *The American religion: The emergence of the post-Christian nation*. Simon & Schuster.

19. Lifton, R. J. (1968). *Death in life: Survivors of Hiroshima*. Random House.

20. Klitzman, R. (2015). *The ethics police?: The struggle to make human research safe*. Oxford University Press.

21. Smidt, C. E., Kellstedt, L. A., & Guth, J. L. (2009). The role of religion in American politics: Explanatory theories and associated analytical and measurement issues. In C. E. Smidt, L. A. Kellstedt, & J. L. Guth (Eds.), *The Oxford handbook of religion and American politics* (pp. 3–42). Oxford University Press.

22. Drescher, E. (2016). *Choosing our religion: The spiritual lives of America's nones* (p. 245). Oxford University Press.

23. Drescher, 2016, p. 216..

24. Bellah, R. N. (2011). *Religion in human evolution*. Harvard University Press.

Chapter 7

1. Freud, S. (1899/1994). *The interpretation of dreams*. Translated from the German by A. A. Brill. Modern Library.

2. Hume, D. (1748). *An enquiry concerning human understanding*. Edited by J. Hill Burton. https://www.gutenberg.org/ebooks/9662 (accessed January 11, 2024).)

3. Hume, D. (1779). *Dialogues concerning natural religion*. https://www.gutenberg.org/files/4583/4583-h/4583-h.htm (accessed January 11, 2024).

4. Popkin, G. (2018, April 25). Einstein's "spooky action at a distance" spotted objects almost big enough to see. *Science*. https://www.science.org/content/article/einst

ein-s-spooky-action-distance-spotted-objects-almost-big-enough-see (accessed January 11, 2024).)

5. Becker, H. (1997). *Outsiders: Studies in the sociology of deviance*. Free Press.

6. Goffman, E. (1961). *Asylums: Essays on the social situation of mental patients and other inmates*. Anchor Books.

7. Watson, G. (1985). "I doubt, therefore I am": St. Augustine and skepticism. *The Maynooth Review/Revieú Mhá Nuad*, *12*, 42–50. https://www.jstor.org/stable/20556991.

8. D'Souza, R. (2002). Do patients expect psychiatrists to be interested in spiritual issues? *Australasian Psychiatry*, *10*(1), 44–47. https://doi.org/10.1046/j.1440-1665.2002.00391.x.

Chapter 8

1. Jung, C. (1951/1966). *Fundamental questions of psychotherapy*. In: Jung, C., *Collected works of C. G. Jung* (2nd ed., Vol. 16). Princeton University Press.

2. Oxford English Dictionary. (2023). "Miracle." https://www.oed.com/search/diction ary/?scope=Entries&q=Miracle (accessed January 22, 2024).

3. Balboni, M. J., Sullivan, A., Enzinger, A. C., Smith, P. T., Mitchell, C., Peteet, J. R., Tulsky, T., VanderWeele J. A., & Balboni, T. A. (2017). US clergy religious values and relationships to end-of-life discussions and care. *Journal of Pain and Symptom Management*, *53*(6), 999–1009. doi:10.1016/j.jpainsymman.2016.12.346.

4. DeLiser, H. M. (2009). A practical approach to the family that expects a miracle. *Chest*, *135*(6), 1643–1647. doi:0.1378/chest.08-280.

Chapter 9

1. Levine, E. G., Aviv, C., Yoo, G., Ewing, C., & Au, A. (2009). The benefits of prayer on mood and well-being of breast cancer survivors. *Supportive Care in Cancer*, *17*(3), 295–306. https://doi.org/10.1007/s0052000804825.

2. Koenig, H. G., George, L. K., & Peterson, B. L. (1998). Religiosity and remission of depression in medically ill older patients. *American Journal of Psychiatry*, *155*(4), 536–542. doi:10.1176/ajp.155.4.536.

3. Steinhauser, K. E., Christakis, N. A., Clipp, E. C., McNeilly, M., McIntyre, L., & Tulsky, J. A. (2000). Factors considered important at the end of life by patients, family, physicians, and other care providers. *JAMA*, *284*(19), 2476–2482. doi:10.1001/jama.284.19.2476.

4. Alcoholics Anonymous. *The origin of our Serenity Prayer*. http://www.aahistory.com/prayer.html (accessed January 12, 2024).

5. Klitzman, R. (2015, August 13). Doctors fail to address patients' spiritual needs. *New York Times*. https://archive.nytimes.com/well.blogs.nytimes.com/2015/08/13/doctors-fail-to-address-patients-spiritual-needs//> (accessed January 22, 2024)).

6. Comment on Klitzman, R. (2015, August 13). Doctors fail to address patients' spiritual needs. *New York Times*. https://archive.nytimes.com/well.blogs.nytimes.com/2015/08/13/doctors-fail-to-address-patients-spiritual-needs/ (accessed January 22, 2024).

7. Hodge, D. R. (2007). A systematic review of the empirical literature on intercessory prayer. In *Database of abstracts of reviews of effects (DARE): Quality-assessed reviews*. University of York Centre for Reviews and Dissemination.

8. Cardeña, E. (2018). The experimental evidence for parapsychological phenomena: A review. *American Psychologist, 73*(5), 663–677. https://doi.org/10.1037/amp0000236.

Chapter 10

1. Stein, G. L., Berkman, C., O'Mahoney, S., Godfrey, D., Javier, N.-M., & Maingi, S. (2020). Experiences of lesbian, gay, bisexual, and transgender patients and families in hospice and palliative care: Perspectives of the palliative care team. *Journal of Palliative Medicine, 23*(6), 817–824. doi:10.1089/jpm.2019.0542.

2. Rando, T. A. (1985). Creating therapeutic rituals in the psychotherapy of the bereaved. *Psychotherapy: Theory, Research, Practice, Training, 22*(2), 236–240. doi:10.1037/h0085500.

3. Centers for Disease Control and Prevention. (2013). *The state of aging & health in America 2013*. U.S. Department of Health and Human Services.

4. Marshal, M. P., Dietz, L. J., Friedman, M. S., Stall, R., Smith, H. A., McGinley, J., Thoma, B. C., Murray, P. J., D'Augelli, A. R., & Brent, D. A. (2011). Suicidality and depression disparities between sexual minority and heterosexual youth: A meta-analytic review. *Journal of Adolescent Health, 49*(2), 115–123. doi:10.1016/j.jadohealth.2011.02.005.

5. Williams Institute at UCLA School of Law. (2020). *Vulnerabilities to COVID-19 among transgender adults in the US*. https://williamsinstitute.law.ucla.edu/publications/transgender-covid-19-risk/ (accessed January 12, 2024).

6. Pew Research Center. (2013, June 13). *Report: A survey of LGBT Americans*. https://www.pewresearch.org/social-trends/2013/06/13/a-survey-of-lgbt-americans/ (accessed January 12, 2024).

7. Lomash, E. F., Brown, T. D., & Galupo, M. P. (2019). "A whole bunch of love the sinner, hate the sin": LGBTQ microaggressions experienced in religious and spiritual context. *Journal of Homosexuality, 66*(10), 1495–1511. doi:10.1080/00918369.2018.1542204.

8. Sandstrom, A., & Schwadel, P. (2019, June 13). Lesbian, gay and bisexual Americans are more critical of churches than straight adults are. Pew Research Center. https://www.pewresearch.org/short-reads/2019/06/13/lesbian-gay-and-bisexual-americans-are-more-critical-of-churches-than-straight-adults-are/ (accessed January 22, 2024).

9. Murphy, C. (2015, May 26). Lesbian, gay and bisexual Americans differ from general public in their religious affiliations. Pew Research Center. https://www.pewresearch. org/short-reads/2015/05/26/lesbian-gay-and-bisexual-americans-differ-from-gene ral-public-in-their-religious-affiliations/ (accessed January 12, 2024).

10. Pew Research Center. (2015, April 2). *The future of world religions: Population growth projections, 2010–2050*.:<https://www.pewresearch.org/religion/2015/04/02/religi ous-projections-2010-2050/ (accessed January 12, 2024).

11. Samari, G., Alcalá, H., & Sharif, M. H. (2018). Islamophobia, health and public health: systematic literature review. *American Journal of Public Health*, *108*(6), e1–e9. doi: 10.2105/AJPH.2018.304402.

12. Gustafson, C., & Lazenby. M. (2019). Assessing the unique experiences and needs of Muslim oncology patients receiving palliative and end-of-life care: An integrative re-view. *Journal of Palliative Care*, *34*(1), 52–61. doi:10.1177/0825859718800496.

13. Gregorian, V. (2003). *Islam: mosaic, not a monolith*. Brookings Institution Press.

Chapter 11

1. Becker, E. (1974/1997). *The denial of death*. Free Press.

2. Romanoff, B. D., & Terenzio, M. (1998). Rituals and the grieving process. *Death Studies*, *22*(8), 697–711. doi:10.1080/074811898201227.

3. Turner, V. (1970). *The ritual process: Structure and anti-structure*. Routledge.

4. van Gennep, A. (1909/2019). *The rites of passage* (2nd ed.). University of Chicago Press.

5. Rando, T. A. (1985). Creating therapeutic rituals in the psychotherapy of the bereaved. *Psychotherapy: Theory, Research, Practice, Training*, *22*(2), 236–240. doi:10.1037/ h0085500.

6. Bolton, C., & Camp, D. J. (1987). Funeral rituals and the facilitation of grief work. *OMEGA—Journal of Death and Dying*, *17*(4), 343–352. doi:10.2190/ VDHT-MFRC-LY7L-EMN7.

7. Oliver, M. (2005). *New and Selected Poems, Volume One*. Random House.

8. Sanders, C. M. (1980). A comparison of adult bereavement in the death of a spouse, child, and parent. *OMEGA—Journal of Death and Dying*, *10*(4), 303–322. https://doi. org/10.2190/X565-HW49-CHR0-FYB4.

9. Yu, H. U., & Chan, S. (2010). Nurses' response to death and dying in an intensive care unit: A qualitative study. *Journal of Clinical Nursing*, *19*(7–8), 1167–1169. doi:10.1111/j.1365-2702.2009.03121.x.

Chapter 12

1. Silveira, M. J., Kim, S. Y., & Langa, K. M. (2010). Advance directives and outcomes of surrogate decision making before death. *New England Journal of Medicine*, *362*(13), 1211–1218. doi:10.1056/NEJMsa0907901.

2. Sommer, S., Marckmann, G., Pentzek, M., Wegscheider, K., Abholz, H. H., & in der Schmitten, J. (2012). Advance directives in nursing homes: Prevalence, validity, significance, and nursing staff adherence. *Deutsches Ärzteblatt International, 109*(37), 577–583. doi:10.3238/arztebl.2012.0577.

3. The Joint Commission. (2022, July 19). Does the Joint Commission specify what needs to be included in a spiritual assessment?. https://www.jointcommission.org/standards/standard-faqs/critical-access-hospital/provision-of-care-treatment-and-services-pc/000001669/ (accessed January 19, 2024).

4. Ehman, J. (2023, July 1 E-dition). References to spirituality, religion, beliefs, and cultural diversity in the Joint Commission's *Comprehensive accreditation manual for hospitals*. https://www.uphs.upenn.edu/pastoral/resed/jcahorefs.pdf (accessed January 19, 2024).

5. Rabbinical Council of America (2009, August 10). *Halachic guidelines to assist patients and their families in making "end-of-life" medical choices.* http://www.rabbis.org/pdfs/hcpi.pdf (accessed January 17, 2024).

6. Jehovah's Witnesses. (2022). https://www.jw.org/en/ (accessed January 17, 2024).

7. Genesis 9:4. *Holy Bible*, King James Version.

8. Leviticus 3:16–17. *Holy Bible*, King James Version.

9. Joint United Kingdom (UK) Blood Transfusion and Tissue Transportation Services Professional Advisory Committee. (2020, January 4). *12:2: Jehovah's Witnesses and blood transfusion.* https://www.transfusionguidelines.org/transfusion-handbook/12-management-of-patients-who-do-not-accept-transfusion/12-2-jehovah-s-witnesses-and-blood-transfusion (accessed January 17, 2024).

10. Gyamfi, C., & Berkowitz, R. L. (2004). Responses by pregnant Jehovah's Witnesses on health care proxies. *Obstetrics and Gynecology, 104*(3), 541–544. doi:10.1097/01.AOG.0000135276.25886.8e.

Chapter 13

1. Piaget, J. (1957). *Construction of reality in the child.* Routledge & Kegan Paul.

Chapter 14

1. Fox, R. C. (1989). *The sociology of medicine: A participant observer's view.* Pearson College Division.

2. Best, M., Washington, J., Condello, M., & Kearney, M. (2020). "This ward has no ears": Role of the pastoral care practitioner in the hospital ward. *Journal of Health Care Chaplaincy, 13*, 1–15. doi:101.10080/08854726.2020.1814089.

3. Williams, J. A., Meltzer, D., Arora, V., Chung, G., & Curlin, F. A. (2011). Attention to inpatients' religious and spiritual concerns: Predictors and association with patient

satisfaction. *Journal of General Internal Medicine*, *26*(11), 265–1271. doi:10.1007/s11606-011-1781-y.

4. Wirpsa, W. J., Johnson, R. E., Bieler, J., Boyken, L., Pugliese, K., Rosencrans, E., & Murphy, P. (2019). Interprofessional models for shared decision making: The role of the healthcare chaplain. *Journal of Health Care Chaplaincy*, *25*(1), 20–44. doi:10.1080/08854726.2018.150113.

5. Handzo, G. F., Flannelly, K. J., Murphy, K. M., Bauman, J. P., Oettinger, M., Goodell, E., Hasan, Y. H., Barrie, D. P., & Jacobs, M. R. (2008). What do chaplains really do? I. Visitation in the New York Chaplaincy Study. *Journal of Health Care Chaplaincy*, *14*(1), 20–38. doi:10.1080/08854720802053838.

6. Lazar, S. G. (2014). The cost-effectiveness of psychotherapy for the major psychiatric diagnoses. *Psychodynamic Psychiatry*, *43*(3), 423–457. https://doi.org/10.1521/pdps.2014.42.3.423.

7. Goode, J., Park, J., Parkin, S., Tompkins, K. A., & Swift, J. K. (2017). A collaborative approach to psychotherapy termination. *Psychotherapy*, *54*(1), 10–14. doi:10.1037/pst0000085.

8. Kälvemark, S., Höglund, A. T., Hansson, M. G., Westerholm, P., & Arnetz, B. (2004). Living with conflicts ethical dilemmas and moral distress in the health care system. *Social Science & Medicine*, *58*(6), 1075–1084. doi:10.1016/s0277-9536(03)00279-x.

9. Hiver, C., Villa, A., & Bellagamba, G. (2022). Burnout prevalence among European physicians: A systematic review and meta-analysis. *International Archives of Occupational and Environmental Health*, *95*, 259–273. https://doi.org/10.1007/s00420-021-01782-z.

10. Maslach, C., & Jackson, S. E. (1981). The measurement of experienced burnout. *Journal of Organizational Behavior*, *2*(2), 99–113. https://doi.org/10.1002/job.4030020205.

11. Maslach, C., & Leiter, M. P. (2008). Early predictors of job burnout and engagement. *Journal of Applied Psychology*, *93*(3), 498–512. doi:10.1037/0021-9010.93.3.498.

12. Hiver, C., Villa, A., & Bellagamba, G. (2022). Burnout prevalence among European physicians: A systematic review and meta-analysis. *International Archives of Occupational and Environmental Health*, *95*, 259–273. doi: https://doi.org/10.1007/s00420-021-01782-z.

13. Duffy, R. D., Dik, B. J., Douglass, R. P., England, J. W., & Velez, B. L. (2018). Work as a calling: A theoretical model. *Journal of Counseling Psychology*, *65*(4), 423–439. doi:10.1037/cou0000276.

Chapter 15

1. Valine, Y. A. (2018). Why cultures fail: The power and risk of Groupthink. *Journal of Risk Management in Financial Institutions*, *11*, 301–307.

2. Frank, A. (1995/2013). *The wounded storyteller: Body, illness and ethics* (2nd ed.). University of Chicago Press.

3. Wiegmann, D. A., von Thaden, T. L., & Gibbons, A. M. (2007). A review of safety culture theory and its potential application to traffic safety. *National Academies of Sciences, Engineering, and Medicine, 113*, 6–7. doi: https://aaafoundation.org/wp-content/uploads/2018/02/ImprovingTrafficSafetyCultureinUSReport.pdf

4. Teague, P., Kraeuter, S., York, S., Scott, W., Furqan, M. F., & Zakaria, S. (2019). The role of the chaplain as a patient navigator and advocate for patients in the intensive care unit: One academic medical center's experience. *Journal of Religion and Health, 58*(5), 1833–1846. doi:10.1007/s10943-019-00865-z.

5. Geer, J., Groot, M., Andela, R., Leget, C., Prins, J., Vissers, K., & Zock, H. (2017). Training hospital staff on spiritual care in palliative care influences patient-reported outcomes: Results of a quasi-experimental study. *Palliative Medicine, 31*(8), 743–753. doi:10.1177/0269216316676648.

Chapter 16

1. Best, M., Washington, J., Condello, M., & Kearney, M. (2020). 'This ward has no ears': Role of the pastoral care practitioner in the hospital ward,' *Journal of Health Care Chaplaincy, 13*, 1–15. doi:101.10080/08854726.2020.1814089.

2. Gomez, S., Nuñez Ba, C., White, B., Browning, J., & DeLisser, H. M. (2021). Chaplain–physician interactions from the chaplain's perspective: A mixed method analysis. *American Journal of Hospice and Palliative Care, 38*(11), 1308–1313. doi:10.1177/1049909120984390.

3. Wirpsa, W. J., Johnson, R. E., Bieler, J., Boyken, L. Pugliese, K., Rosencrans, E., & Murphy, P. (2019). Interprofessional models for shared decision making: The role of the healthcare chaplain. *Journal of Health Care Chaplaincy, 25*(1), 20–44. doi:10.1080/08854726.2018.150113.

4. Damen, A., Labuschagne, D., Fosler, L., O'Mahony, S., Levine, S., & Fitchett, G. (2019). What do chaplains do: The views of palliative care physicians, nurses, and social workers. *American Journal of Hospice and Palliative Care, 36*(5), 396–401. doi:10.1177/1049909118807123.

5. U.S. Department of Veterans Affairs. (2020, July 16). VA health care first to have Centers for Medicare & Medicaid services codes for chaplain care. https://www.va.gov/opa/pressrel/pressrelease.cfm?id = 5488 (accessed January 10, 2024).

6. Spiritual Care Association (2024). Approval of HCPCS Codes for Chaplains, https://www.spiritualcareassociation.org/approval-of-hcpcs-codes-for-chaplains/ (accessed January 10, 2024).

7. Weiner, S. (2017, November 20). Is there a chaplain in the house? Hospitals integrate spiritual care. AAMC News. https://www.aamc.org/news/there-chaplain-house-hospitals-integrate-spiritual-care (accessed January 10, 2024).

8. Damen, A., Murphy P., Fullam, F., Mylod. D., Shah, R. C., & Fitchett, G. (2020). Examining the association between chaplain care and patient experience. *Journal of Patient Experience, 7*(6), 1174–1180. doi:10.1177/2374373520918723.

9. Robinson, K. A., Cheng, M.-R., Hansen, P. D., & Gray, R. J. (2017). Religious and spiritual beliefs of physicians. *Journal of Religion and Health, 56*(1), 205–225. doi:10.1007/s10943-016-0233-8.

10. Jeuland, J., Fitchett, G., Schulman-Green, D., & Kapo, J. (2017). Chaplains working in palliative care: Who they are and what they do. *Journal of Palliative Medicine, 20*(5), 502–508. doi:10.1089/jpm.2016.0308.

11. Timmins, F., Caldeira, S., Murphy, M., Pujol, N., Sheaf, G., Weathers, E., Whelan, J., & Flanagan, B. (2018). The role of the healthcare chaplain: A literature review. *Journal of Health Care Chaplaincy, 24*(3), 87–106. doi:10.1080/08854726.2017.1338048.

12. Stewart, K. (2022, June 25). How the Christian right took over the judiciary and changed America. *The Guardian.* https://www.theguardian.com/world/2022/jun/25/roe-v-wade-abortion-christian-right-america (accessed January 10, 2024)).

13. Medicare.gov. *Hospice care.* https://www.medicare.gov/coverage/hospice-care (accessed January 10, 2024).

14. Medicaid.gov. *Hospice benefits.* https://www.medicaid.gov/medicaid/benefits/hospice-benefits/index.html (accessed January 10, 2024).

15. Williams, J. A., Meltzer, D., Arora, V., Chung, G., & Curlin, F. A. (2011). Attention to inpatients' religious and spiritual concerns: Predictors and association with patient satisfaction. *Journal of General Internal Medicine, 26*(11), 265–1271. doi:10.1007/s11606-011-1781-y.

16. Cadge, W., Freese, J., & Christakis, N. A. (2008). The provision of hospital chaplaincy in the United States: A national overview. *Southern Medical Journal, 101*(6), 626–630. doi:10.1097/SMJ.0b013e3181706856.

17. VandeCreek, L., Siegel, K., Gorey, E., Brown, S., & Toperzer, R. (2001). How many chaplains per 100 inpatients? Benchmarks of health care chaplaincy departments. *Journal of Pastoral Care, 55*(3), 289–301. doi:10.1177/002234090105500307.

18. Cadge, W. (2012). *Paging God: Religion in the halls of medicine.* University of Chicago Press.

19. Hasselbacher, L. A., Hebert, L. E., Liu, Y., & Stulberg, D. B. (2020). "My hands are tied": Abortion restrictions and providers' experiences in religious and nonreligious health care systems. *Perspectives on Sexual and Reproductive Health, 52*(2), 107–115. doi:10.1363/psrh.12148.

20. Birkmeyer, J. D., Siewers, A. E., Finlayson, E. V., Stukel, T. A., Lucas, F. L., Batista, I., Welch, H. G., & Wennberg, D. E. (2002). Hospital volume and surgical mortality in the United States. *New England Journal of Medicine, 346*(15), 1128–1137. doi:10.1056/NEJMsa012337.

21. Finks, J. F., Osborne, N. H., & Birkmeyer, J. D. (2011). Trends in hospital volume and operative mortality for high-risk surgery. *New England Journal of Medicine, 364*(22), 2128–2137. doi:10.1056/NEJMsa1010705.

22. Norman, J. (2018, April 6). The religious regions of the U.S. Gallup. https://news.gallup.com/poll/232223/religious-regions.aspx (accessed January 10, 2024).

Chapter 17

1. Swensen, S., Shanafelt, T., & Mohta, N. S. (2016). Leadership survey: Why physician burnout is endemic, and how health care must respond. *NEJM Catalyst, 2*(6). https://catalyst.nejm.org/doi/full/10.1056/CAT.16.0572.

2. Shanafelt, T., Boone, S., Tan, L., Dyrbye, L. N., Sotile, W., Satele, D., West, C. P., Sloan, J., & Oreskovich, M. R. (2012). Burnout and satisfaction with work-life balance among US physicians relative to the general US population. *Archives of Internal Medicine, 172*, 1377–1385. doi:10.1001/archinternmed.2012.3199.

3. Granqvist, P., Mikulincer, M., & Shaver, P. R. (2010). Religion as attachment: Normative processes and individual differences. *Personality and Social Psychology Review, 14*(1), 49–59. https://doi.org/10.1177/1088868309348618.

4. Sedikides, C., & Gebauer, J. E. (2021). Do religious people self-enhance? *Current Opinion in Psychology, 40*, 29–33. https://doi.org/10.1016/j.copsyc.2020.08.002.

5. Soler, J. K., Yaman, H., Esteva, M., Dobbs, F., Asenova, R. S., Katić, M., Ožvačić Z., Desgranges J.P., Moreau, A., Lionis C., Kotányi, P., Carelli, F., Nowak, P. R., de Aguiar, Z., Azeredo, S., Marklund, E., Churchill, D., Ungan, M., & the European General Practice Research Network Burnout Study Group (2008). Burnout in European family doctors: The EGPRN study. *Family Practice, 25*(4), 245–265. doi:10.1093/fampra/cmn038.

6. Kumar, S. (2016). Burnout and doctors: Prevalence, prevention and intervention. *Healthcare (Basel), 4*(3), 37. doi:10.3390/healthcare4030037.

7. Anders, R. L. (2021). Patient safety time for federally mandated registered nurse to patient ratios. *Nursing Forum, 56*(4), 1038–1043. doi:10.1111/nuf.12625.

8. McLernon, L. M. (2020, November 30). Covid-related nursing shortages hit hospitals nationwide. CIDRAP. https://www.cidrap.umn.edu/covid-19/covid-related-nursing-shortages-hit-hospitals-nationwide (accessed January 16, 2024).

9. Wan, W. (2021, April 22). Burned out by the pandemic, 3 in 10 health-care workers consider leaving the profession. *Washington Post.* https://www.washingtonpost.com/health/2021/04/22/health-workers-covid-quit/ (accessed January 16, 2024).

10. Melnikow, J., Padovani, A., & Miller, M. (2022). Frontline physician burnout during the COVID-19 pandemic: National survey findings. *BMC Health Services Research, 22*(1), 365. doi:10.1186/s12913-022-07728-6.

11. Norman, S. B., Feingold, J. H., Kaye-Kauderer H., Kaplan, C. A., Hurtado, A., Kachadourian, L., Feder, A., Murrough, J. W., Charney, D., Southwick, S. M., Ripp, J., Peccoralo, L., & Pietrzak. R. H. (2021). Moral distress in frontline healthcare workers in the initial epicenter of the COVID-19 pandemic in the United States: Relationship to PTSD symptoms, burnout, and psychosocial functioning. *Depression and Anxiety, 38*(10), 1007–1017. doi:10.1002/da.23205.

12. Fox, R. C. (1989). *The sociology of medicine: A participant observer's view.* Pearson College Division.

13. Tata, B., Nuzum, D., Murphy, K., Karimi, L., & Cadge, W. (2021). Staff-care by chaplains during COVID-19. *Journal of Pastoral Care and Counseling, 75*(1 suppl), 24–29. doi:10.1177/1542305020988844.

14. Kwak, J., Rajagopal, S., Handzo, G., Hughes, B. P., & Lee, M. (2021). Perspectives of board-certified healthcare chaplains on challenges and adaptations in delivery of spiritual care in the COVID-19 era: Findings from an online survey. *Palliative Medicine, 36*(1), 105–113. https://doi.org/10.1177/02692163211043373.

15. Snowden A. (2021). What did chaplains do during the covid pandemic? An international survey. *Journal of Pastoral Care and Counseling, 75*(1_suppl), 6–16. doi:10.1177/1542305021992039.

16. Romanoff, B. D., & Terenzio, M. (1998). Rituals and the grieving process. *Death Studies, 22*(8), 697–711. doi:10.1080/074811898201227.

17. Turner, V. (1970). *The ritual process: Structure and anti-structure.* Routledge.

18. van Gennep, A. (1909/2019). *The rites of passage* (2nd ed.). University of Chicago Press.

19. Rando, T. A. (1985). Creating therapeutic rituals in the psychotherapy of the bereaved. *Psychology and Psychotherapy, 22*(2), 236–240. doi:10.1037/h0085500.

20. Bolton, C., & Camp, D. J. (1987). Funeral rituals and the facilitation of grief work. *OMEGA—Journal of Death and Dying, 17*(4), 343–352. doi:10.2190/VDHT-MFRC-LY7L-EMN7.

21. Stone, R. S. B. (2018). Code Lavender: A tool for staff support. *Nursing, 48*(4), 15–17. doi:10.1097/01.NURSE.0000531022.93707.08.

Chapter 18

1. Geer, J. V., Visser, A., Zock, H., Leget, C., Prins, J., & Vissers, K. (2018). Improving spiritual care in hospitals in the Netherlands: What do health care chaplains involved in an action research study report? *Journal of Health Care Chaplaincy, 24*(4), 151–173. doi:10.1080/08854726.2017.1393039.

2. Zollfrank, A. A., Trevino, K. M., Cadge, W., Balboni, M. J., Thiel, M. M., Fitchett, G., Gallivan, K., VanderWeele, T., & Balboni, T. A. (2015). Teaching health care providers to provide spiritual care: A pilot study. *Journal of Palliative Medicine, 18*(5), 408–414. doi:10.1089/jpm.2014.030.

3. Koenig, H. G., Hooten, E. G., Lindsay-Calkins, E., & Meador, K. G. (2010). Spirituality in medical school curricula: Findings from a national survey. *The International Journal of Psychiatry in Medicine, 40*(4), 391–398. doi:10.2190/PM.40.4.

4. Puchalski, C. M. (2001). The role of spirituality in health care. *Proceedings (Baylor University Medical Center), 14*(4), 352–357. doi:10.1080/08998280.2001.11927788.

5. Paal, P., Helo, Y., & Frick, E. (2015). Spiritual care training provided to healthcare professionals: A systematic review. *The Journal of Pastoral Care and Counseling, 69*(1), 19–30. doi:10.1177/1542305015572955.

6. Balboni, M. J., Sullivan, A., Enzinger, A. C., Epstein-Peterson, Z. D., Tseng, Y. D., Mitchell, C., Niska, J., Zollfrank, A., VanderWeele, T. J., & Balboni, T. A. (2014). Nurse and physician barriers to spiritual care provision at the end of life. *Journal of Pain and Symptom Management, 48*, 400–410. doi:10.1016/j.jpainsymman.2013.09.020.

7. Nursing Times Contributor. (2009, February 24). A Christian nurse suspended for offering to pray has sparked health care and religion debate. *Nursing Times*. https://www.nursingtimes.net/archive/a-christian-nurse-suspended-for-offering-to-pray-has-sparked-health-care-and-religion-debate-24-02-2009/ (accessed January 17, 2024).

8. U.S. Health and Human Services Department. (2019, January 26). *Protecting statutory conscience rights in health care; delegations of authority*. https://www.federalregister.gov/documents/2019/05/21/2019-09667/protecting-statutory-conscience-rights-in-health-care-delegations-of-authority (accessed January 17, 2024).

9. World Population Review. (2024). *Hindu countries 2024*. https://worldpopulationreview.com/country-rankings/hindu-countries (accessed January 17, 2024).

10. Lawrence, R. J. (2002). The witches' brew of spirituality and medicine. *Annals of Behavioral Medicine*, 24(1), 74–76. doi:10.1207/S15324796ABM2401_09.

11. Sloan, R. P., Bagiella, E., VandeCreek, L., Hover, M., Casalone, C., Jinpu Hirsch, T., Hasan, Y., Kreger, R., & Poulos, P. (2000, June 22). Should physicians prescribe religious activities? *The New England Journal of Medicine*, 342(25), 1913–1916. doi:10.1056/NEJM200006223422513.

12. The Joint Commission. (2022, July 19). Does the Joint Commission specify what needs to be included in a spiritual assessment?. https://www.jointcommission.org/standards/standard-faqs/critical-access-hospital/provision-of-care-treatment-and-services-pc/000001669/ (accessed January 17, 2024).

13. Choi, P. J., Curlin, F. A., & Cox, C. E. (2019). Addressing religion and spirituality in the intensive care unit: A survey of clinicians. *Palliative & Supportive Care*, 17(2), 159–164. doi:10.1017/S147895151800010X.

Chapter 19

1. Cadge, W., Freese, J., & Christakis, N. A. (2008). The provision of hospital chaplaincy in the United States: A national overview. *Southern Medical Journal*, 101(6), 626–630. doi:10.1097/SMJ.0b013e3181706856.

2. Damen, A., Murphy P., Fullam, F., Mylod. D., Shah, R. C., & Fitchett, G. (2020). Examining the association between chaplain care and patient experience. *Journal of Patient Experience*, 7(6), 1174–1180. doi:10.1177/2374373520918723.

3. Aristotle. (350 BCE/2004). *The Nicomachean Ethics*. Translated from the Greek by J. A. K. Thomson. Penguin Classics.

4. Bishop, J. P. (2009). Biopsychosociospiritual medicine and other political schemes. *Christian Bioethics*, 15(3), 254–276. doi:10.1093/cb/cbp017.

5. Best, M., Leget, C., Goodhead, A., & Paal, P. (2020). An EAPC white paper on multi-disciplinary education for spiritual care in palliative care. *BMC Palliative Care*, 19(1), 9. doi:10.1186/s12904-019-0508-4.

6. Best, M., Washington, J., Condello, M., & Kearney, M. (2020). 'This ward has no ears': Role of the pastoral care practitioner in the hospital ward. *Journal of Health Care Chaplaincy*, 13, 1–15. doi:101.10080/08854726.2020.1814089.

7. Gibbons, J., Thomas, J., VandeCreek, L., & Jessen, A. K. (1991). The value of hospital chaplains: Patient perspectives. *Journal of Pastoral Care, 45*(2), 117–125. doi:10.1177/002234099104500203.

8. Marin, D. B., Sharma, V., Sosunov, E., Egorova, N., Goldstein, R., & Handzo, G. F. (2015). Relationship between chaplain visits and patient satisfaction. *Journal of Health Care Chaplaincy, 21*(1), 14–24. doi:10.1080/08854726.2014.981417.

9. Szilagyi, C., Vandenhoeck, A., Best, M. C., Desjardins, C. M., Drummond, D. A., Fitchett, G., Harrison, S., Haythorn, T., Holmes, C., Muthert, H., Nuzum, D., Verhoef, J. H. A., & Willander, E. (2022). Chaplain leadership during COVID-19: An international expert panel. *Journal of Pastoral Care and Counseling, 76*(1), 56–65. doi:10.1177/15423050211067724.

10. Oxford English Dictionary. (2023). Chaplain. https://www.oed.com/search/diction ary/?scope=Entries&q=chaplain (accessed January 17, 2024).

Chapter 20

1. St. Ignatius of Loyola. (1522–1524/2021). *The spiritual exercises of St. Ignatius: Based on studies in the language of the autograph* (2nd ed.). Edited and translated by Louis J. Puhl, SJ. Loyola Press.

2. Teehan, J. (2006). The evolutionary basis of religious ethics. *Journal of Religion and Science, 41*(3), 747–774. https://doi.org/10.1111/j.1467-9744.2005.00772.x.

3. Suk Gersen, J. (2022, December 26). A year of dominance and defiance at the Supreme Court. *The New Yorker*. https://www.newyorker.com/culture/2022-in-review/a-year-of-dominance-and-defiance-at-the-supreme-court (accessed January 18, 2024.).

4. Politico. (2023, June 29). Read the dissents in the Supreme Court ruling against affirmative action. https://www.politico.com/news/2023/06/29/sotomayor-brown-jackson-supreme-court-affirmative-action-00104193 (accessed January 18, 2024).

5. Russell, B. (1957/1967). *Why I am not a Christian and other essays on religion and related subjects.* Touchstone.

6. Brosnan, S. F. (2013, June 18). Justice- and fairness-related behaviors in nonhuman primates. *Proceedings of the National Academy of Sciences of the United States of America, 110 Suppl 2*(Suppl 2), 10416-10423. doi: https://doi.org/10.1073/pnas.1301194110.

7. Russell, 1957, preface, p. v.

8. Russell, B. (1925/2004), *What I believe* (2nd ed.). Routledge Classics.

9. Plato. (circa 375 BCE/2007). *The Republic.* Translated from the Greek by D. Lee. Penguin Classics.

10. Montaigne, M. (1580/2003). On cannibals. In *Michel de Montaigne: The complete essays.* Translated by M. A. Screech. Penguin Classics, 228–242.

11. Harris, S. (2004). *The end of faith: Religion, terror, and the future of reason.* W.W. Norton & Company.

12. Harris, S. (2005). *Letter to a Christian nation.* Vintage.

13. Harris, S. (2014). *Waking up: A guide to spirituality without religion.* Simon & Schuster.

14. Bellah, R. N. (2011/2017). *Religion in human evolution: From the Paleolithic to the Axial Age.* Harvard University Press.

15. Ponzetti, J. (2014). Renewal in Catholic community life and new monasticism: The way of a contemporary religious communal movement. *Journal for the Sociological Integration of Religion and Society, 4*(2), 35–50.

16. Pew Research Center. (2004, April 7). 64% of online Americans have used the Internet for religious or spiritual purposes. *Pew Research Center Internet & Technology.* https://www.pewresearch.org/internet/2004/04/07/64-of-online-americans-have-used-the-internet-for-religious-or-spiritual-purposes/ (accessed July 22, 2022).

17. James, W. (1902/1984). *The varieties of religious experiences.* Penguin American Library.

18. Scarry, E. (1985). *The body in pain.* Oxford University Press.

Appendix B

1. Guest, G., Bunce, A., & Johnson, L. (2006). How many interviews are enough? An experiment with data saturation and variability. *Field Methods, 18*, 59–82. http://dx.doi.org/10.1177/1525822X05279903.

2. Geertz, C. (1973). *The interpretation of cultures: Selected essays.* Basic Books.

3. Klitzman, R. (2008). *When doctors become patients.* New York: Oxford University Press.

4. Klitzman, R. (1997). *Being positive: The lives of men and women with HIV.* Ivan R. Dee.

5. Klitzman, R. (2012). *Am I my genes?: Confronting fate and family secrets in the age of genetic testing.* Oxford University Press.

6. Klitzman, R. (2019). *Designing babies: How technology is changing the ways we create children.* New York: Oxford University Press.

7. Corbin, J., & Strauss, A. (2008). *Basics of qualitative research: Techniques and procedures for developing grounded theory* (3rd ed.). SAGE Publications, Inc.

Index